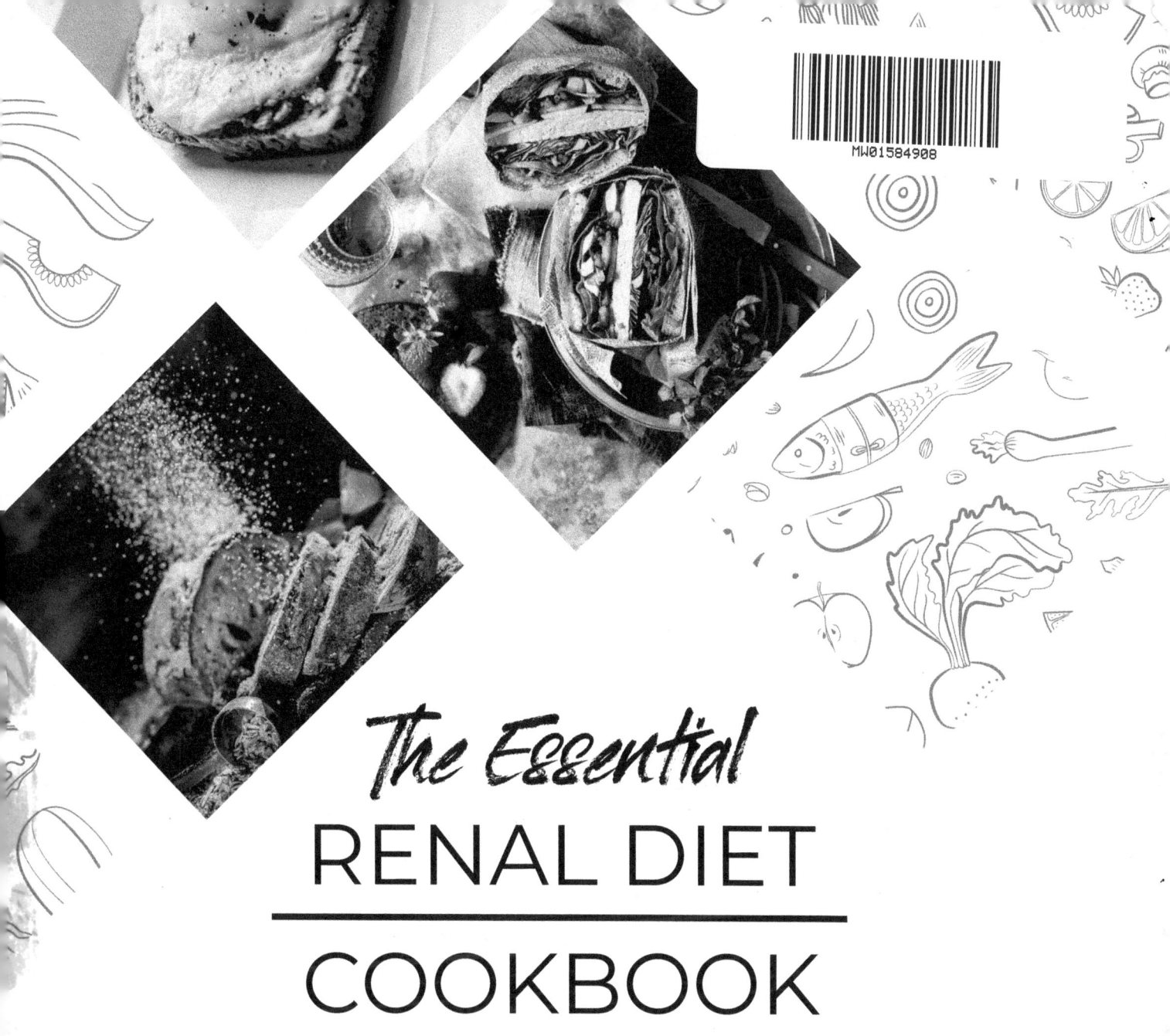

The Essential
RENAL DIET
COOKBOOK

201 Quick, Healthy, and Easy-to-Follow Recipes to Raise Your Sodium, Potassium, and Phosphorus Level. Avoid Dialysis with This 4-Week Meal Plan

Sidney Low

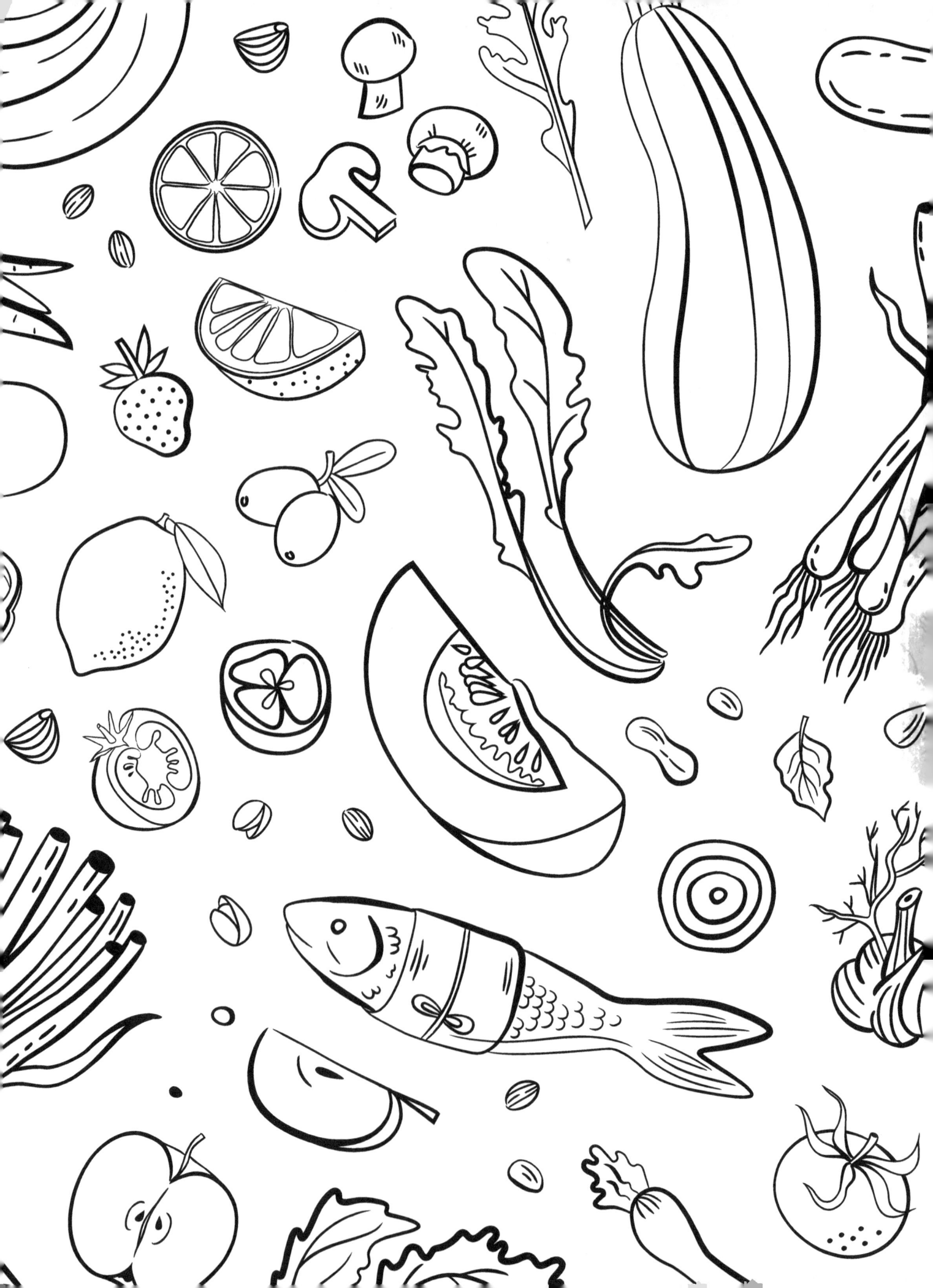

Copyright 2020 - All rights reserved.

The content contained within this book may not be reproduced, duplicated or transmitted without direct written permission from the author or the publisher.

Under no circumstances will any blame or legal responsibility be held against the publisher, or author, for any damages, reparation, or monetary loss due to the information contained within this book. Either directly or indirectly.

Legal Notice:

This book is copyright protected. This book is only for personal use. You cannot amend, distribute, sell, use, quote or paraphrase any part, or the content within this book, without the consent of the author or publisher.

Disclaimer Notice:

Please note the information contained within this document is for educational and entertainment purposes only. All effort has been executed to present accurate, up to date, and reliable, complete information. No warranties of any kind are declared or implied. Readers acknowledge that the author is not engaging in the rendering of legal, financial, medical or professional advice. The content within this book has been derived from various sources. Please consult a licensed professional before attempting any techniques outlined in this book.

By reading this document, the reader agrees that under no circumstances is the author responsible for any losses, direct or indirect, which are incurred as a result of the use of information contained within this document, including, but not limited to, - errors, omissions, or inaccuracies.

TABLE OF CONTENTS

INTRODUCTION 13
    Kidney Diseases and Illnesses 14
    Causes and Risk Factors 17

CHAPTER 1 • What Do You Need to Know About Kidney Disease......17
    Symptoms of Kidney Disease.. 18
    Risk Factors and Chronic Kidney Disease 19
    Five Stages of Chronic Kidney Disease 23

CHAPTER 2 • Five Stages 23
    Dietary Choices for a Healthier Lifestyle 25

CHAPTER 3 • The Healthier Lifestyle for People Affected by CKD.....25
    Healthy Dietary Choices 26
    How Can Diet Affect Symptoms of Kidney Disease?........................... 29

CHAPTER 4 • Key Nutritional Concerns 29
    What to Eat and Avoid in the Renal Diet 31
    List of Juices and Drinks for the Renal Diet 33

CHAPTER 5 • Meal Plan 35
    Week 1.. 36
    Week 2 37
    Week 3 38
    Week 4 39

BREAKFAST RECIPES..41
    1. Green Breakfast Soup... 42
    2. Peach Berry Parfait 43
    3. Open-Faced Bagel Breakfast Sandwich.. 44
    4. Cauliflower Rice and Coconut 45
    5. Kale and Garlic Platter 46
    6. Blistered Beans and Almond 47
    7. Lemon and Broccoli Platter 48
    8. Chicken Liver Stew 49

9. Garlic and Butter-Flavored Cod 50
10. Egg White and Pepper Omelet 51
11. Turkey Breakfast Sausage 52
12. Italian Apple Fritters 53
13. Tofu and Mushroom Scramble 54
14. Egg Fried Rice 55
15. Cottage Cheese Pancakes 56
16. Asparagus Bacon Hash 57
17. Parmesan Zucchini Frittata 58
18. Mexican Baked Beans and Rice 59
19. Quick Thai Chicken and Vegetable Curry 60
20. Cajun Stuffed Peppers 61
21. Stuffed Zucchini 62

SMOOTHIES AND DRINKS 63

22. Sunny Pineapple Breakfast Smoothie 64
23. Blueberry Burst Smoothie 65
24. Blueberry Smoothie Bowl 66
25. Cucumber Spinach Green Smoothie 67
26. Watermelon Kiwi Smoothie 68
27. Mint Lassi 69
28. Fennel Digestive Cooler 70
29. Cinnamon Horchata 71
30. Vanilla Chia Smoothie 72
31. Berry Mint Water 73
32. Homemade Rice Milk 74
33. Ginger & Lemon Green Iced-Tea 75
34. Lemon Smoothie 76
35. Tropical Juice 77
36. Mixed Fruit Anti-Inflammatory Smoothie 78
37. Banana Apple Smoothie 79
38. Winter Berry Iced Milkshake 80
39. Aloha Cocktail 81

SNACKS AND SIDES 83

40. Savory Collard Chips 84
41. Roasted Red Pepper Hummus 85
42. Thai-Style Eggplant Dip 86
43. Coconut Pancakes 87
44. Spiced Peaches 88
45. Pumpkin Cheesecake Bar 89
46. Blueberry and Vanilla Mini Muffins 90
47. Puffy French Toast 91
48. Puff Oven Pancakes 92
49. Savory Muffins with Protein 93
50. European Pancakes 94
51. Easy and Fast Mac-n-Cheese 95
52. Sandwich with Chicken Salad 96
53. Celery and Arugula Salad 97
54. Chicken, Charred Tomato, and Broccoli Salad 98
55. Easy Baked Shepherd's Pie 99
56. Crunchy Potato Croquettes 100
57. Vegetarian Summer Rolls 101

SOUPS 103

58. Tofu Soup 104
59. Onion Soup 105
60. Roasted Carrot Soup 106
61. Mushroom Cream Soup 107
62. Garlic Soup 108
63. Pesto Green Vegetable Soup 109
64. Cucumber Soup 110
65. Tangy Orange Shrimp 111
66. Shrimp and Greens 112
67. Seared Herbed Scallops 113
68. Almond-Crusted Sole 114
69. Breaded Baked Sole 115

70. Roasted Tilapia with Garlic Butter 116
71. Pesto-Crusted Tilapia 117
72. Lime Baked Haddock 118
73. Fish Tacos with Vegetable Slaw 119
74. Eggplant and Red Pepper Soup 120
75. Chicken Pho 121
76. Herbed Cabbage Stew 122
77. Vegetable Lentil Soup 123
78. French Onion Soup 124
79. Creamy Broccoli Soup 125

SALAD 127

80. Cucumber Salad 128
81. Thai Cucumber Salad 129
82. Red Potato Salad 130
83. Broccoli-Cauliflower Salad 131
84. Macaroni Salad 132
85. Green Bean and Potato Salad 133
86. Eggplant Salad 134
87. Spinach Salad with Orange Vinaigrette 135
88. Mixed Green Leaf and Citrus Salad 136
89. Roasted Beet Salad 137
90. Appealing Green Salad 138
91. Mango with Avocado Salad 139
92. Avocado and Lettuce Salad 140
93. Rocket Salad with Mango, Avocado, and Cherry Tomatoes 141
94. Chickpea Salad 142
95. Bulgur and Broccoli Salad 143
96. Pear and Watercress Salad 144
97. Tropical Chicken Salad 145
98. Chicken and Grape Salad 146
99. Fresh Berry Salad 147
100. Cauliflower Mash 148

101. Asian Cucumber Salad 149

102. Garden Fresh Salad 150

103. Avocado Boats with Shrimp Salad and Crostinis 151

VEGETABLES 153

104. Curried Veggie Stir-Fry 154

105. Chilaquiles 155

106. Roasted Veggie Sandwiches 156

107. Roasted Peach Open-Face Sandwich 157

108. Pasta Fagioli 158

109. Spinach Alfredo Lasagna Rolls 159

110. Spicy Corn and Rice Burritos 160

111. Crust less Cabbage Quiche 161

112. Creamy Veggie Casserole 162

113. Vegetable Green Curry 163

114. Zucchini Bowl 164

115. Nice Coconut Haddock 165

116. Vegetable Rice Casserole 166

117. Vegetable Confetti Relish 167

118. Braised Cabbage 168

119. Raw Vegetables. Chopped Salad 169

120. Broccoli Soup, Green Leaves, And Beans 170

121. Pumpkin Filled With Vegetables and Quinoa 171

122. Vegan Vegetable Mini Tortillas 172

123. Vegetarian Recipe 173

124. White Bean Veggie Burgers 174

125. Spicy Tofu and Broccoli Stir-Fry 175

126. Barley and Roasted Vegetable Bowl 176

127. Fragrant Egg Fried Rice 177

128. Pumpkin Filled With Vegetables and Quinoa 178

SEAFOOD 179

129. Corn and Shrimp Quiche 180

130. Ginger Shrimp with Snow Peas 181

131. Roasted Cod with Plums 182
132. Family Hit Curry 183
133. Homemade Tuna Nicoise 184
134. Cajun Crab 185
135. Creamy Crab Soup 186
136. Spicy Lime Shrimp 187
137. Seafood Casserole 188
138. Tilapia Ceviche 189
139. Fish Tacos 190
140. Jambalaya 191
141. Asparagus Shrimp Linguini 192
142. Tuna Noodle Casserole 193
143. Oven-Fried Southern Style Catfish 194
144. Cilantro-Lime Cod 195
145. Shrimp Quesadilla 196
146. Maryland Crab Cakes 197
147. Citrus Grilled Glazed Salmon 198
148. Omega-3 Rich Salmon 199
149. Wholesome Salmon Meal 200
150. Succulent Tilapia 201
151. Festive Tilapia 202

POLTRY AND MEAT 203

152. Curried Chicken Stir-Fry 204
153. Thai-Style Chicken Salad 205
154. Flavorful Pork Chop 206
155. Creamy Chicken 207
156. Fabulous Chicken 208
157. Divine Ground Chicken 209
158. Comforting Chicken Chili 210
159. Simple Lamb Chops 211
160. Beer Pork Ribs 212
161. Mexican Steak Tacos 213

162. Mexican Chorizo Sausage 214

163. Caribbean Turkey Curry 215

164. Lemon and Fruit Pork Kebabs 216

165. Chicken Stew 217

166. Asian Style Pan-Fried Chicken 218

167. Curried Chicken with Cauliflower 219

168. Red and Green Grapes Chicken Salad with Curry 220

169. Grilled Chicken Pizza 221

170. Chicken Breast and Bok Choy 222

171. Baked Herbed Chicken 223

172. Chicken and Cabbage Stir-Fry 224

173. Herb Crusted Pork Tenderloin 225

174. Pork and Plum Tenderloin 226

175. Exceptional Steak 227

176. Chicken and Leek Salad 228

DESSERT 229

177. Buttery Pound Cake 230

178. Pudding Glass with Banana and Whipped Cream 231

179. Chocolate Beet Cake 232

180. Strawberry Pie 233

181. Grape Skillet Galette 234

182. Pumpkin Cheesecake 235

183. Small Chocolate Cakes 236

184. Strawberry Whipped Cream Cake 237

185. Sweet Cracker Pie Crust 238

186. Old-Fashioned Apple Kuchen 239

187. Carob Angel Food Cake 240

188. Elegant Lavender Cookies 241

189. Gingerbread Loaf 242

190. Rhubarb Crumble 243

191. Honey Bread Pudding 244

192. Vanilla-Infused Couscous Pudding 245

193. Raspberry Brûlée	246
194. Sweet Cinnamon Custard	247
195. Raspberry Mousse	248
196. Honey Ginger Cookies	249
197. Honey Baked Pear	250
198. Watermelon Sorbet	251
199. Aunt Tula's Carrot Cake	252
200. Turnover Delights	253
201. Peaches and Cream Puffs	254

CHAPTER 15 • Frequently Asked Questions 255

Best Advice to Avoid Dialysis 257

APPENDIX A • Measurement and Conversion 259

Volume 259

Metric Cups Conversion 260

Weight 261

Oven Temperatures 262

APPENDIX B • Dirty Dozen and Clean Fifteen 263

CONCLUSION 265

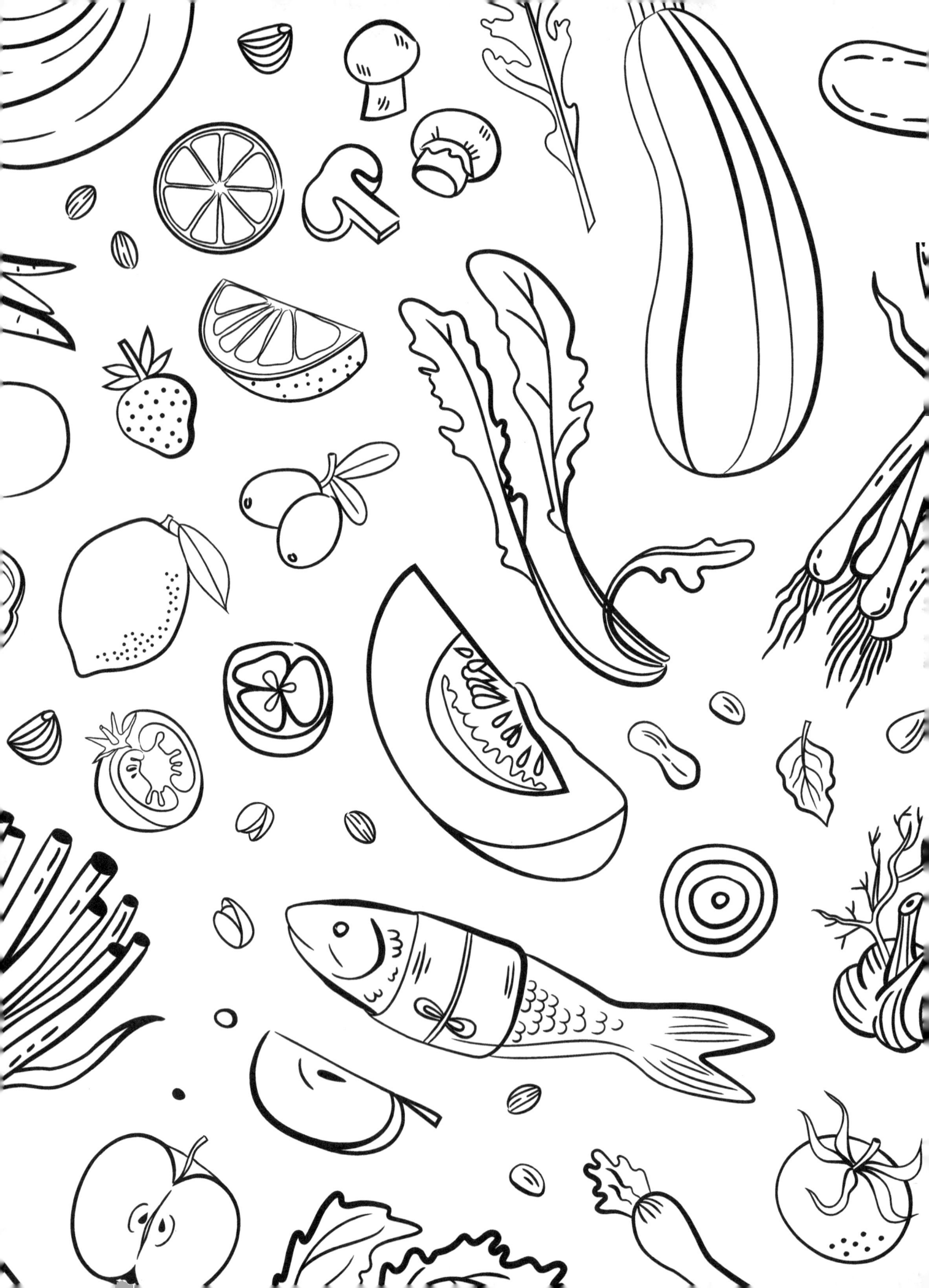

INTRODUCTION

Kidney disease is infrequently thought about by people unless they have been diagnosed with it themselves. Yet, while many Americans go on their way, unaware an estimated thirty-seven million adults have been diagnosed with the condition. Not only that, but a person can feel fine and seem healthy and still be at a high risk of developing this disease if they don't take care of themselves, as millions of Americans are at risk. Thankfully, if a person is aware of the risk of kidney disease and the condition is detected early, it can help prevent the progression of the disease and potential kidney failure. Therefore, early diagnosis, treatment, and understanding of kidney disease and kidney health are vital.

People who are at the highest risk of developing chronic kidney disease are those with a family history of kidney failure, diabetes, and high blood pressure. The elderly, Latinx people, Native people, Pacific Islanders, and black people are also at an increased risk of developing kidney disease.

If your doctor suspects you might have kidney disease or that you are at an increased risk of developing kidney problems, they will check your blood pressure, urine albumin, and serum creatinine. Increased markers on these three tests usually result in a kidney disease diagnosis, but your doctor who is familiar with your individual case will be able to know for sure and officially diagnose you. Keep in mind that nobody but your doctor can diagnose you with kidney disease, even if your test results indicate you might have one.

If you are worried that you or someone you care about may have developed kidney disease, then see your doctor right away, they will be able to run the necessary test to either confirm or deny whether you have the condition. Usually, both kidneys will be affected by the disease. As the kidneys become damaged, they will be unable to properly filter your blood, resulting in excess fluid and waste within your body. While there are often no symptoms present until the late stages of the disease, it is possible to experience side effects.

And, of course, you should be more careful of kidney disease if there is any history of it in your family. If you are concerned about an increased risk of developing the disease, ask your doctor about a plan to monitor your kidney health in the future to prevent any damage going unchecked.

Kidney Diseases and Illnesses

There are many different conditions that can cause kidney disease or overall poor kidney health. However, one of the most common and dangerous of these conditions is chronic kidney disease, also known as kidney failure. With this condition, a person's kidneys slowly lose their ability to function. If the person takes good care of their health, follows the treatment plans given to them by their doctors, and follows kidney health guidelines, they will hopefully be able to halt the progression of their kidney disease. On the other hand, if a person practices poor kidney health choices and goes without treatment, their kidneys will slowly deteriorate until they reach kidney failure.

When a person reaches kidney failure, the most severe stage of chronic kidney disease, the kidneys will be unable to function without medical intervention. In order to survive, people with kidney failure must either receive a kidney transplant or regular dialysis. Thankfully, healthy individuals are able to donate part of one of their kidneys or even a whole kidney to those in need without generally becoming sick themselves. This allows family members and friends to help their loved ones who are in dire need of a kidney transplant, and even kindhearted strangers who want to improve the world and do a good deed. If you are interested in donating part of your kidney, know that it is a common practice and is one of the most common surgeries in the United States, making it a relatively safe procedure. If you are interested in donating a kidney or part of a kidney, talk to your doctor, as they will know if your kidney is a good candidate for donation. They will also be able to discuss the safety and risks of your specific situation.

There are many conditions that can cause kidney diseases, such as inflammation of the kidneys, urinary tract obstructions, high blood pressure, and type I and type II diabetes. Kidney cancer is also extremely common, with it being the seventh most common type of cancer in the United States. There are also multiple types of kidney cancer, with renal cell carcinoma being the most common.

Kidney stones are extremely common and very painful, but generally, don't cause any damage. These stones are formed from minerals and acid found within the kidneys, usually making them a hard rock-like substance made of concentrated urine. Kidney stones usually pass on their own as long as you stay well hydrated. If you suspect you have a kidney stone and are unable to pass it on your own or worry that it might have caused rare damage contact your doctor, and they can direct you further.

Another form of kidney illness is an infection of the kidneys. Usually, kidney infections are caused by bacteria that entered the body through the urethra, traveled through the bladder, and into the kidneys. Kidney infections can easily be treated, but if left untreated, they can cause permanent damage. Therefore, if you might have a kidney infection, seek medical attention immediately.

Along with chronic kidney disease, cancer, stones, and infections, there are some other kidney conditions, as well. If you suspect you have a kidney disorder that is not one of the ones mentioned above, your doctor will be able to discuss the possibilities with you and make a plan to figure out whether your kidneys have any problems.

Two-thirds of the cases of chronic kidney disease are caused by high blood pressure and diabetes. The reason for this is because diabetes, which occurs when your blood sugar is overly high, causes damage to your body. This results in damage to the kidneys and blood vessels, as well as the heart.

When a person has high blood pressure, known as hypertension, the blood in your veins pushes against the walls of the blood vessels. When left poorly controlled or uncontrolled, it can result in not only heart attacks and stroke but also kidney disease. Along with high blood pressure causing kidney disease, kidney disease itself can also cause high blood pressure.

While two-thirds of the cases of chronic kidney disease may be caused by diabetes and high blood pressure, there are other causes as well. This includes repeated kidney infections, glomerulonephritis disorders, obstructions caused by kidney stones or tumors, polycystic kidney disease, and other inherited diseases, Lupus, and malformations of a baby developing in a person's womb which results in pressure on the kidneys.

While there is no way to know for sure whether you have kidney disease without an official diagnosis from your doctor, there are some symptoms to keep an eye out for. It is important to understand our own bodies so that we can seek medical attention whenever there is a cause for concern. By knowing and understanding these symptoms, you can inform your doctor of any concerns, which they can then keep an eye on to ensure you are in the best of health. After all, you will have the highest rate of success with treatment and lower risk of kidney failure if you get diagnosed and start treatment early.

CHAPTER 1

What Do You Need to Know About Kidney Disease

Kidneys may be small, but they do have important functions in the body. These bean-shaped organs work hard, but they may experience injuries and other problems that prevent them from functioning properly. But the question is, what causes kidney disease and how to detect it?

Causes and Risk Factors

What many of us are not aware of is that the cause of kidney disease doesn't necessarily have to occur in kidneys themselves. Problems affecting our overall health and well-being can also induce damage to the kidneys. In the same way, common health problems can also impair the function of these organs. The most frequent causes of kidney disease are hypertension and diabetes.

High blood pressure, which affects 75 million people in the US or one in three adults, can damage blood vessels in the kidney and thereby impair their function. In other words, damage to blood vessels in the kidneys due to hypertension doesn't allow them to remove wastes and extra fluid from your body. This leads to a vicious cycle as an accumulation of waste and extra fluid increases blood pressure. Besides damaging filtering units in kidneys, high blood pressure can also reduce the flow of blood to these organs. As you're already aware, without a blood supply, organs cannot function properly.

About 30.3 million people, or 9.4% of the population in the United States, have diabetes, which can cause several complications. Just like hypertension, diabetes also damages small blood vessels in the kidneys. As a result, the body retains more salt and water than it should. Moreover, diabetes also causes damage to the nerves in the body, which can make it difficult for you to empty the bladder. The pressure from a full bladder can back up and damage or injure kidneys. Let's also not forget the fact that if urine remains in the body for a long time, it can lead to an infection from the fast growth of bacteria and high blood sugar levels. Estimates show that 30% of patients with type 1 diabetes and 10% to 40% of people with type 2 diabetes will eventually experience kidney failure.

Besides diabetes and hypertension, other causes of kidney disease include:

- Infection
- Renal artery stenosis
- Heavy metal poisoning
- Lupus
- Some drugs
- Prolonged obstruction of the urinary tract from conditions such as kidney stones, enlarged prostate, some cancers

Symptoms of Kidney Disease

Signs and symptoms of kidney disease don't appear suddenly, and they develop over time. Many people don't even know they have kidney disease until it reaches late stages because they are unable to identify some warning signs. Symptoms of kidney diseases may vary from one person to another as well as their severity. But generally speaking, the most common signs of kidney disease include:

- Nausea and vomiting
- Hypertension that is difficult to control
- Loss of appetite
- Shortness of breath

- Chest pain
- Weakness or fatigue
- Sleep disturbances
- Persistent itching
- Changes in how much a patient urinates
- Swollen feet and ankles
- Reduced mental sharpness
- Muscle cramps and twitching
- Blood in urine or foamy urine

It is worth mentioning that symptoms of kidney disease can be non-specific as they are greatly influenced by causes of these conditions and underlying diseases.

Risk Factors and Chronic Kidney Disease

Non-modifiable risk factors, advanced age, male sex, low birth weight, race or ethnicity, genetic and hereditary factors predispose to an increased risk of CKD development. However, it must be recognized that the racial factor is sometimes difficult to analyze as it is probably associated with a genetic predisposition but also environmental and socio-economic factors such as inequalities of access to care, nutritional intake, and low birth weight.

Unmodifiable Risk Factors

- Advanced age
- Sex (masculine/feminine)
- Race/ethnicity (African Americans, Native Americans, Hispanics, Whites, African Blacks)
- Low birth weight
- Genetics/family

Modifiable Risk Factors

- Hypertension (I & P)
- Diabetes mellitus (I & P)
- Obesity (I & P)
- Proteinuria (P)
- Dyslipidemia (I & P)
- Hyperuricemia (I & P)
- Smoking (I & P)
- Alcohol consumption (I)
- Infections (I)
- Autoimmune diseases (I)
- Drug/plant poisoning/analgesic abuse (I)
- Obstructive lithiasis/uropathies (I)
- Low socio-economic class (I & P)

Abbreviations: I = initiation; P = progression

As the main emunctory, the kidney is potentially exposed to many aggressions. Although the parenchyma has an extraordinary ability to adapt and regenerate, the CKD is able to progressively destroy the functional structures of the kidney: glomeruli, tubes, interstitium, and vessels. Moreover, whatever the cause or the various and multiple underlying pathophysiological mechanisms, it has a common functional consequence: chronic kidney disease (CKD). This one is likely to evolve inexorably towards the terminal stage corresponding to the renal death. The latter results in serious consequences for the entire organism that has lost the constancy of the internal environment, related to uremic intoxication, on the one hand, and failures of renal, endocrine functions on the other hand.

Family history of chronic kidney disease, low birth weight, smoking, and alcoholism

CKD risk factors reported elsewhere, such as HF-CKD, low birth weight, smoking, and alcoholism, did not emerge as an independent determinant of

CKD. This lack of association could be explained by the difference in methodology and probably the relatively small size of the sample and the low frequency of the factors mentioned above in this work.

The frequency of HF-CKD varied between 5 and 9% according to the cross-sectional studies composing this dissertation. Among some subjects who knew their birth weight, they were, respectively, 3% (mass screening campaign), 6% (study in CSS), and 7% (household survey).

With regard to HF-CKD and low birth weight, lack of knowledge of the CKD and its association with HF-CKD or birth weight by both patients and the general population could partly explain this lack of association of HF-CKD or low birth weight and the CKD.

However, low birth weight is well-known, associated with a reduction in nephron mass in utero, with increased risk of diabetes mellitus, hypertension, and progressive renal impairment in adulthood. In addition, the nephron deficit would also increase the susceptibility of the kidneys to various assaults, such as hypertension, diabetes mellitus, and HIV infection.

In populations with low socio-economic levels, such as those of different African or Afro-American black ethnic groups, birth weight is frequently lower. We also believe that low birth weight has not been properly researched in this work. According to several authors, the term low birth weight should not be limited to the universal birth weight threshold < 2.5 Kg. For these authors, low birth weight or better, fetal hypotrophy should be defined as a small weight for the gestational age in reference to a birth weight below the 5th or 10th percentile of weight distributions by age and sex gestation. These data were not available in this memory and can, in principle, only be correctly gathered in longitudinal studies.

As for smoking, its frequency was between 7 and 10% in the various surveys carried out in this work. Previous studies have clearly shown the role of tobacco in the initiation and progression of the CKD. In this respect, the incidence of IRT in non-diabetic subjects is multiplied by 5.9 in heavy smokers (> 15 packets/year). Another study had shown that the risk of development of albuminuria was multiplied by 3 in heavy smokers (> 20 packets/year) compared to non-smokers. The possible mechanism by which tobacco may contribute to renal impairment includes stimulation of the sympathetic nervous system, glomerular capillary hypertension, endothelial damage, and direct tubular toxicity of nicotine. The reason for the lack of association between proteinuria and smoking in all our work is unclear and requires a longitudinal study. It is possible, however, that some of the subjects studied did not admit this intoxication.

With regard to alcoholism, its frequency was respectively 28%, 20%, and 8% in the mass screening campaign, in the general population (household study), and in the health structures (among the subjects at risk of alcoholism). The possible role of alcohol in the pathogenesis of the CKD remains a controversial subject. A case study control found a significant association between IRT and consumption of > 2 glasses of alcohol/day, while another similar study did not confirm this association. Taking alcohol can increase the risk of CKD through initiation and/or promotion of risk factors.

CHAPTER 2

Five Stages

There are five stages of renal or chronic kidney disease, each differentiated by the amount of kidney damage and glomerular filtration rate, a measure of how well the kidneys are working. Stage 1 is the least severe and comes the closest to healthy kidney function, while stage 5 requires dialysis or a kidney transplant. Your physician will determine your treatment based on which stage of kidney disease you have. Talk to your doctor if you have any questions about your stage of kidney disease or treatment.

Five Stages of Chronic Kidney Disease

STAGE	DESCRIPTION	GLOMERULAR FILTRATION RATE (GFR)
Normal kidney function	Healthy kidneys	90 mL/min or more
Stage 1	Kidney damage with normal or high GFR	90 mL/min or more
Stage 2	Kidney damage with a mild decrease in GFR	60–89 mL/min
Stage 3	Moderate decrease in GFR	30–59 mL/min
Stage 4	Severe decrease in GFR	15–29 mL/min
Stage 5	Kidney failure	< 15 mL/min or receiving dialysis

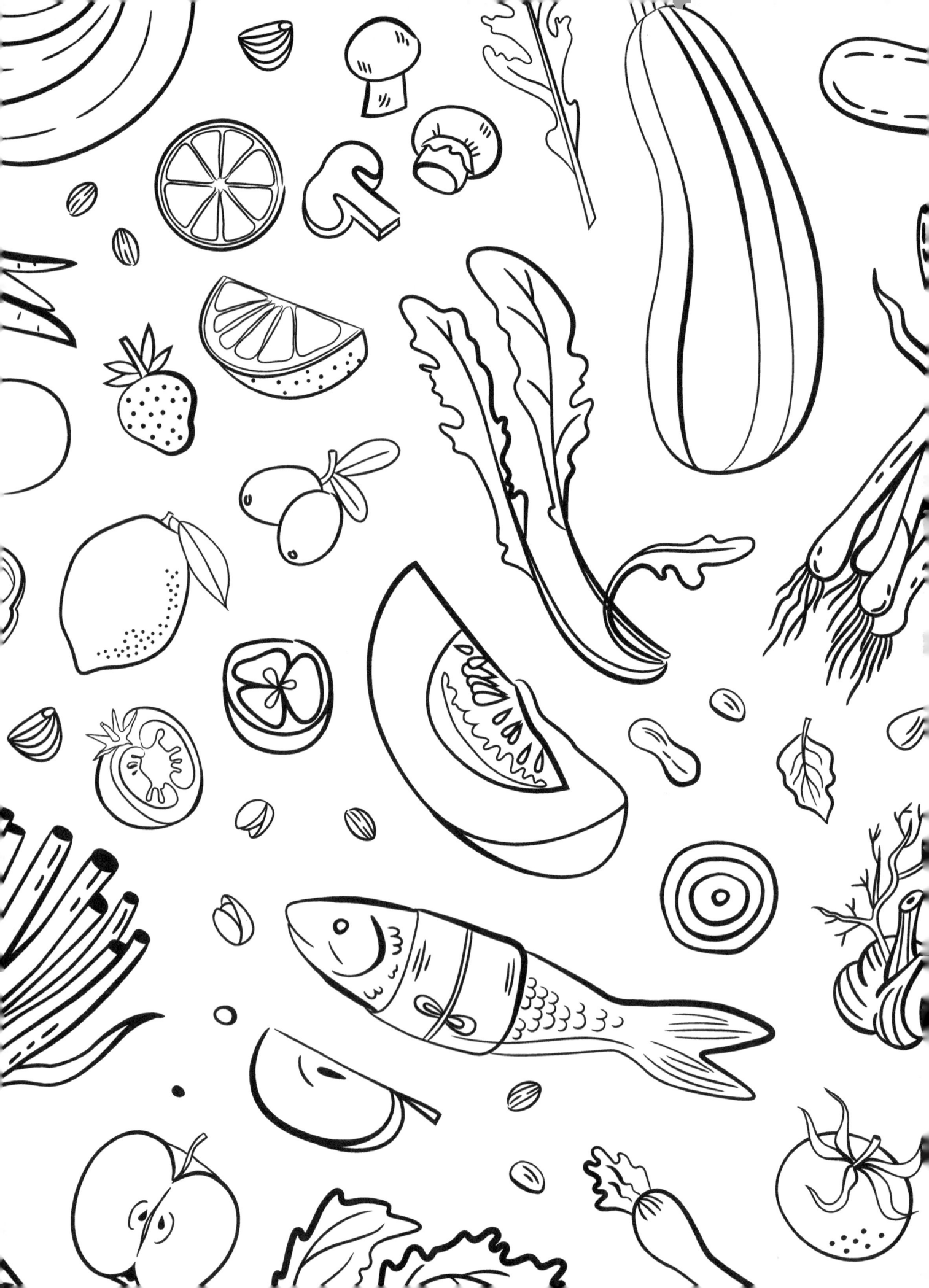

CHAPTER 3

The Healthier Lifestyle for People Affected by CKD

Dietary Choices for a Healthier Lifestyle

Your choices in your diet and lifestyle can make a huge difference to your daily life, the symptoms you experience, and in the early stages of kidney disease, the rate at which this develops. Changes can even prevent your kidneys from deteriorating, give you more energy, help you maintain a healthy weight, and prevent illnesses and infections.

Overall there are four main elements that you should be focusing on within your diet: phosphorous, potassium, sodium, and protein intake should be limited, and by making these changes in the early stages of the disease, you may even be able to prevent a far stricter diet in the later stages of the disease.

Unfortunately, the diet many of us consume in the US and other western countries is not beneficial to our health. What nutritionists have termed the 'Standard American Diet' is unhealthy in many different respects: whilst including high levels of saturated fats, processed foods, and animal fats, it is also light on complex carbohydrates, fiber, fruits, and vegetables. All of this leads to a dramatically increased chance of stroke, heart disease, obesity, cancer, and, of course, kidney disease.

One of the main issues in this diet is processed food, which is when chemicals have been added to food in order to preserve and make readily available to the consumer. In addition to these chemicals, processed foods include upwards of four times as much sugar as their natural counterparts. Excessive sugar levels increase the risk of type 2 diabetes, raise cholesterol levels, and creates a build-up of fat around the liver. As the liver works alongside the kidneys to remove toxins from the body, it is clear how these dietary choices can drastically increase the risk of kidney disease.

Always consult your doctor and nutritionist because it is the best thing to devise a meal plan specifically suited to your needs and the stage of the disease you are in. It is also important that you monitor and control your calorie intake as a loss of appetite is commonly experienced as a side effect of the disease, and therefore weight loss needs to be carefully monitored.

Healthy Dietary Choices

This section will cover the choices you can make to ensure a healthy diet and the best treatment for your kidneys. Advice and guidance will differ according to what stage of the disease you're in; however, the principles remain similar throughout. Check with your doctor or nutritionist to ensure your diet plans are the best for you. Healthy food types and recommendations are outlined, as well as food types and groups to consider avoiding or cutting down.

Carbohydrates and Fiber: Although carbohydrates may be difficult to process at later stages of kidney disease, they provide a vital source of energy that can combat the feelings of lethargy. As a low protein diet is recommended, carbohydrates can also help to replace calories. Some carbohydrates are also sources of fiber. It is recommended that you eat at least 25 grams of fiber per day, even when suffering from stage 5 kidney disease and undergoing dialysis. You may become frustrated when trying to count your fiber levels as many high fibrous foods are also high in potassium, phosphorous, and fluid (all of which are restricted). The food lists are a useful starting point for ingredients and their various nutritional values.

Fats: Fats often get a bad reputation as we don't often distinguish between healthy and unhealthy fats. Polyunsaturated and monounsaturated fats are healthy when consumed in moderation, whereas trans fats and saturated fats should be avoided.

If you need to consume extra calories because of weight loss, these 'good' types of fat are great as part of a balanced diet. Too much fat, particularly trans fats, can lead to a rapid increase in cholesterol, worsening symptoms experienced, and also increasing your risk of heart disease. This is, in turn, linked to diabetes and high blood pressure, so it is always advised that you consume healthy fats in moderation and steer clear of the unhealthy fats altogether if possible. Oily fishes like tuna, salmon, and mackerel are excellent sources of these good fats. Choose oils for cooking and dressing such as coconut oil, canola oil, and olive oil instead of sesame and vegetable oils.

Protein: Although bodybuilders usually come to mind when we think of protein, it is actually an essential component of our diets and vital for repairing tissues, keeping infections at bay, and, of course, building muscle, even in the most exercise-phobic of us! If you have chronic kidney disease in the first few stages, it is still usually advised to consume protein for up to 15% of your daily diet, with carbohydrates and fats making up 85%. This is the same amount recommended for an average adult's daily intake. At stage 4, this recommendation usually decreases to only 10% protein. During stage 5, and if you are on dialysis, the dialysis will filter out the waste toxins from your body as well as protein; therefore, it is crucial for you to include protein as part of your diet. Please note that you must follow your doctor's advice on how much protein you should be consuming at each stage, as it depends on various factors such as your height, weight, and which stage of the disease you have. Always consult a professional for individual guidance before making any changes to your diet.

Phosphorus and Calcium: Phosphates are salt compounds that include salt as well as other minerals; they work, as it does calcium, to strengthen and keep our bones healthy. Extra phosphorous in the blood is usually removed by our kidneys, but kidney disease will prevent this process from functioning as it should. Unfortunately, it's not as simple as just removing all phosphates from your diet as they are pretty much in most foods, but we can look out for those high in phosphorous. A list of foods and identifies whether they are low, medium, or high in phosphorous. You should typically stay away from processed foods as these often contain additives. Too much phosphorus can also lead to a calcium deficit, which can, in turn, lead to the extreme bouts of itchiness that many chronic kidney disease sufferers report. If low calcium levels persist, this can lead to further pain, a general weakening of the bones, and even bone disease. It might be that your doctor will recommend taking a calcium supplement if your phosphorus levels remain too high. After this, medicines known as phosphorous binders may be required but always consult a professional.

Fluids: As the kidneys start to decrease in functionality, waste toxins and excess liquids are not removed from the body as they should be. This may lead to your doctor recommending you limit the liquids you consume. Foods with high liquid content also need to be considered as well as the drinks you consume, for instance, fruits such as apples and pears, milk, soups, ice creams, etc. This is more likely during the later stages of kidney disease, and you should consult a professional for specific advice.

Potassium: Is a mineral that has an essential role in keeping your heart healthy as well as regulating water levels in the body. Again, this is another mineral that is usually removed when in excess through the kidney filtration system. Too much of one particular mineral is problematic as the kidneys just cannot remove it in the way they can when they are completely healthy. That being said, extremely low levels of potassium are also harmful, and kidney disease sufferers may experience either extreme. This is unique to you, so it will need to be monitored by a professional. Potassium is commonly found in many fruits and vegetables—stick with watermelon, tangerines, pineapple, berries, apples, cherries, pears, grapes, and peaches as low potassium fruits.

Iron: Anyone whose chronic kidney disease has resulted in anemia will need extra iron in their diet. Options that are high in iron include iron-fortified cereals, kidney beans, lima beans, chicken, pork, beef, and liver. As some iron-rich sources may conflict with other dietary considerations such as protein, ensure you find out from your doctor which sources of iron you can have.

CHAPTER 4

Key Nutritional Concerns

How Can Diet Affect Symptoms of Kidney Disease?

Changing your diet and lifestyle can go a long way in helping to control your kidney disease and prevent the later stages of kidney disease. This chapter will explore the different food and nutrient groups that you should familiarize yourself with if you have kidney disease. Always ask for your doctor's advice before changing your diet.

Carbohydrates: Should make up the majority of your diet, as they're the primary source of energy for your body.

Complex and simple are the two types of carbohydrates. An example of a simple carbohydrate is fruit. Fruit is packed with the fiber, vitamins, and energy that your body needs. Examples of complex carbohydrates are grains, bread and vegetables. All these carbohydrates provide minerals and vitamins as well as energy and fiber. Carbohydrates also play a vital role in balancing blood-sugar levels.

Protein: Repairs tissue and builds muscle. Your body also uses protein to build antibodies. These are your body's defense against disease. Animal foods are the primary sources of protein, such as milk, beef, eggs, chicken, and pork.

Protein can also be found in some plants. Legumes, nuts, and soybean products are all good sources of proteins. Vegetables also contain small amounts of protein. Protein is essential for good health; however, in later stages of chronic kidney disease, your renal dietitian may have you cut back on protein intake to help reduce stress on the kidneys.

Fats: Transport vitamins K, E, D, and A to your cells. They produce the hormones testosterone and estrogen. Some fats contain fatty acids that are good for your skin. These fatty acids also make up the linings of cells in the body and help with the transmission of nerves. However, too much fat or the wrong kind of fat in your diet can cause weight gain, leading to heart disease and many other problems with your health.

There are two types of fats: unsaturated and saturated. Meat and dairy products are saturated fats. Too much of these fats can elevate your cholesterol; this cholesterol is what causes heart disease and clogged arteries. The food and drug administration recommends reducing your saturated fat intake. Nuts, fish, and certain oils are good sources of unsaturated fats and all help to reduce cholesterol. Trans fats will raise cholesterol levels, just like saturated fats. The FDA suggests you choose food that is low in trans fats and saturated fats. Processed foods usually contain trans fats.

Sodium, potassium, and phosphorus: These are the three main minerals balanced by the kidneys. As chronic kidney disease gets worse, some foods will need to be avoided as your kidneys are already unable to remove the excess from these minerals. Blood tests will be conducted to monitor the levels of these minerals.

Sodium: In the early stages of kidney disease, a low sodium diet may be all you need if you have high blood pressure. Your kidneys cannot get rid of excess fluid and sodium from your body whilst experiencing kidney disease. To help identify salt in foods, look for ingredients on the label such as baking powder, sodium, or brine. Generally, children and adults should eat less than 2,300 mg of sodium a day.

Kidney disease stage 1 and 2 = 1–3.5g per day

Kidney disease stage 3 - 4 = 1–2.5g per day

Kidney disease stage 5 = 1–2g per day

Potassium: Kidneys usually get rid of excess potassium in your urine to maintain normal levels in your blood. When experiencing kidney disease, they can no longer do this effectively.

Hyperkalemia (or high potassium levels) occurs in the later stages of kidney disease. Symptoms of high potassium are a slow pulse, numbness, weakness, and nausea.

Kidney disease stage 1 and 2 = 2–5g per day

Kidney disease stage 3 - 4 =2–4g per day

Kidney disease stage 5 = 2–2.5 per day

Phosphorus: Since your kidneys can no longer remove phosphorus from your blood and urine, hyperphosphatemia or high phosphorus may become a problem during stage 4 or 5 kidney disease.

Kidney disease stage 1 and 2 = up to 1000mg per day

Kidney disease stage 3–4 (GFR of 25–90+) = p to 1000mg per day

Kidney disease stage 4 (GFR of 15–25) = up to 750mg per day

Kidney disease stage 4 (GFR of 5–15) = up to 7mg per kg of body weight

What to Eat and Avoid in the Renal Diet

As specified above, some nutrients should be limited in the renal diet, e.g., phosphorus, potassium, and thus any foods that contain high amounts of these should be taken only in low amounts and not on a daily basis. The foods that should be limited are:

- Bananas
- Avocadoes
- Beetroots
- Dried beans
- Dried fruit
- Mangos
- Melons

- Molasses
- Nuts and seeds
- Oranges
- Parsnips
- Spinach
- Potatoes
- Fish
- Low-fat yogurt

Be attentive! The following foods have a high amount of sodium, and their consumption should be limited:

- Salty snacks, e.g., pretzels, potato chips, packed popcorn etc.
- Savory pies, e.g., cheese pies, sausage rolls, and Greek spinach pies
- Processed meats, e.g., luncheon meat, salami, sausages
- Pickled foods in salt brine
- Condiments, e.g., ketchup, mustard, and mayo
- Soy sauce
- Canned soups and sauces

Now, here are the top foods you can consume without any (strict) restrictions, as they are naturally low in potassium, phosphorus, and sodium:

- Cabbage
- Cucumber
- Broccoli
- Cauliflower
- Brussels sprouts
- Onions
- Garlic
- Apples
- Berries (blueberries, cranberries, berries, strawberries)

- Cherries
- Red grapes
- Egg whites
- Wild-caught fish
- Olive oil
- Bulgur wheat
- Oatmeal
- Skinless chicken and turkey
- Arugula
- Macadamia Nuts
- Radishes
- Shiitake mushrooms
- Pineapple
- Grapefruits
- Kale
- Ginger
- All spices and herbs

Red meat and dairy can also be consumed in moderation, but they should not be combined with high phosphorus, potassium, or sodium foods as they contain moderate amounts of these alone.

List of Juices and Drinks for the Renal Diet

If you wish sufficiently hydrate yourself without increasing your sodium, phosphorus, or potassium intake, there are a few drinks and juices you can drink on a regular basis:

- Freshly made apple juice
- Berry juices
- Red wine (limited to two glasses a day)

- Grape juice
- Filtered drinking water
- Pineapple juice
- Cucumber juice
- Lemon juice diluted
- Most unsweetened herbal tea, e.g., green tea, mint, ginger, cinnamon, etc.
- Coffee (in moderation)

During the late stages of renal dysfunction and particularly from stage 3, as usual, physicians recommend the limitation of fluids up to 1500 mg/day (which is equal to 5–6 glasses of liquids per day). However, this is something that you'd better discuss with your doctor as adjusting the amount yourself may lead to fluid imbalance.

CHAPTER 5

Meal Plan

Whether you are going to prepare your meals in advance or not, planning is essential. If you don't plan out your meals, then you will have difficulty shopping for what you need and cooking with what you have on hand. By first planning out what you will eat for the week, you will be able to seamlessly shop for and prepare your meals with ease. I will provide you with a four-week menu plan for your renal diet.

Here's a 4-week meal plan:

Week 1

DAY	BREAKFAST	LUNCH	DINNER	SNACKS
1	Green Breakfast Soup	Mediterranean Green Beans Recipe	Zesty Orange Tilapia	Savory Collard Chips
2	Peach Berry Parfait	Raw Vegetables, Chopped Salad	Curried Chicken Stir-Fry	Open-Faced Steak and Onion Sandwich
3	Open-Faced Bagel Breakfast Sandwich	Broccoli Soup, Green Leaves, and Beans	Thai-Style Chicken Salad	Roasted Red Pepper Hummus
4	Cauliflower Rice and Coconut	Pumpkin Filled with Vegetables and Quinoa	Chili Rice With Beef	Coconut Pancakes
5	Kale and Garlic Platter	Vegan Vegetable Mini Tortillas	Salisbury Steak	Spiced Peaches
6	Blistered Beans and Almond	Vegetarian Recipe	Swedish Meatballs	Pumpkin Cheesecake Bar
7	Lemon and Broccoli Platter	White Bean Veggie Burgers	Taco Stuffing	Blueberry and Vanilla Mini Muffins

The Essential Renal Diet Cookbook

Week 2

DAY	BREAKFAST	LUNCH	DINNER	SNACKS
1	Chicken Liver Stew	Spicy Tofu and Broccoli Stir-Fry	Basic Meat Loaf	Puffy Oven Pancakes
2	Garlic and Butter-Flavored Cod	Barley and Roasted Vegetable Bowl	Turkey and Noodles	Savory Muffins with Protein
3	Egg White and Pepper Omelet	Corn and Shrimp Quiche	Barbecue Cups	European Pancakes
4	Turkey Breakfast Sausage	Ginger Shrimp with Snow Peas	Simple Lamb Chops	Easy and Fast Mac-n-Cheese
5	Italian Apple Fritters	Roasted Cod with Plums	Beer Pork Ribs	Sandwich with Chicken Salad
6	Tofu and Mushroom Scramble	Seafood Croquettes	Mexican Steak Tacos	Acorn Squash Baked with Pineapple Recipe
7	Sunny Pineapple Breakfast Smoothie	Homemade Tuna Nicoise	Mexican Chorizo Sausage	Super Moist Chocolate Brownies Recipe

Week 3

DAY	BREAKFAST	LUNCH	DINNER	SNACKS
1	Egg Fried Rice	Cajun Crab	Caribbean Turkey Curry	Roast Pork Loin with Sweet and Tart Apple Stuffing
2	Cottage Cheese Pancakes	Spicy Lime Shrimp	Lemon and Fruit Pork Kebabs	Hawaiian-Style Slow Cooked Pulled Pork Recipe
3	Asparagus Bacon Hash	Seafood Casserole	Chicken Stew	Parslied Onions and Pinto Beans Recipe
4	Parmesan Zucchini Frittata	Tilapia Ceviche	Asian Style-Fried Chicken	Spaghetti Squash Boats Recipe
5	Curried Veggie Stir-Fry	Fish Tacos	Curried Chicken with Cauliflower	Sauce-less BBQ Baby Back Ribs Recipe
6	Chilaquiles	Jambalaya	Red and Green Grapes Chicken Salad with Curry	Butternut Squash, Cauliflower, and Beef Shepherd's Pie
7	Roasted Peach Open-Face Sandwich	Asparagus Shrimp Linguini	Grilled Chicken Pizza	Vegan Quinoa Chili Recipe

Week 4

DAY	BREAKFAST	LUNCH	DINNER	SNACKS
1	Pasta Fagioli	Tuna Noodle Casserole	Chicken Breast and Bok Choy	Chicken, Charred Tomato, and Broccoli Salad
2	Spinach Alfredo Lasagna Rolls	Tilapia Ceviche	Baked Herbed Chicken	Easy Baked Shepherd's Pie
3	Spicy Corn and Rice Burritos	Oven-Fried Southern Style Catfish	Chicken and Cabbage Stir Fry	Tofu Soup
4	Crustless Cabbage Quiche	Cilantro-Lime Cod	Herb Crusted Pork Tenderloin	Onion Soup
5	Creamy Veggie Casserole	Shrimp Quesadilla	Simple Lamb Chops	Roasted Carrot Soup
6	Vegetable Rice Casserole	Maryland Crab Cakes	Chili Rice With Beef	Mushroom Cream Soup
7	Vegetable Confetti Relish	Citrus Grilled Glazed Salmon	Ginger Shrimp with Snow Peas	Garlic Soup

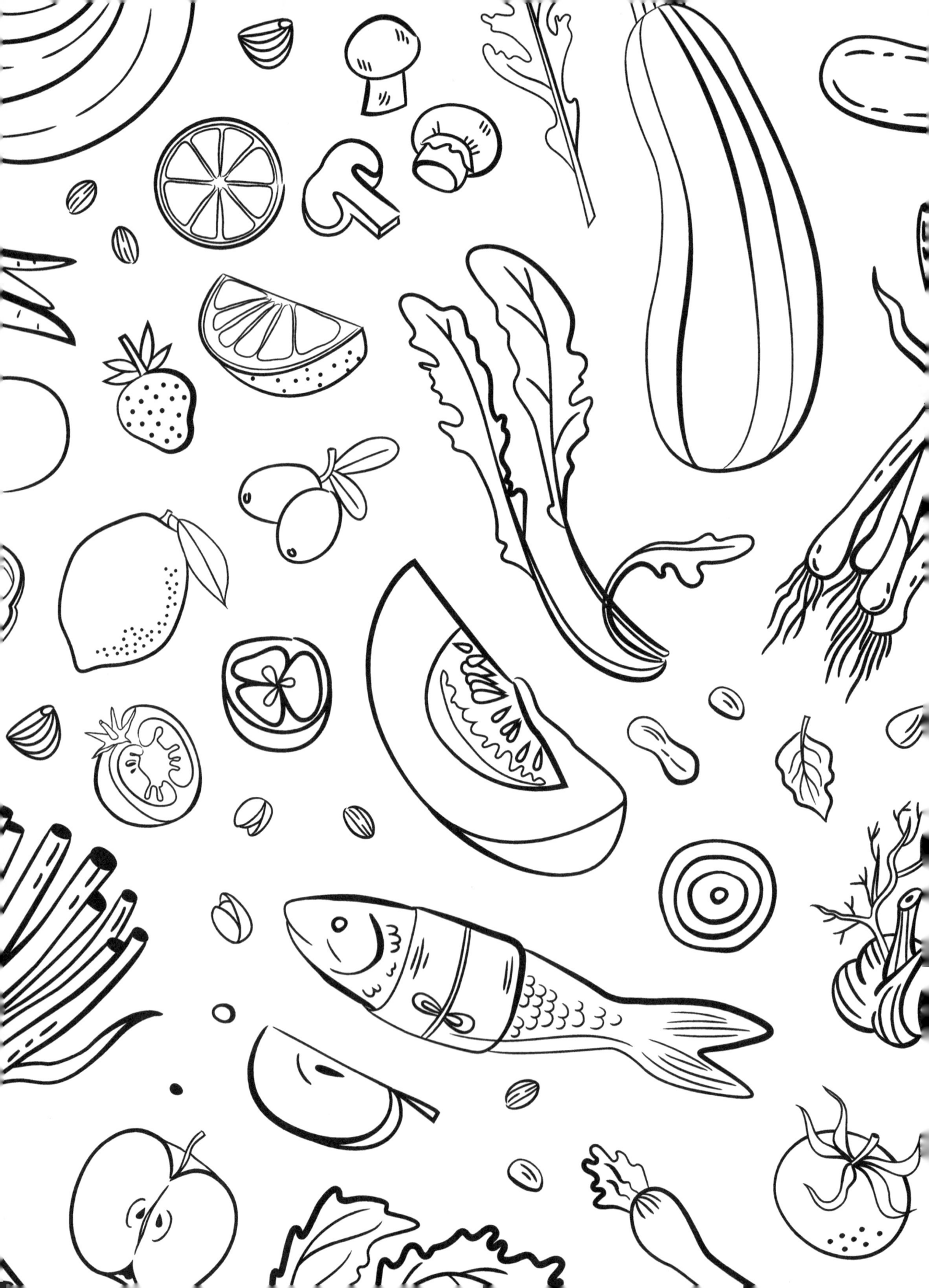

Chapter 6

BREAKFAST RECIPES

1. Green Breakfast Soup

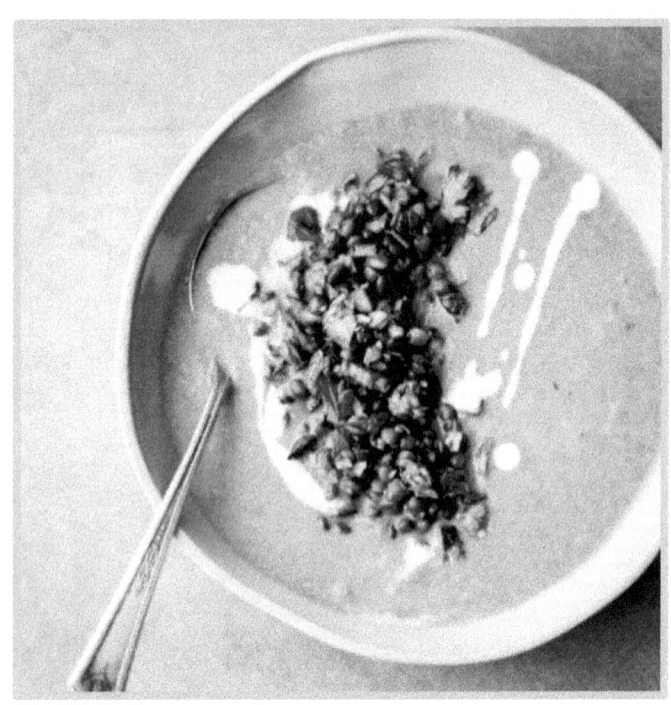

NUTRITION

Calories: 221
Total Fat: 18g
Saturated Fat: 3g
Cholesterol: 0mg
Carbohydrates: 15g
Fiber: 10g
Protein: 5g
Phosphorus: 58mg
Potassium: 551mg
Sodium: 170mg

PREP TIME
5 min

COOK TIME
5 min

SERVING
2 people

DIRECTIONS

1. Using a food processor, add the spinach, avocado, broth, coriander, cumin, and turmeric. Process until smooth.
2. Transfer the mixture to a small saucepan over medium heat, and cook until heated through, 2 to 3 minutes—season with pepper.

Lower sodium tip: If you want to lower the sodium further, consider making your own Simple Chicken Broth for more control over the ingredients. Freeze the broth in 2-cup portions so you can make quick soups when needed.

INGREDIENTS

- 2 cups of spinach
- 1 avocado, halved
- 2 cups of low-sodium vegetable or chicken broth (lower sodium)
- 1 teaspoon of ground coriander
- 1 teaspoon of ground cumin
- 1 teaspoon of ground turmeric
- Freshly ground black pepper

2. Peach Berry Parfait

PREP TIME
5 min

COOK TIME
5 min

SERVING
2 people

NUTRITION

Calories: 191

Total Fat: 10g

Saturated Fat: 3g

Cholesterol: 15mg

Carbohydrates: 14g

Fiber: 14g

Protein: 12g

Phosphorus: 189mg

Potassium: 327mg

Sodium: 40mg

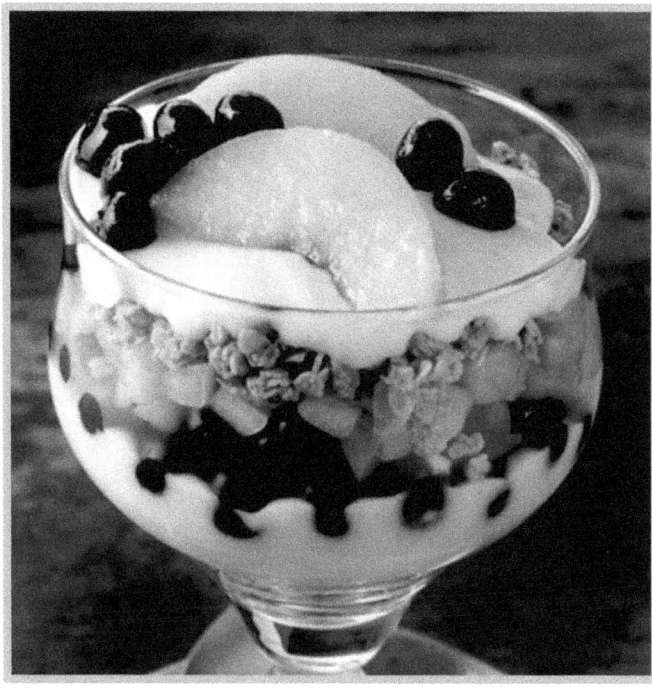

INGREDIENTS

- 1 cup of plain, unsweetened yogurt, divided
- 1 teaspoon of vanilla extract
- 1 small peach, diced
- ½ cup of blueberries
- 2 tablespoons of walnut pieces

DIRECTIONS

1. Add the yogurt and vanilla in a bowl together, then add 2 tablespoons of yogurt to each of 2 cups. Divide the diced peach and the blueberries between the cups, and top with the remaining yogurt.
2. Sprinkle each cup with 1 tablespoon of walnut pieces.

Cooking tip: Make these up to three days in advance, cover, and refrigerate until ready to eat.

3. Open-Faced Bagel Breakfast Sandwich

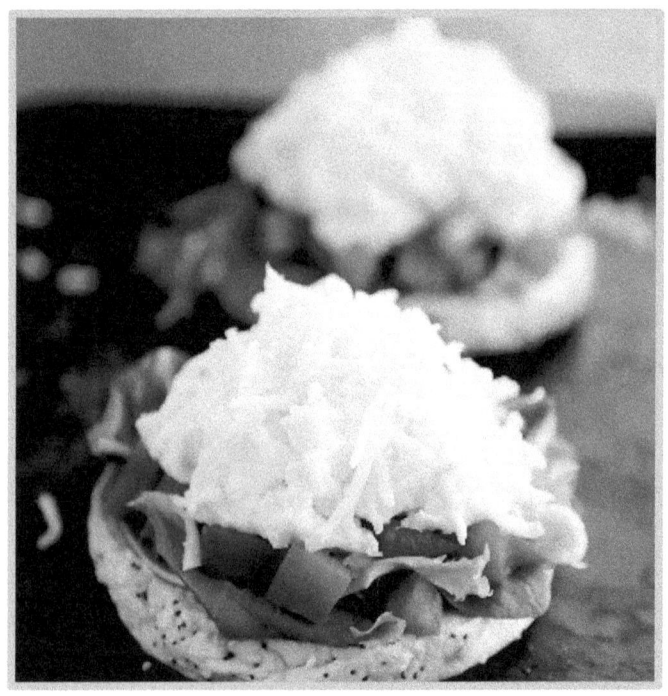

NUTRITION

Calories: 156
Total Fat: 6g
Saturated Fat: 3g
Cholesterol: 18mg
Carbohydrates: 22g
Fiber: 3g
Protein: 5g
Protein: 5g
Phosphorus: 98mg
Potassium: 163mg
Sodium: 195mg

PREP TIME 5 min

COOK TIME 5 min

SERVING 2 people

DIRECTIONS

1. Toast the bagel in a toaster lightly.
2. Spread the cream cheese on each of the bagel halves, then top each half with 1 slice of tomato and a couple of onion rings.
3. Season with the black pepper.
4. Top each half with ½ cup of microgreens and serve.

INGREDIENTS

- 1 multigrain bagel, halved
- 2 tablespoons cream cheese, divided
- 2 slices tomato
- 1 slice red onion
- Freshly ground black pepper
- 1 cup microgreens

4. Cauliflower Rice and Coconut

PREP TIME 20 min

COOK TIME 20 min

SERVING 4 people

NUTRITION

Calories: 95

Fat: 7g

Carbohydrates: 4g

Protein: 1g

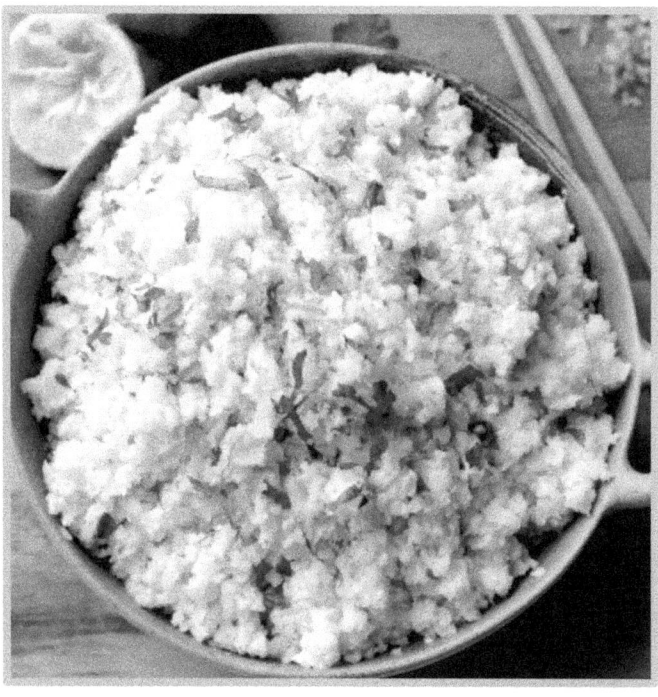

INGREDIENTS

- 3 cups of cauliflower, riced
- 2/3 cups of full-fat coconut milk
- 1-2 teaspoons of sriracha paste
- ¼- ½ teaspoon of onion powder
- Salt as needed
- Fresh basil for garnish

DIRECTIONS

1. Take a pan and place it over medium-low heat.
2. Add all of the ingredients and stir them until fully combined.
3. Cook for about 5–10 minutes, making sure that the lid is on.
4. Remove the lid and keep cooking until there's no excess liquid.
5. Once the rice is soft and creamy, enjoy it!

5. Kale and Garlic Platter

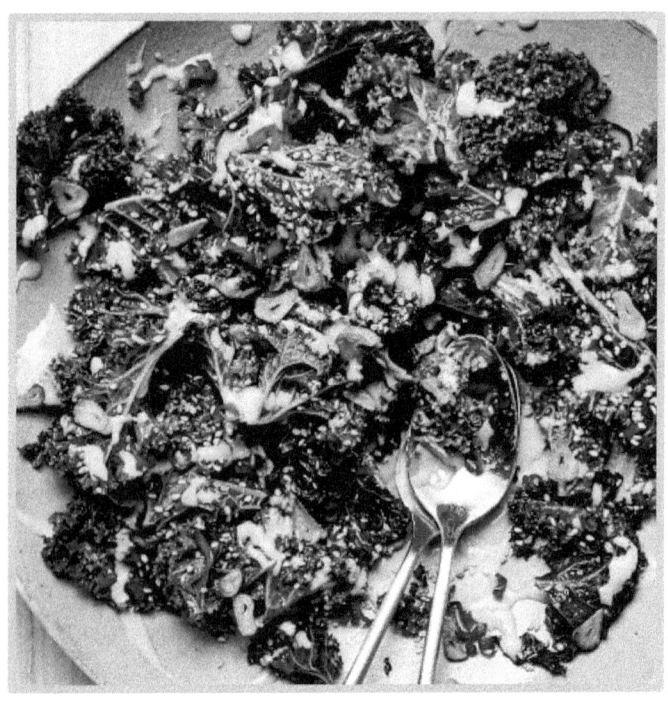

NUTRITION

Calories: 121

Fat: 8g

Carbohydrates: 5g

Protein: 4g

PREP TIME
5 min

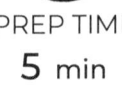

COOK TIME
10 min

SERVING
4 people

DIRECTIONS

1. Carefully tear the kale into bite-sized portions, making sure to remove the stem.
2. Discard the stems.
3. Take a large-sized pot and place it over medium heat.
4. Add olive oil and let it heat up.
5. Add garlic and stir for 2 minutes.
6. Add kale and cook for 5–10 minutes.
7. Serve!

INGREDIENTS

- 1 bunch of kale
- 2 tablespoons of olive oil
- 4 garlic cloves, minced

6. Blistered Beans and Almond

PREP TIME 10 min

COOK TIME 20 min

SERVING 4 people

NUTRITION

Calories: 347

Fat: 16g

Carbohydrates: 6g

Protein: 45g

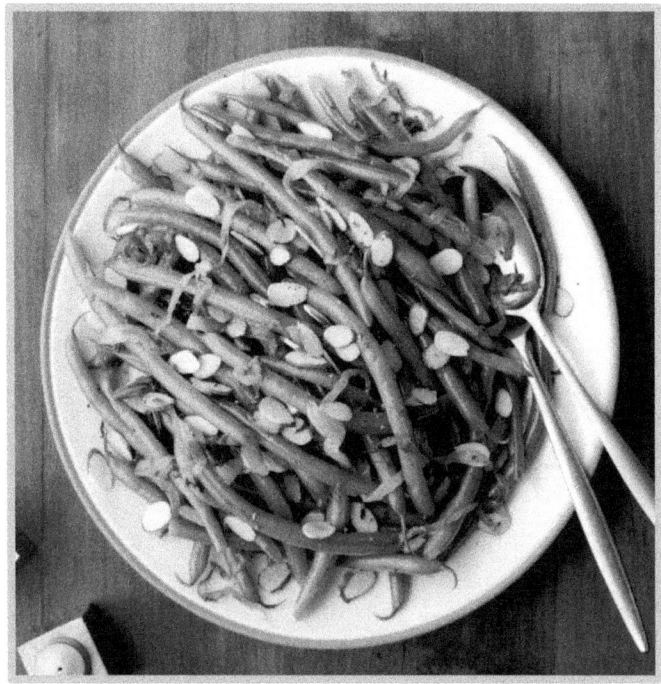

INGREDIENTS

- 1 pound of fresh green beans, ends trimmed
- 1 ½ tablespoon of olive oil
- ¼ teaspoon of salt
- 1 ½ tablespoon of fresh dill, minced
- Juice of 1 lemon
- ¼ cup of crushed almonds
- Salt as needed

DIRECTIONS

1. Preheat your oven to 400°F.
2. Add in the green beans with your olive oil and also the salt.
3. Then spread them in one single layer on a large-sized sheet pan.
4. Roast for 10 minutes and stir nicely, then roast for another 8–10 minutes.
5. Remove it from the oven and keep stirring in the lemon juice alongside the dill.
6. Top it with crushed almonds, some flaky sea salt and serve.

7. Lemon and Broccoli Platter

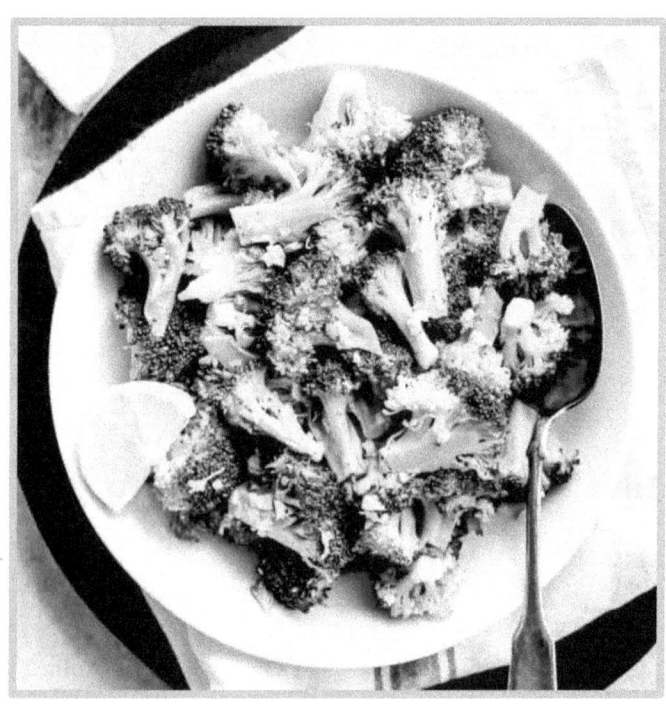

NUTRITION

Calories: 49

Fat: 1.9g

Carbohydrates: 7g

Protein: 3g

PREP TIME
10 min

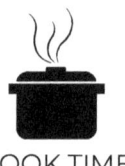

COOK TIME
15 min

SERVING
6 people

DIRECTIONS

1. Preheat your oven to 400°F.
2. Take a large-sized bowl and add broccoli florets.
3. Drizzle olive oil and season with pepper, salt, and garlic.
4. Spread the broccoli out in a single even layer on a baking sheet.
5. Bake for 15–20 minutes until fork tender.
6. Squeeze lemon juice on top.
7. Serve and enjoy!

INGREDIENTS

- 2 heads of broccoli, separated into florets
- 2 teaspoons of extra virgin olive oil
- 1 teaspoon of salt
- ½ teaspoon of black pepper
- 1 garlic clove, minced
- ½ teaspoon of lemon juice

8. Chicken Liver Stew

PREP TIME
10 min

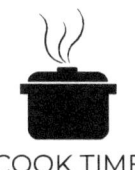
COOK TIME
20 min

SERVING
2 people

NUTRITION

Calories: 146
Fat: 9g
Carbohydrates: 2g
Protein: 15g

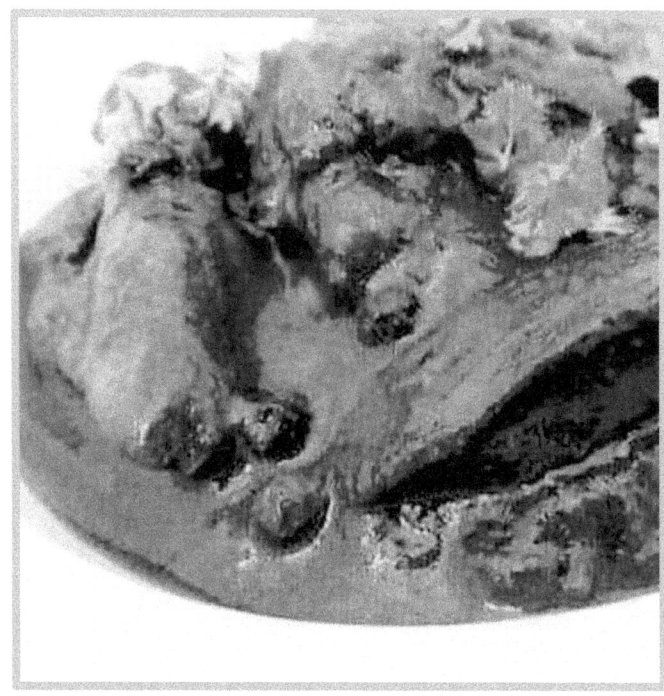

INGREDIENTS

- 10 ounces of chicken livers
- 1 ounce of onion, chopped
- 2 ounces of sour cream
- 1 tablespoon of olive oil
- Salt to taste

DIRECTIONS

1. Take a pan and place it over medium heat.
2. Add oil and let it heat up.
3. Add onions and fry until just browned.
4. Add livers and season with salt.
5. Cook until livers are half cooked.
6. Transfer the mix to a stew pot.
7. Add sour cream and cook for 20 minutes.
8. Serve and enjoy!

9. Garlic and Butter-Flavored Cod

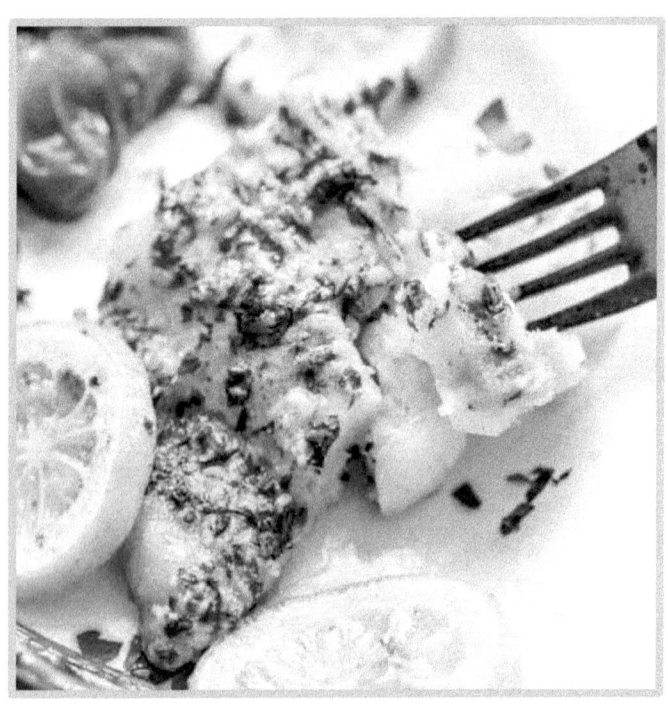

NUTRITION

Calories: 355
Fat: 21g
Carbohydrates: 3g
Protein: 37g

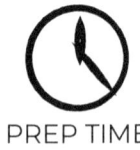

PREP TIME
5 min

COOK TIME
20 min

SERVING
3 people

DIRECTIONS

1. Preheat your oven to 400°F.
2. Cut 3 sheets of aluminum foil (large enough to fit fillet).
3. Place cod fillet on each sheet and add butter and garlic on top.
4. Add bok choy, season with pepper and salt.
5. Fold packet and enclose them in pouches.
6. Arrange on the baking sheet.
7. Bake for 20 minutes.
8. Let it cool.
9. Enjoy!

INGREDIENTS

- 3 Cod fillets, 8 ounces each
- ¾ pound of baby bok choy halved
- 1/3 cup of almond butter, thinly sliced
- 1 ½ tablespoon of garlic, minced
- Salt and pepper to taste

10. Egg White and Pepper Omelet

PREP TIME
5 min

COOK TIME
5 min

SERVING
1-2 people

NUTRITION

Calories: 165
Carbohydrate: 3.8g
Protein: 9.2g
Sodium: 797mg
Potassium: 193mg
Phosphorus: 202.5mg
Dietary Fiber: 0.7g
Fat: 15.22g
Kidney Disease Stage: 2

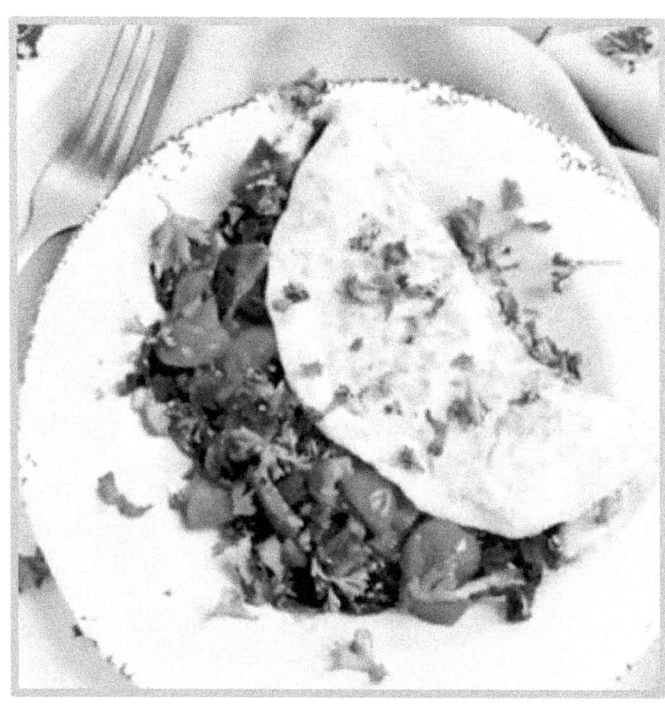

INGREDIENTS

- 4 egg whites, lightly beaten
- 1 red bell pepper, diced
- 1 tsp. of paprika
- 2 tbsp. of olive oil
- ½ tsp. of salt
- Pepper

DIRECTIONS

1. In a shallow pan (around 8 inches), heat the olive oil and sauté the bell peppers until softened.
2. Add the egg whites and the paprika and fold the edges into the fluid center with a spatula and let omelet cook until eggs are fully opaque and solid—season with salt and pepper.

11. Turkey Breakfast Sausage

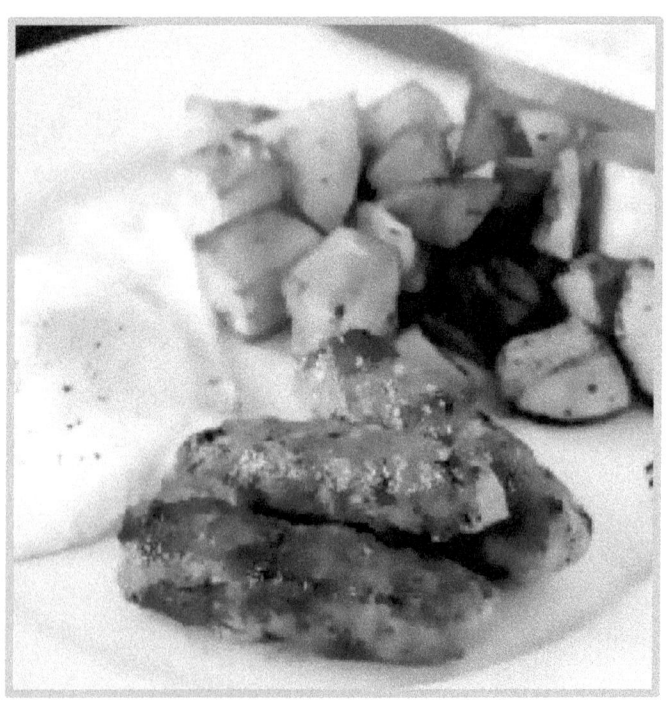

NUTRITION

Calories: 74
Carbohydrate: 0.1g
Protein: 7g
Sodium: 121.9mg
Potassium: 89.5mg
Phosphorus: 75mg
Dietary Fiber: 0g
Fat: 5.16g
Kidney Disease Stage 2

PREP TIME
5 min

COOK TIME
6 min

SERVING
12 people

DIRECTIONS

1. Combine all the ingredients apart from the vegetable oil in a mixing bowl.
2. Form into long and flat (around 4 inch-long) patties.
3. Heat the vegetable oil in a medium frying pan.
4. Add 3-4 patties at a time and cook for approx. 3 minutes on each side. Repeat until you cook all patties.
5. Serve warm.

INGREDIENTS

- (12 patties per recipe)
- 1 pound of lean ground turkey
- 1 tsp. of fennel seed
- ¼ tsp. of garlic powder
- ¼ tsp. of onion powder
- ¼ tsp. of salt
- 2 tbsp. of vegetable oil
- Pepper

12. Italian Apple Fritters

PREP TIME
5 min

COOK TIME
8 min

SERVING
4 people

NUTRITION

Calories: 183

Carbohydrate: 17.9g

Protein: 0.3g

Sodium: 2g

Potassium: 100mg

Phosphorus: 12.5mg

Dietary Fiber: 1.4g

Fat: 14.17g

Kidney Disease Stage 3

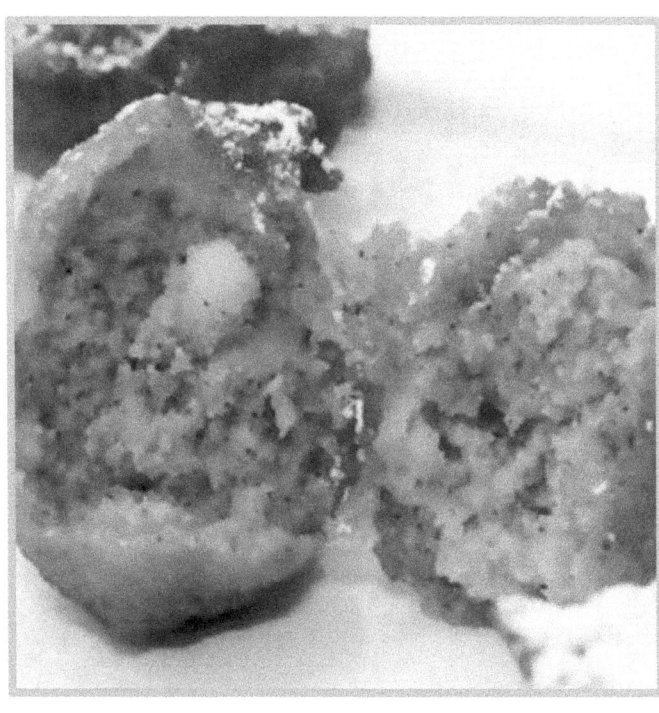

INGREDIENTS

- 2 large apples, seeded, peeled, and thickly sliced in round circles
- 3 tbsp. of cornflour
- ½ tsp. of water
- 1 tsp. of sugar
- 1 tsp. of cinnamon
- Vegetable oil (for frying)
- Sprinkle of icing sugar or honey

DIRECTIONS

1. Combine the cornflour, water, and sugar to make your batter in a small bowl.
2. Deep the apple rounds into the cornflour mix.
3. Heat enough vegetable oil to cover half of the pan's surface over medium to high heat.
4. Add the apple rounds into the pan and cook until golden brown.
5. Transfer into a shallow dish with absorbing paper on top and sprinkle with a bit of cinnamon and icing sugar.

13. Tofu and Mushroom Scramble

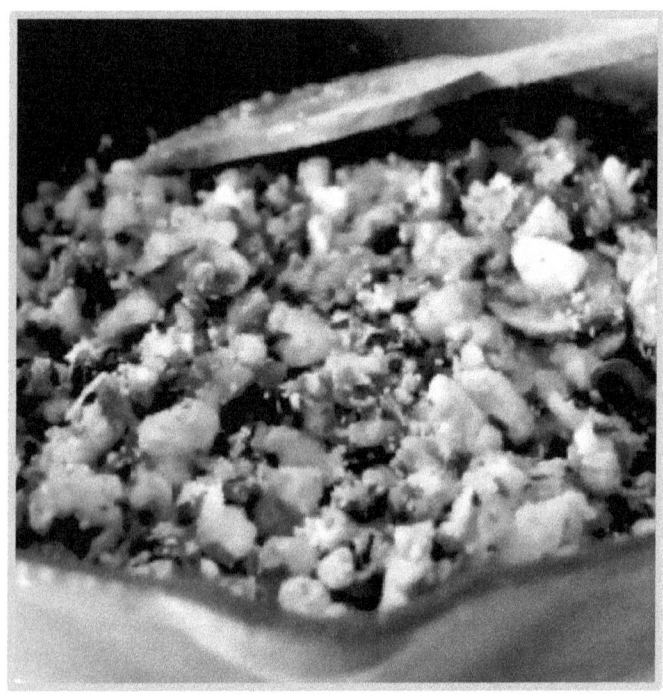

NUTRITION

Calories: 220
Carbohydrate: 2.59g
Protein: 3.2g
Sodium: 288 mg
Potassium: 133.5mg
Phosphorus: 68.5mg
Dietary Fiber: 1.7g
Fat: 23.7g
Kidney Disease Stage 3

PREP TIME
5 min

COOK TIME
4 min

SERVING
2 people

DIRECTIONS

1. Heat the oil frying pan, set it on a medium, and saute the sliced mushrooms with the shallots until softened (around 3–4 minutes) over medium to high heat.
2. Add the tofu pieces and toss in the spices and the garlic salt. Toss lightly until tofu and mushrooms are nicely combined together.
3. Serve warm.

INGREDIENTS

- ½ cup of sliced white mushrooms
- ⅓ cup of medium-firm tofu, crumbled
- 1 tbsp. of chopped shallots
- ⅓ tsp. of turmeric
- 1 tsp. of cumin
- ⅓ tsp. of smoked paprika
- ½ tsp. of garlic salt
- Pepper
- 3 tbsp. of vegetable oil

14. Egg Fried Rice

PREP TIME
10 min

COOK TIME
20 min

SERVING
6 people

NUTRITION

Calories: 204
Total fat: 6g
Saturated fat: 1g
Cholesterol: 141mg
Sodium: 223mg
Carbohydrates: 29g
Fiber: 1g
Phosphorus: 120mg
Potassium: 147mg
Protein: 8g
Kidney Disease Stage 5

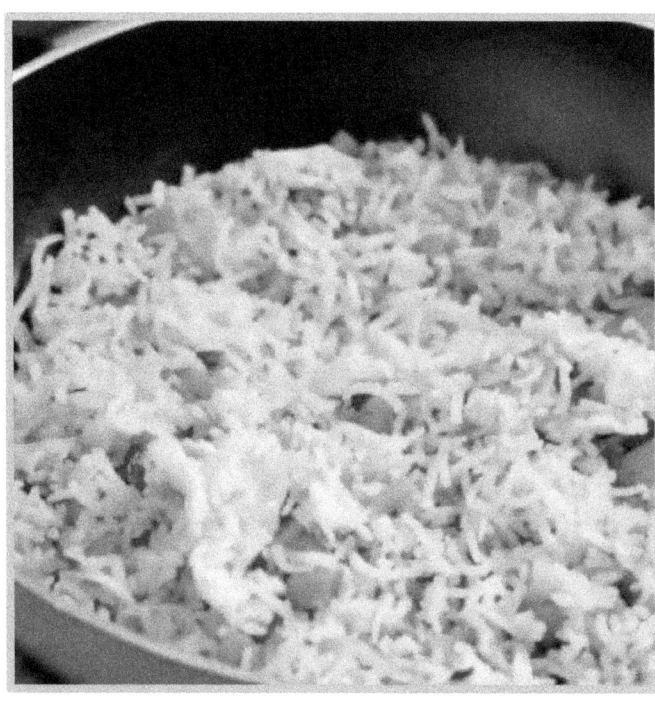

INGREDIENTS

- 1 tablespoon of olive oil
- 1 tablespoon of grated peeled fresh ginger
- 1 teaspoon of minced garlic
- 1 cup of chopped carrots
- 1 scallion, white and green parts, chopped
- 2 tablespoons of chopped fresh cilantro
- 4 cups of cooked rice
- 1 tablespoon of low-sodium soy sauce
- 4 eggs, beaten

DIRECTIONS

1. In a large skillet over medium-high heat, heat the olive oil.
2. Add the ginger and garlic, and sauté until softened, about 3 minutes.
3. Add the carrots, scallion, and cilantro, and sauté until tender, about 5 minutes.
4. Stir in the rice and soy sauce, and sauté until the rice is heated through about 5 minutes.
5. Move the rice over to one side of the skillet, and pour the eggs into the empty space.
6. Scramble the eggs, then mix them into the rice. Serve hot.

Low-sodium tip: Soy sauces, even low-sodium versions, are very salty. If you have the time, making your own substitution sauce is simple and effective, even if it does not taste quite the same. There are many versions of this diet-friendly sauce online, with ingredients like vinegar, molasses, garlic, and herbs.

15. Cottage Cheese Pancakes

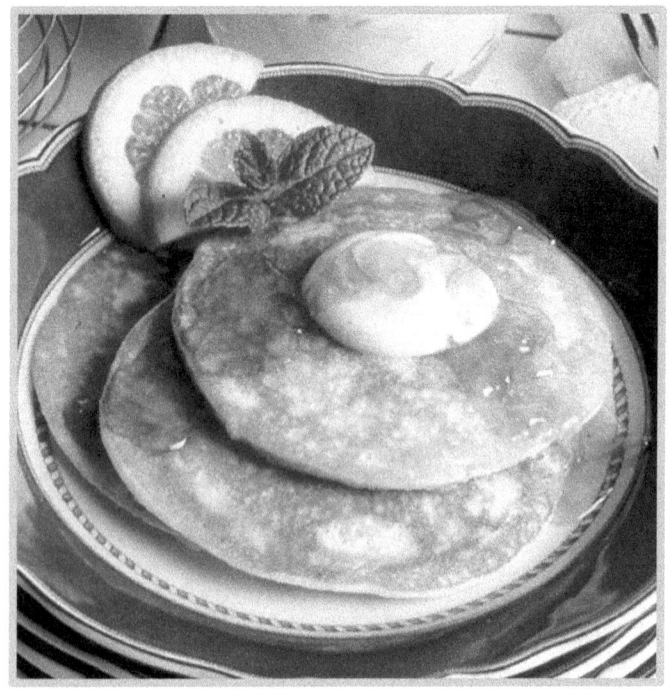

NUTRITION

Calories: 196
Total Fat: 11.3g
Saturated Fat: 3.1g
Cholesterol: 127mg
Sodium: 276mg
Carbohydrate: 10.3g
Dietary Fiber: 0.3g
Sugars: 0.5g
Protein: 13g
Calcium: 58mg
Phosphorous: 187mg
Potassium: 110mg

PREP TIME
10 min

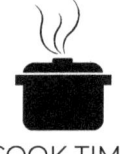

COOK TIME
10 min

SERVING
4 people

DIRECTIONS

1. Begin by beating the eggs in a suitable bowl then stir in the cottage cheese.
2. Once it is well mixed, stir in the flour.
3. Pour a teaspoon of vegetable oil in a non-stick griddle and heat it.
4. Add ¼ cup of the batter in the griddle and cook for 2 minutes per side until brown.
5. Cook more of the pancakes using the remaining batter.
6. Serve.

INGREDIENTS

- 1 cup of cottage cheese
- 1/3 cup of all-purpose flour
- 2 tablespoons of vegetable oil
- 3 eggs, lightly beaten

16. Asparagus Bacon Hash

PREP TIME
10 min

COOK TIME
27 min

SERVING
4 people

NUTRITION

Calories: 290
Total Fat: 17.9g
Saturated Fat: 6.1g
Cholesterol: 220mg
Sodium: 256mg
Carbohydrate: 11.6g
Dietary Fiber: 5.1g
Sugars: 5.3g
Protein: 23.2g
Calcium: 121mg
Phosphorous: 247mg
Potassium: 715mg

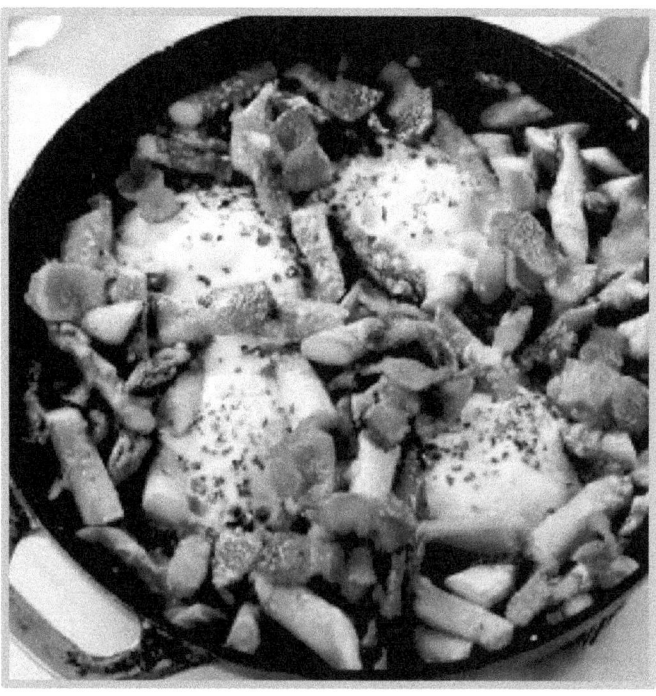

INGREDIENTS

- 6 slices of bacon, diced
- 1/2 onion, chopped
- 2 garlic cloves, sliced
- 2 lb. of asparagus, trimmed and chopped
- Black pepper, to taste
- 2 tablespoons of Parmesan, grated
- 4 large eggs
- 1/4 teaspoon of red pepper flakes

DIRECTIONS

1. Add the asparagus and a tablespoon of water to a microwave-proof bowl.
2. Cover the veggies and microwave them for 5 minutes until tender.
3. Set a suitable non-stick skillet over moderate heat and layer it with cooking spray.
4. Stir in the onion and sauté for 7 minutes, then toss in the garlic.
5. Stir for 1 minute, then toss in the asparagus, eggs, and red pepper flakes.
6. Reduce the heat to low and cover the vegetables in the pan. Top the eggs with Parmesan cheese.
7. Cook for approximately 15 minutes, then slice to serve.

17. Parmesan Zucchini Frittata

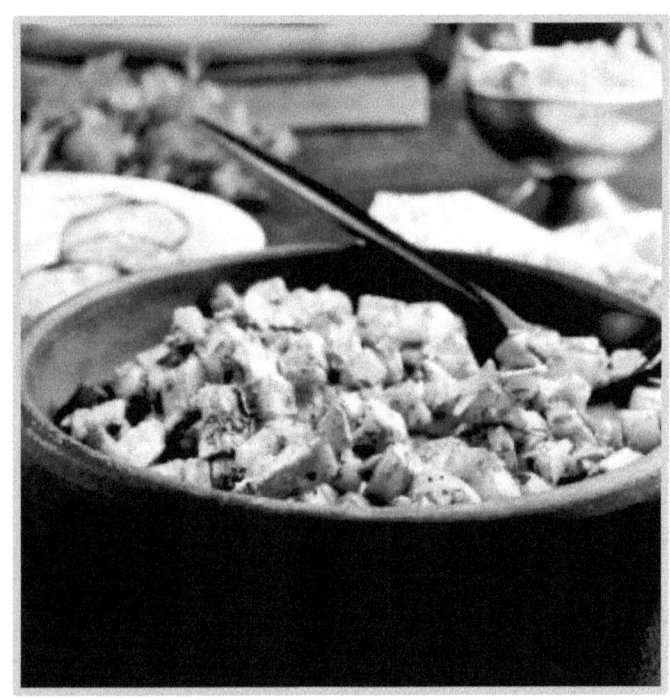

NUTRITION

Calories: 142
Total Fat: 9.7g
Saturated Fat: 2.8g
Cholesterol: 250mg
Sodium: 123mg
Carbohydrate: 4.7g
Dietary Fiber: 1.3g
Sugars: 2.4g
Protein: 10.2g
Calcium: 73mg
Phosphorous: 375mg
Potassium: 286mg

PREP TIME
10 min

COOK TIME
35 min

SERVING
6 people

DIRECTIONS

1. Toss the zucchinis with the onion, parsley, and all other ingredients in a large bowl.
2. Pour this zucchini-garlic mixture in an 11x7 inches pan and spread it evenly.
3. Bake the zucchini casserole for approximately 35 minutes at 350°F.
4. Cut in slices and serve.

INGREDIENTS

- 1 tablespoon of olive oil
- 1 cup of yellow onion, sliced
- 3 cups of zucchini, chopped
- ½ cup of Parmesan cheese, grated
- 8 large eggs
- ½ teaspoon of black pepper
- ⅛ teaspoon of paprika
- 3 tablespoons of parsley, chopped

18. Mexican Baked Beans and Rice

NUTRITION

PREP TIME
20 min

COOK TIME
60 min

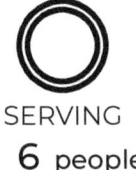
SERVING
6 people

Calories: 264
Carbs: 22g
Protein: 27g
Fat: 9g
Phosphorus: 353mg
Potassium: 682mg
Sodium: 280mg

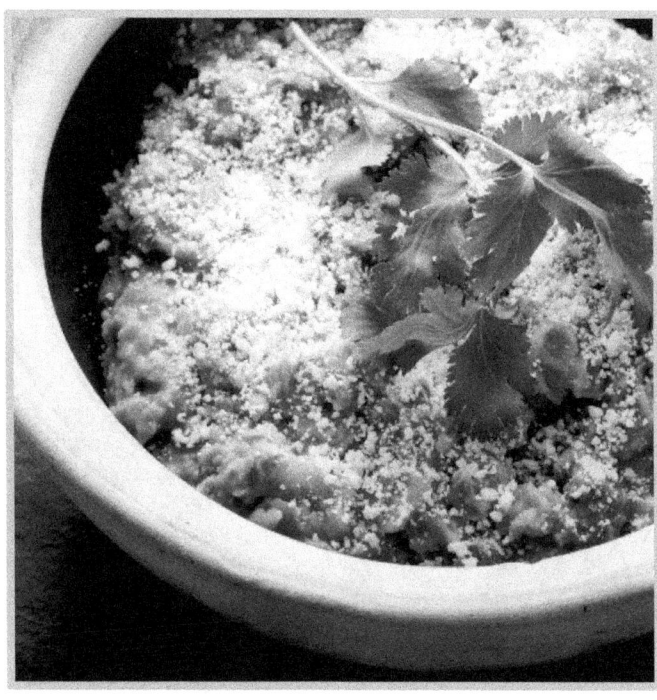

INGREDIENTS

- 1 cup of shredded reduced-fat Monterey Jack cheese
- 4 garlic cloves, crushed
- 1 tbsp. of cumin
- 1 tbsp. of chili powder
- 1 cup of chopped poblano pepper
- 1 cup of chopped red bell pepper
- 1 cup of frozen yellow corn
- Black beans, (15-oz, no-salt-added) drained and rinsed
- 2 (14.5-oz.) cans of no-salt-added tomatoes, diced or crushed
- 1 lb. of chicken breast, skinless, boneless, cubed
- 1 ½ cups of cooked brown rice

DIRECTIONS

1. With cooking spray, grease a ¾ shallow casserole and Preheat oven to 400°F. Spread cooked brown rice at the bottom of the casserole. Layer chicken on top of brown rice.

2. Mix well garlic, seasonings, peppers, corn, beans, and tomatoes in a medium bowl. Evenly spread bean mixture on top of chicken. Sprinkle cheese on top of beans and pop into the oven. Set to bake until cooked (about 45 minutes). Switch off the oven and serve.

19. Quick Thai Chicken and Vegetable Curry

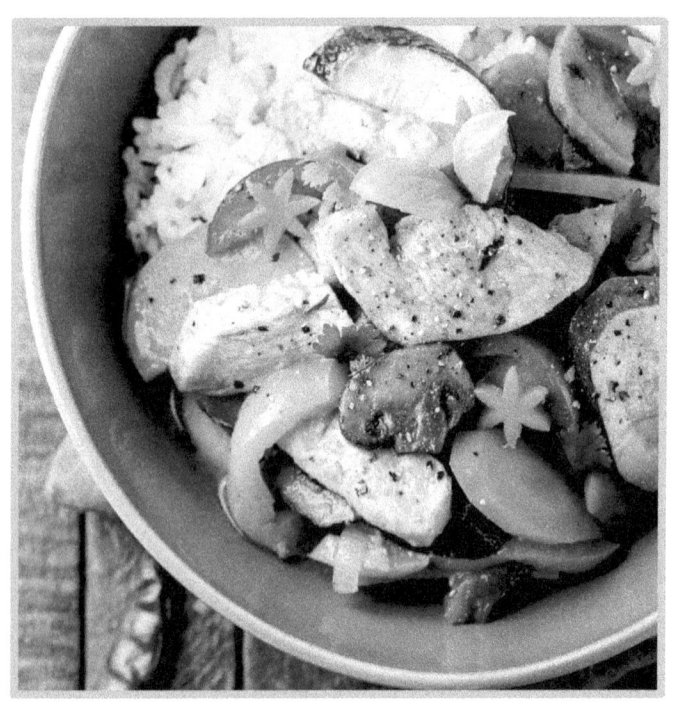

NUTRITION

Calories: 394

Carbs: 11g

Protein: 29g

Fat: 28g

Phosphorus: 316mg

Potassium: 745mg

Sodium: 252mg

PREP TIME
15 min

COOK TIME
20 min

SERVING
4 people

DIRECTIONS

1. Heat oil in a skillet over a medium-high flame. Sauté the onion and bell pepper for four minutes or until soft.
2. Add the ginger, garlic, and curry paste. Mix then add the chicken. Sauté for two minutes before adding the coconut milk, broth, brown sugar, and fish sauce.
3. Add the cauliflowers and reduce the heat to medium-low. Simmer and stir the mixture occasionally until the chicken is cooked through.
4. Add the spinach and lime juice and cook until the spinach has wilted.
5. Serve immediately with lime wedges.

INGREDIENTS

- 1 ½ cups cauliflower florets
- 1 clove garlic, minced
- 1 cup light coconut milk
- 1 cup low sodium chicken broth
- 1 lb chicken breasts
- 1 medium bell pepper, julienned
- 1 medium onion, halved and sliced
- 1 tbsp fish sauce or low sodium soy sauce
- 1 tbsp fresh ginger, minced
- 1 tbsp lime juice
- 1 tsp light brown sugar
- 1 tsp red curry paste
- 2 cups baby spinach
- 2 tsp canola oil
- Lime wedges

20. Cajun Stuffed Peppers

PREP TIME
10 min

COOK TIME
45 min

SERVING
6 people

NUTRITION

Calories: 173.5

Protein: 8.8g

Sodium: 27.7mg

Phosphorus: 8.0mg

Potassium: 166.1mg

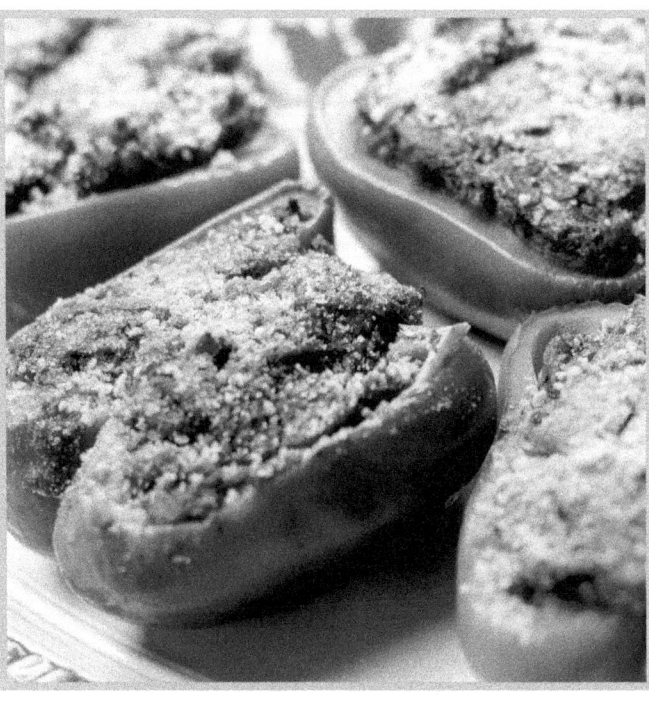

INGREDIENTS

- 1 cup of chopped roasted red peppers
- 6 fresh bell peppers
- 1/2 lb. of ground beef
- 1/2 lb. of ground pork
- 1/4 cup of hot water
- 1 medium onion chopped
- 3 cups of cooked white rice
- 1/2 tsp. of black pepper
- 1/2 tsp. of lemon pepper
- 1 tbsp. of dried thyme
- 1 tbsp. of minced garlic

DIRECTIONS

1. Preheat oven to 350°F.
2. Bring a large pot of water to a boil and drop in the bell peppers.
3. Boil the peppers for 5 minutes. Remove and drain.
4. Prepare the peppers by removing the stem and removing the seeds.
5. In a large skillet, cook the ground meat over medium heat until it is browned.
6. Add the hot water, roasted red peppers, onions, garlic, and spices.
7. Cook for 5 minutes.
8. Add rice and stir to combine and cook for 3 minutes. Remove from the heat and stuff the bell peppers. Put the stuffed peppers in a baking sheet and bake, uncovered, for 30 minutes.
9. Serve with a garnish of roasted red peppers.

21. Stuffed Zucchini

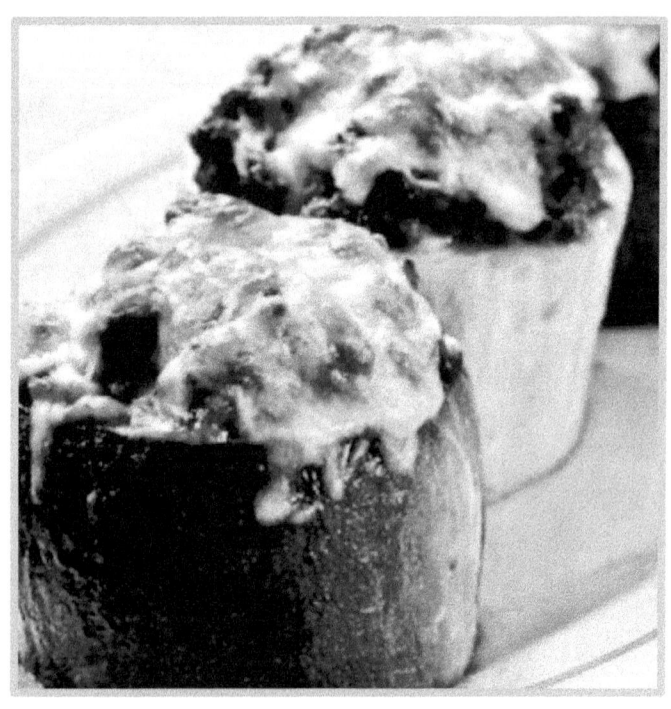

NUTRITION

Calories: 157.0

Protein: 9.5g

Sodium: 49.0mg

Phosphorus: 4.4mg

Potassium: 236.1mg

PREP TIME
20 min

COOK TIME
45 min

SERVING
8 people

DIRECTIONS

1. Preheat oven to 350°F.
2. Slice zucchini in half, lengthwise, and scoop out insides leaving ¼ inch zucchini on skins.
3. Reserve the insides.
4. Place zucchini halves skin-side down on the baking sheet.
5. In a large skillet over medium heat, warm the oil.
6. Add the onion and sauté for 3 minutes.
7. Add the zucchini insides, the rest of the veggies, the matzo, and the spices.
8. Sauté for 2 minutes.
9. Add the chicken and mix well.
10. Remove from heat and stuff the zucchini with the mixture.
11. Bake for 30 minutes.

INGREDIENTS

- 4 large zucchini
- 2 tbsp. of canola oil
- 1 diced onion
- 1 red bell pepper diced
- 1 cup of shredded carrots
- 1 summer squash diced
- 4 matzo broken into pieces
- 1 tsp. of dried oregano
- 2 tsp. of minced garlic
- 1 tsp. of ground pepper
- 1 lb. of ground chicken, cooked

Chapter 7

SMOOTHIES AND DRINKS

22. Sunny Pineapple Breakfast Smoothie

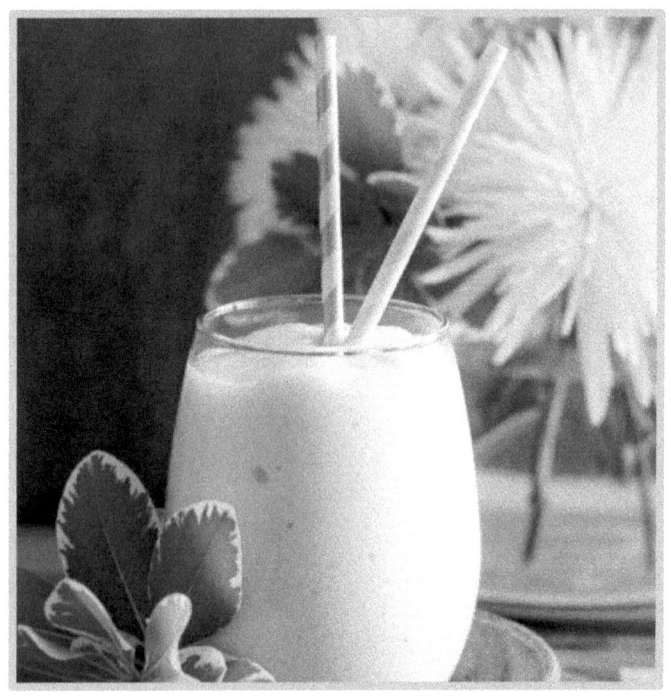

NUTRITION

Calories: 186
Carbohydrate: 43.7g
Protein: 2.28g
Sodium: 130mg
Potassium: 135mg
Phosphorus: 18mg
Dietary Fiber: 2.4g
Fat: 2.3g
Kidney Disease Stage 2

PREP TIME
5 min

COOK TIME
1 min

SERVING
1 people

DIRECTIONS

1. Blend everything in a blender until nice and smooth (around 30 seconds).
2. Transfer into a tall glass or mason jar.
3. Serve and enjoy.

INGREDIENTS

- ½ cup of frozen pineapple chunks
- ⅔ cup of almond milk
- ½ tsp. of ginger powder
- 1 tbsp. of agave syrup

23. Blueberry Burst Smoothie

PREP TIME
5 min

COOK TIME
0 min

SERVING
2 people

NUTRITION

Calories: 131
Total Fat: 6g
Saturated Fat: 0g
Cholesterol: 0mg
Carbohydrates: 19g
Fiber: 3g
Protein: 3g
Phosphorus: 51mg
Potassium: 146mg
Sodium: 60mg

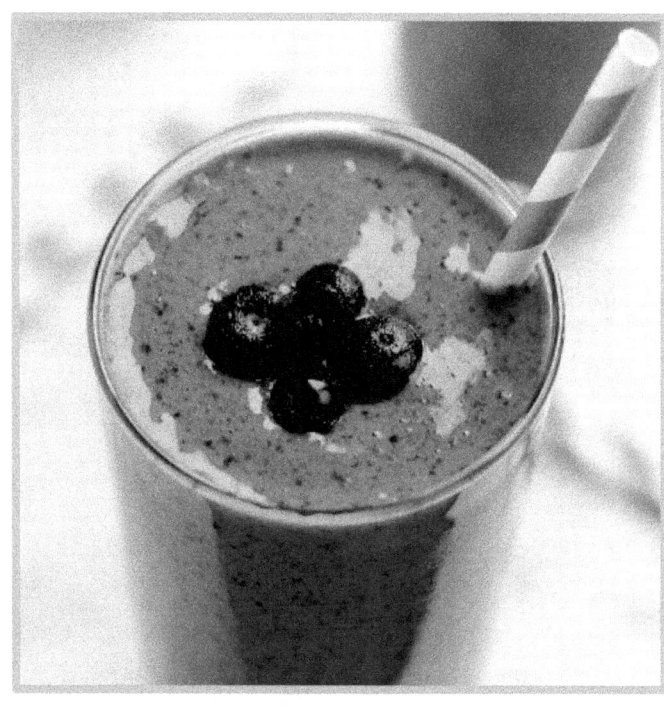

INGREDIENTS

- 1 cup of blueberries
- 1 cup of chopped collard greens
- 1 cup of Homemade Rice Milk or unsweetened store-bought rice milk
- 1 tablespoon of almond butter
- 3 ice cubes

DIRECTIONS

1. In a blender, combine the blueberries, collard greens, milk, almond butter, and ice cubes.
2. Process until smooth, and serve.

Nutrition tip: Collard greens are a nutrient-dense food loaded with anticarcinogenic, antiviral, antibiotic, and antioxidant properties. Because collard greens are much lower in potassium than kale, they are a great substitute in recipes that call for its cruciferous cousin.

24. Blueberry Smoothie Bowl

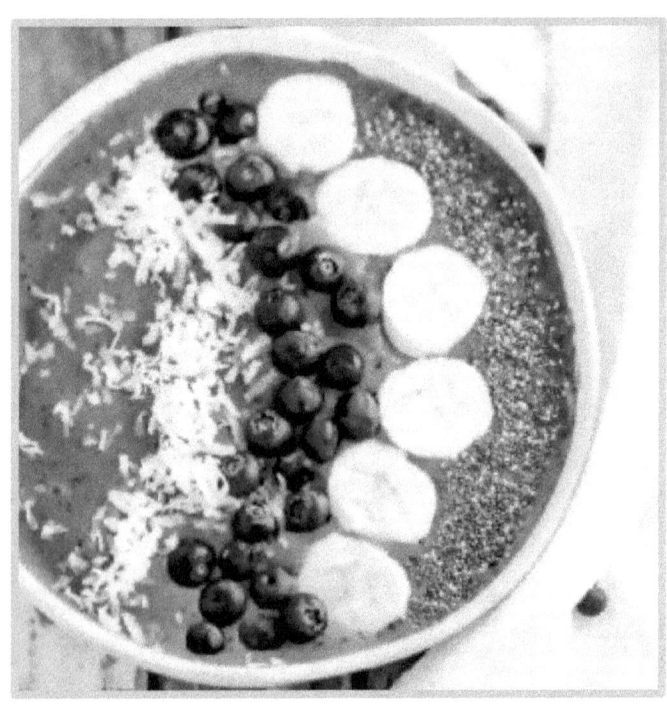

NUTRITION

Calories: 278.5
Carbohydrate: 38.72g
Protein: 1.3g
Sodium: 76.33mg
Potassium: 229.1mg
Phosphorus: 59.2mg
Dietary Fiber: 7.4g
Fat: 6g
Kidney Disease Stage 1

PREP TIME
5 min

COOK TIME
0 min

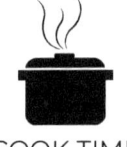

SERVING
1 people

DIRECTIONS

1. Put all the ingredients in the blender except chia seeds, and blend until smooth. You should end up with a thick smoothie paste.
2. Transfer into a cereal bowl and top with chia seeds on top.

INGREDIENTS

- ½ cup of frozen blueberries
- ½ cup of vanilla-flavored almond milk
- 1 tbsp. of agave syrup
- 1 tsp. of chia seeds

25. Cucumber Spinach Green Smoothie

PREP TIME
5 min

COOK TIME
0 min

SERVING
2 people

NUTRITION

Calories: 75
Total Fat: 2g
Saturated Fat: 0g
Cholesterol: 0mg
Carbohydrates: 14g
Fiber: 2g
Protein: 1g
Phosphorus: 34mg
Potassium: 313mg
Sodium: 81mg

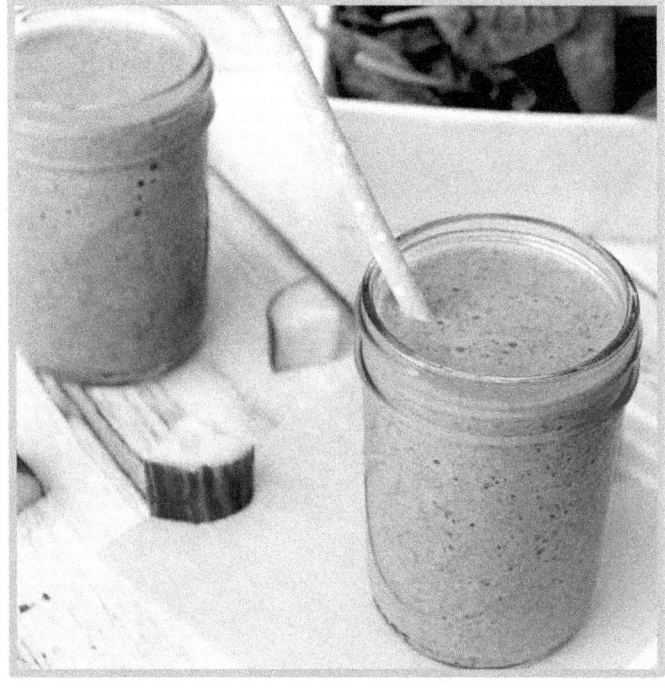

INGREDIENTS

- ½ cucumber, peeled and roughly chopped
- ½ green apple, roughly chopped
- 1 cup of Homemade Rice Milk or unsweetened store-bought rice milk
- 2 cups of spinach
- 3 ice cubes

DIRECTIONS

1. In a blender, combine the cucumber, apple, milk, spinach, and ice.
2. Process until smooth, and serve.

Substitution tip: A tart green apple is lovely in this smoothie, as it creates a subtle sweetness. However, if you prefer, other apples, such as Fuji, Red Delicious, or McIntosh, can be used. If you are using a thick-skinned apple, peel it first for a nicer texture in the finished smoothie.

26. Watermelon Kiwi Smoothie

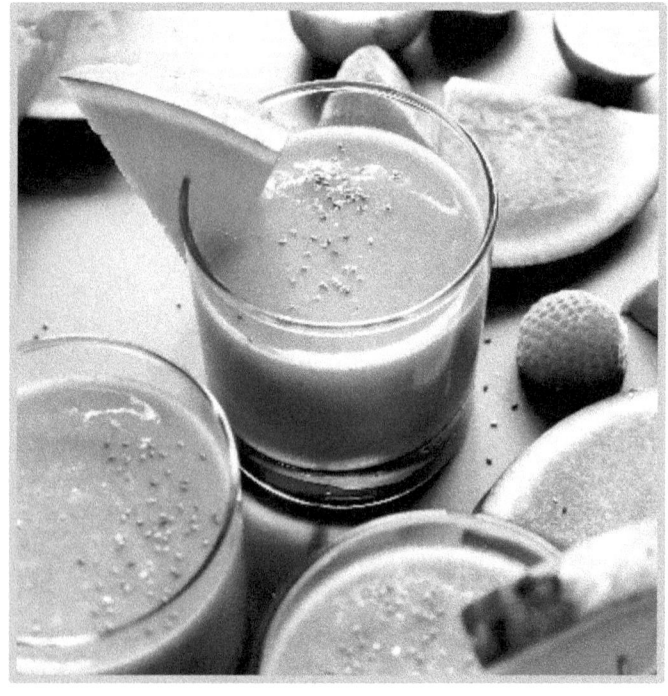

NUTRITION

Calories: 67
Total Fat: 0g
Saturated Fat: 0g
Cholesterol: 0mg
Carbohydrates: 17g
Fiber: 2g
Protein: 1g
Phosphorus: 28mg
Potassium: 278mg
Sodium: 3mg

PREP TIME
5 min

COOK TIME
0 min

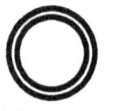

SERVING
2 people

DIRECTIONS

1. In a blender, combine the watermelon, kiwi, and ice.
2. Process until smooth.

Nutrition tip: While watermelon tastes particularly sweet, it has only half the sugar of an apple. Because sugar is the main taste-producing element, it stands out the most. The other primary ingredient in watermelon is water.

INGREDIENTS

- 2 cups of watermelon chunks
- 1 kiwifruit, peeled
- 1 cup of ice

27. Mint Lassi

PREP TIME
5 min

COOK TIME
0 min

SERVING
2 people

NUTRITION

Calories: 114
Total Fat: 6g
Saturated Fat: 3g
Cholesterol: 15mg
Carbohydrates: 5g
Fiber: 0g
Protein: 10g
Phosphorus: 158mg
Potassium: 179mg
Sodium: 43mg

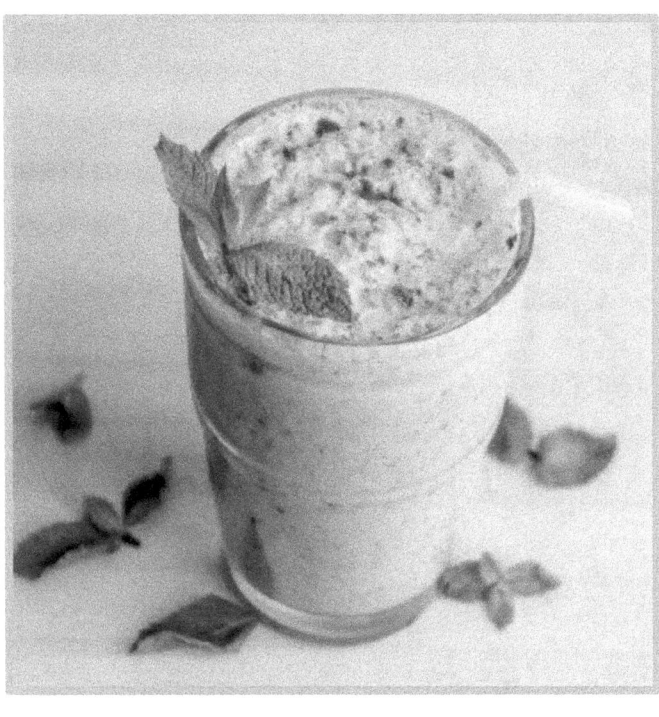

INGREDIENTS

- 1 teaspoon of cumin seeds
- ½ cup of mint leaves
- 1 cup of plain, unsweetened yogurt
- ½ cup of water

DIRECTIONS

1. In a skillet, toast cumin seeds until fragrant, 1 to 2 minutes in medium heat.
2. Transfer the seeds to a blender, along with the mint, yogurt, and water, and process until smooth.

Substitution tip: If you prefer the flavor of cilantro over mint, try it here instead. Another great substitute is to use ½ cup of strawberries along with ¼ teaspoon of ground cardamom instead of the mint.

28. Fennel Digestive Cooler

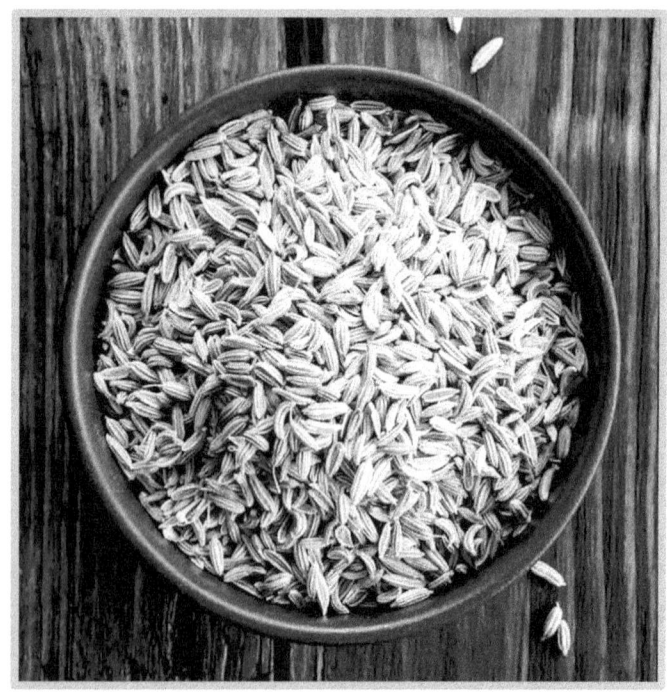

NUTRITION

Calories: 163
Total Fat: 2g
Saturated Fat: 0g
Cholesterol: 0mg
Carbohydrates: 30g
Fiber: 5g
Protein: 3g
Phosphorus: 57mg
Potassium: 205mg
Sodium: 141mg

PREP TIME
5 min

COOK TIME
15 min

SERVING
2 people

DIRECTIONS

1. In a blender, combine the milk, fennel seeds, cloves, and honey.
2. Process until smooth, and let rest for 30 minutes.
3. Pour over a wire mesh strainer lined with cheesecloth or over a coffee filter set over a glass or jar.
4. Serve.

Nutrition tip: Fennel is a warming herb that is supportive of treating indigestion, gas, and hypertension. High in quercetin, an antioxidant flavonoid, fennel fights inflammation and inhibits the development of cancer, among other benefits.

INGREDIENTS

- 2 cups Homemade Rice Milk or unsweetened store-bought rice milk
- ¼ cup fennel seeds, ground
- ¼ teaspoon ground cloves
- 1 tablespoon honey

29. Cinnamon Horchata

PREP TIME
5 min

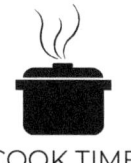
COOK TIME
0 min

SERVING
5 people

NUTRITION

Calories: 123
Total Fat: 2g
Saturated Fat: 0g
Cholesterol: 0mg
Carbohydrates: 26g
Fiber: 0g
Protein: 1g
Phosphorus: 34mg
Potassium: 78mg
Sodium: 32mg

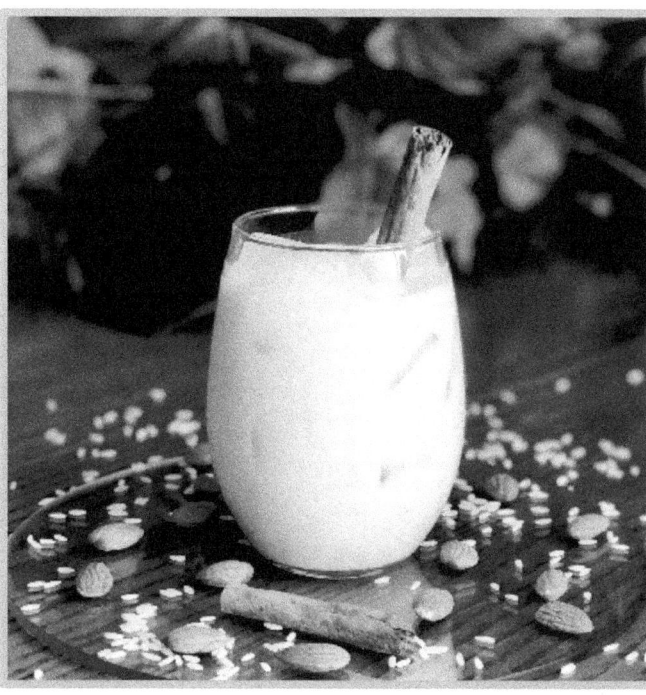

INGREDIENTS

- 1 cup of long-grain white rice
- 4 cups of water
- 1 cinnamon stick, broken into pieces
- 1 cup of Homemade Rice Milk or unsweetened store-bought rice milk
- 1 teaspoon of vanilla extract
- 1 teaspoon of ground cinnamon
- ⅓ cup of granulated sugar

DIRECTIONS

1. Using a blender, mix the rice, water, and cinnamon-stick pieces. For about 1 minute, blend until the rice begins to break up. Let stand at room temperature for at least 3 hours or overnight.
2. Place a wire mesh strainer over a pitcher, and pour the liquid into it. Discard the rice.
3. Add the milk, vanilla, ground cinnamon, and sugar. Stir to combine.
4. Serve over ice.

Variation tip: For an even richer flavor, add 1 tablespoon of unsweetened cocoa powder to the horchata with the ground cinnamon in Step 3.

30. Vanilla Chia Smoothie

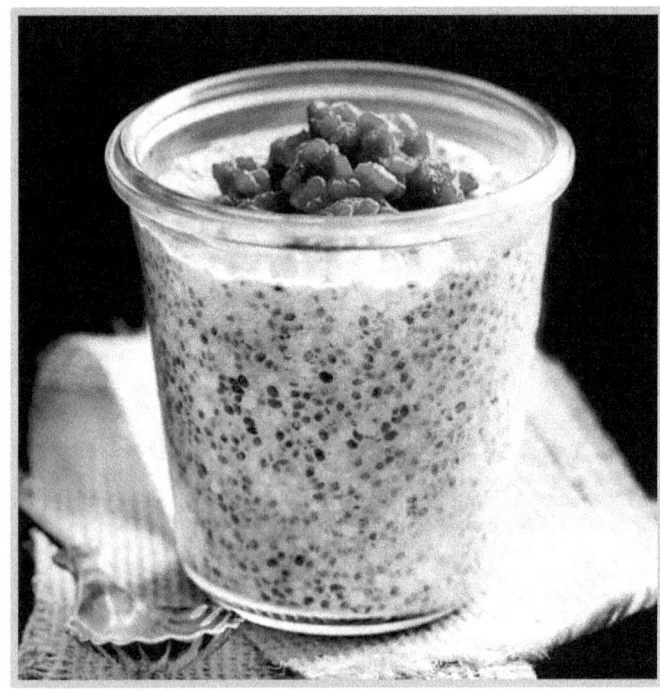

NUTRITION

Calories: 143
Total Fat: 5g
Saturated Fat: 1g
Cholesterol: 0mg
Carbohydrates: 19g
Fiber: 6g
Protein: 3g
Phosphorus: 3mg
Potassium: 93mg
Sodium: 73mg

PREP TIME
5 min

COOK TIME
5 min

SERVING
2 people

DIRECTIONS

1. In a small pan, heat the rice milk to just steaming. Steep the tea bags for 5 minutes, then discard.
2. In a blender, combine the rice milk, vanilla, ice, honey, chia seeds, cinnamon, ginger, cardamom, and cloves. Process until smooth, and serve.

Substitution tip: To make this ahead, complete Step 1 and refrigerate the milk tea in an airtight container. When ready to make the smoothie, proceed as directed, reducing the ice to ½ cup and adding ¼ cup of water.

INGREDIENTS

- 1 cup of Homemade Rice Milk or unsweetened store-bought rice milk
- 2 black tea bags
- 1 teaspoon of vanilla extract
- 1 cup of ice
- 1 teaspoon of honey
- 2 tablespoons of chia seeds
- ½ teaspoon of ground cinnamon
- ½ teaspoon of ground ginger
- ¼ teaspoon of ground cardamom
- ¼ teaspoon of ground cloves

31. Berry Mint Water

PREP TIME
5 min

COOK TIME
0 min

SERVING
8 people

NUTRITION

Calories: 7
Total Fat: 0g
Saturated Fat: 0g
Cholesterol: 0mg
Carbohydrates: 2g
Fiber: 1g
Protein: 0g
Phosphorus: 4mg
Potassium: 28mg
Sodium: 0mg

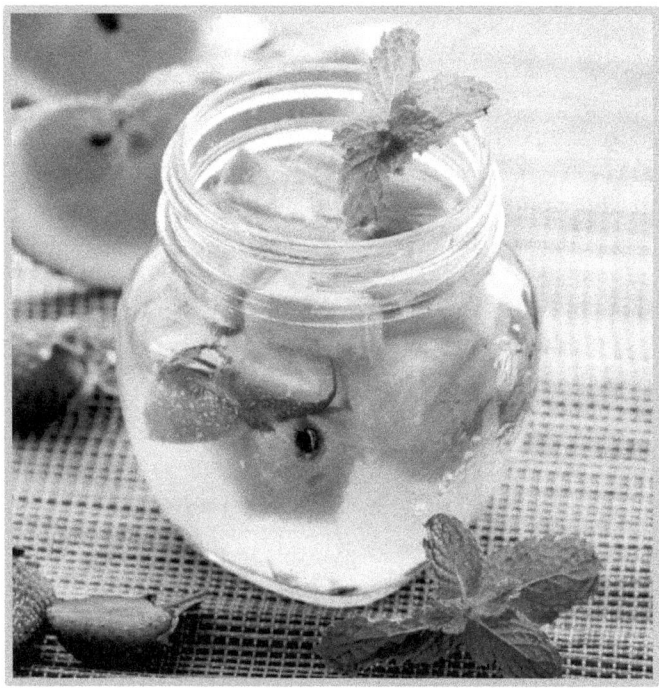

INGREDIENTS

- 8 cups of water
- ½ cup of strawberries
- ½ cup of blackberries
- 3 mint sprigs

DIRECTIONS

1. In a large pitcher, mix the water, strawberries, blackberries, and mint.
2. Cover and chill for at least 1 hour before drinking.
3. Store in the refrigerator for up to two days.

Substitution tip: Substitute any of your favorite fruits in this recipe to create your own flavored water. You can also try out different herbs to add bold and complementary flavors. Some additional herbs that taste nice paired with fruit include cilantro, basil, rosemary, and thyme. Ginger root is another favorite water flavor enhancer that stimulates digestion and cleanses the kidneys.

32. Homemade Rice Milk

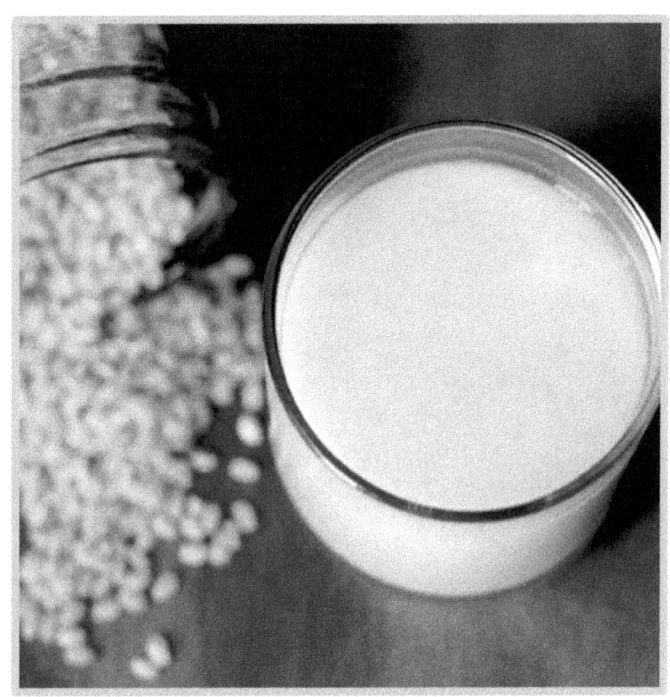

NUTRITION

Calories: 112
Total Fat: 0g
Saturated Fat: 0g
Cholesterol: 0mg
Carbohydrates: 24g
Fiber: 0g
Protein: 0g
Phosphorus: 0mg
Potassium: 55mg
Sodium: 80mg

PREP TIME
5 min

COOK TIME
0 min

SERVING
4 people

DIRECTIONS

1. In a dry skillet, set at medium heat, toast the rice until lightly browned, about 5 minutes.
2. Transfer the rice to a jar or bowl, and add the water. Cover, refrigerate and soak overnight.
3. In a blender, add the rice and water, along with the vanilla (if using), and process until smooth.
4. Place a fine-mesh strainer over a glass jar or bowl, and pour the milk into it. Serve immediately, or cover, refrigerate and serve within three days. Shake before using it.

Substitution tip: Rice milk can be substituted in most recipes calling for whole milk or another nut milk as a low-fat, low-phosphorus, and low-potassium alternative. Use an equal amount of rice milk in place of other milk products, and proceed as directed in the recipe.

INGREDIENTS

- 1 cup of long-grain white rice
- 4 cups of water
- ½ teaspoon of vanilla extract (optional)

33. Ginger & Lemon Green Iced-Tea

PREP TIME
5 min

COOK TIME
0 min

SERVING
2 people

NUTRITION

Calories: 20

Fat: 0g

Carbohydrates: 5g

Phosphorus: 9mg

Potassium: 106mg

Sodium: 4mg

Protein: 1g

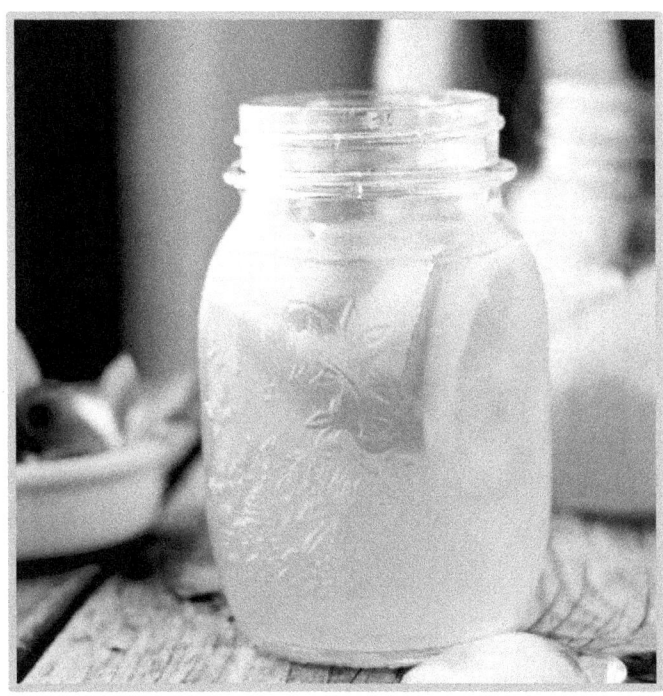

INGREDIENTS

- 2 cups of concentrated green or matcha tea, served hot
- 1 lemon, cut into wedges
- 1/4 cup of crystallized ginger, chopped into fine pieces

DIRECTIONS

1. Get a glass container and mix the tea with the ginger and then cover and chill for 3 hours.
2. Strain and pour into serving glasses on top of ice if you wish.
3. Garnish with a wedge of lemon to serve.

34. Lemon Smoothie

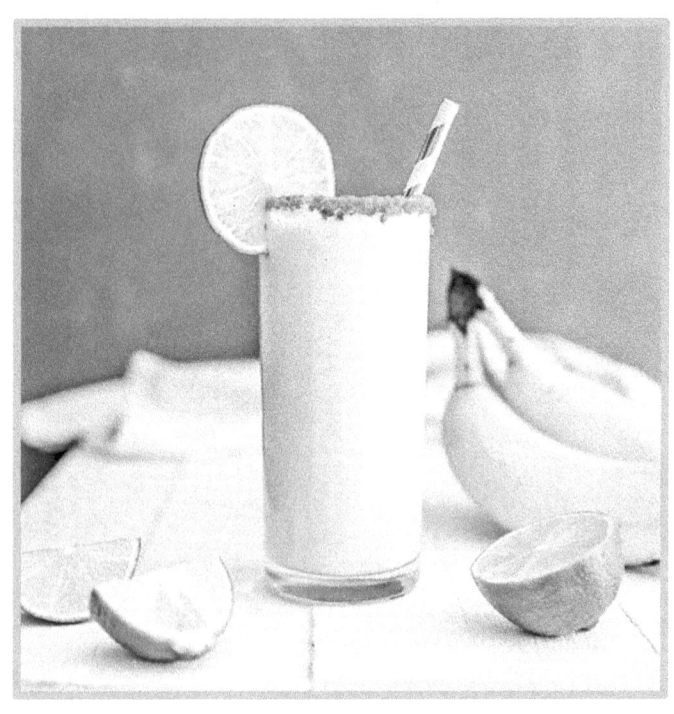

NUTRITION

Calories: 4
Fat: 0g
Carbohydrates: 5g
Phosphorus: 10mg
Potassium: 112mg
Sodium: 110mg
Protein: 8g

PREP TIME
5 min

COOK TIME
0 min

SERVING
2 people

DIRECTIONS

1. In a blender, combine all the ingredients. Process until smooth.
2. Garnish with a slice of lemon.

INGREDIENTS

- 2 tbsp. of lemon juice
- 2 tbsp. of brown sugar or stevia
- 4 pasteurized liquid egg whites

35. Tropical Juice

PREP TIME
5 min

COOK TIME
0 min

SERVING
2 people

NUTRITION

Calories: 55
Fat: 9g
Carbohydrates: 6g
Phosphorus: 11mg
Potassium: 129mg
Sodium: 111mg
Protein: 7g

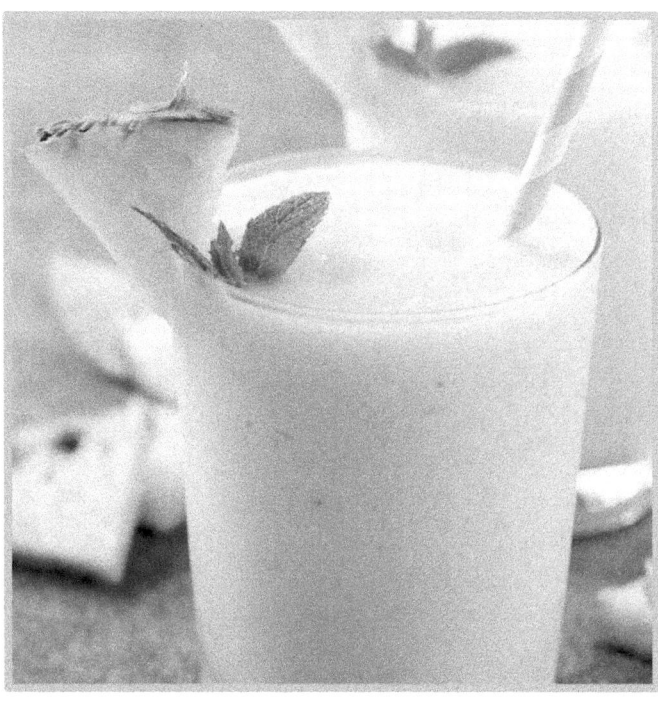

INGREDIENTS

- 2 cups of pineapple, chunks.
- 1/2 cup of low-fat coconut milk
- 1 cup of water

DIRECTIONS

1. In a blender, combine all the ingredients. Process until smooth.
2. Serve immediately.

Tip: Check with your doctor or dietitian as to whether you can still have coconut milk. Alternatively, use non-dairy milk, such as almond.

36. Mixed Fruit Anti-Inflammatory Smoothie

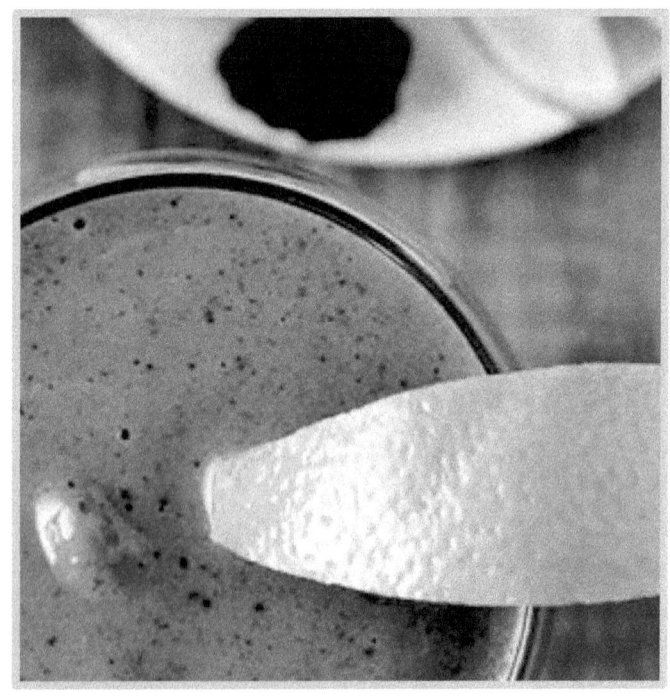

NUTRITION

Calories: 48

Fat: 0g

Carbohydrates: 12g

Phosphorus: 17mg

Potassium: 203mg

Sodium: 6mg

Protein: 1g

PREP TIME

5 min

COOK TIME

0 min

SERVING

4 people

DIRECTIONS

1. In a blender, combine all the ingredients. Process until smooth.
2. Serve immediately in tall glasses.
3. Tear mint with fingers and serve with smoothies (optional).

INGREDIENTS

- 1 cup of red or white grapes
- 1 cup of sliced frozen or fresh peaches
- 1 cup of chopped cabbage
- 1/2 cup of ice cubes
- 1/2 cup of water
- 1 sprig of fresh mint

37. Banana Apple Smoothie

PREP TIME
5 min

COOK TIME
0 min

SERVING
4 people

NUTRITION

Calories: 182

Fat: 14g

Carbohydrates: 16g

Phosphorus: 70mg

Potassium: 300mg

Sodium: 14mg

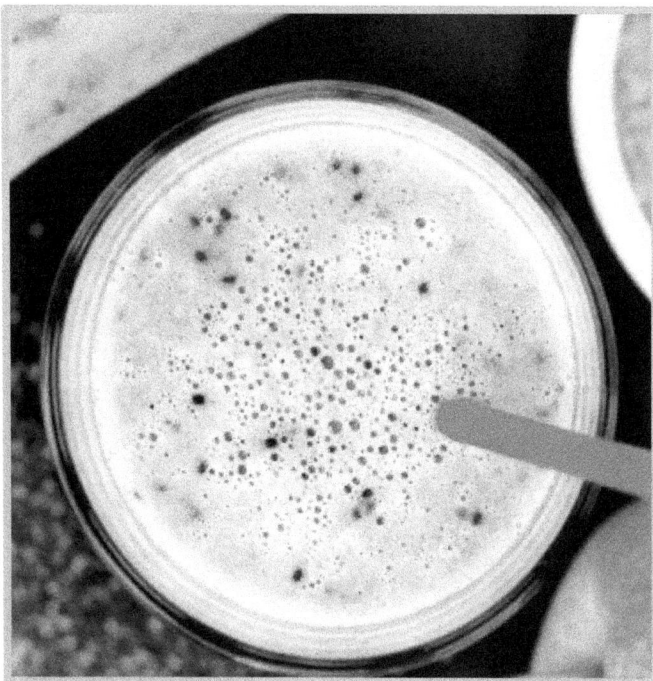

INGREDIENTS

- 1 banana
- 1 apple, cored and peeled
- 2 cups of filtered water
- 1 tbsp. of stevia
- 1 cup of low-fat coconut milk

DIRECTIONS

1. Take a food processor and add all of the ingredients, processing until smooth.
2. Serve over ice.

Tip: Check with your doctor or dietitian as to whether you can still have coconut milk. Alternatively, use non-dairy milk, such as almond.

38. Winter Berry Iced Milkshake

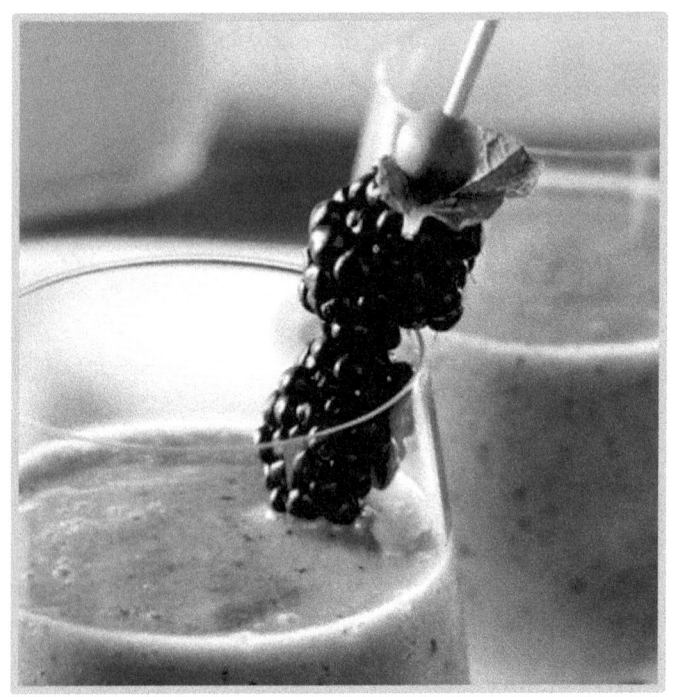

NUTRITION

Calories: 45
Fat: 1g
Carbohydrates: 7g
Phosphorus: 33mg
Potassium: 118mg
Sodium: 29mg
Protein: 2g

PREP TIME
5 min

COOK TIME
0 min

SERVING
4 people

DIRECTIONS

1. Add ingredients together in a blender, blending until smooth, and then serve in tall glasses.

INGREDIENTS

- 1 cup of rice milk, unenriched
- 1/2 cup of organic blueberries (or washed if non-organic)
- 1/2 cup of blackberries
- Ice cubes to the desired concentration

39. Aloha Cocktail

PREP TIME
10 min

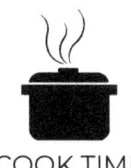
COOK TIME
0 min

SERVING
2 people

NUTRITION

Calories: 63.5

Protein: 0.4g

Sodium: 5.4mg

Phosphorus: 0.8mg

Potassium: 110.4mg

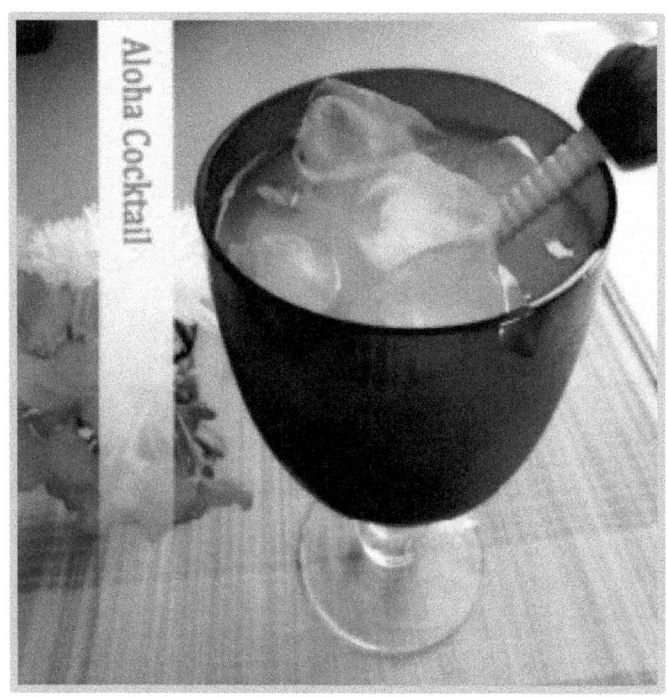

INGREDIENTS

- 1 cup of fresh pineapple cubes
- 1 lime cut in half and juiced
- ½ cup of ginger ale
- Ice cubes

DIRECTIONS

1. Place pineapple, lime juice, and ginger ale in the blender.
2. Blend until smooth.
3. Pour into a glass filled with ice.

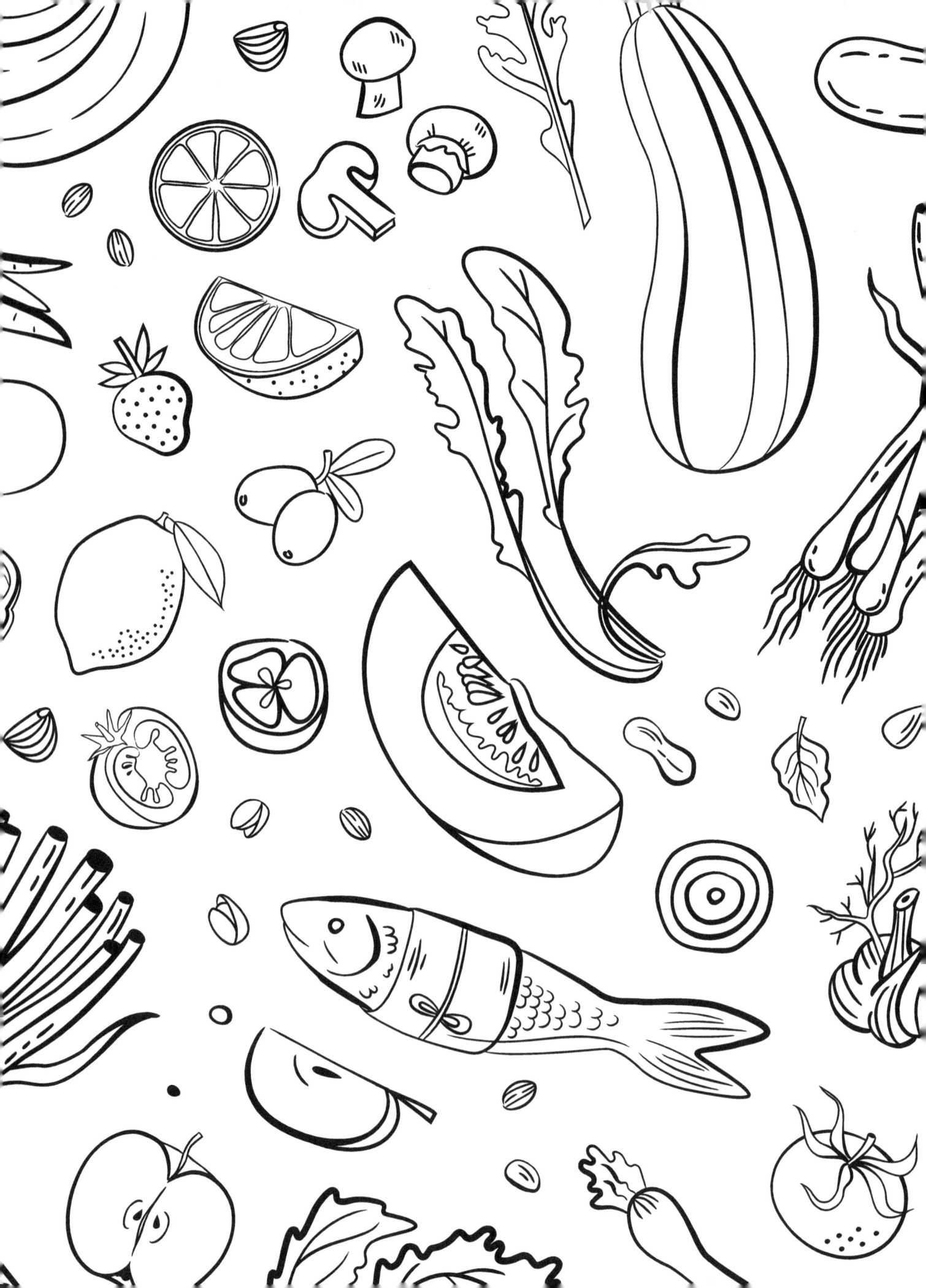

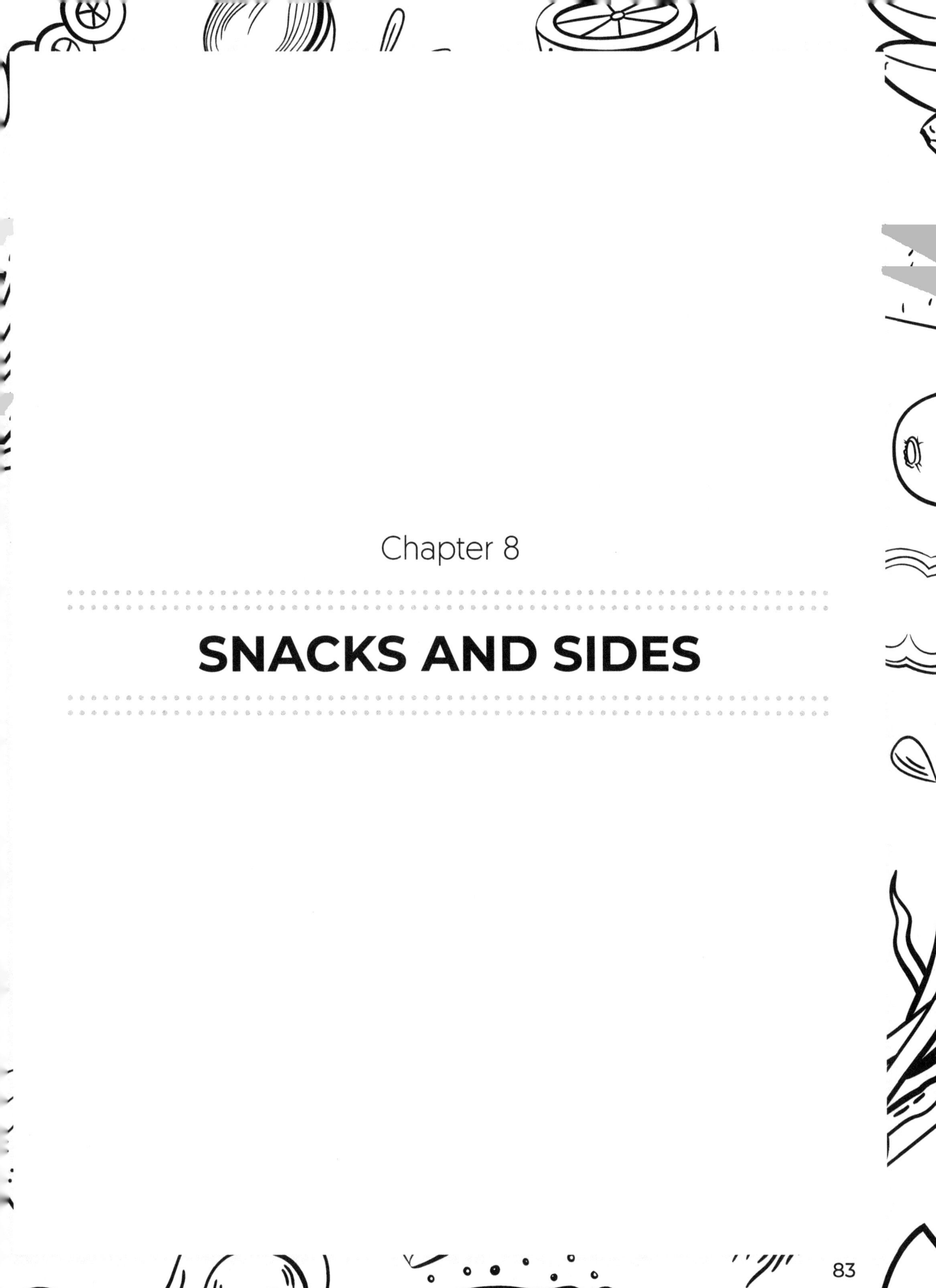

Chapter 8

SNACKS AND SIDES

40. Savory Collard Chips

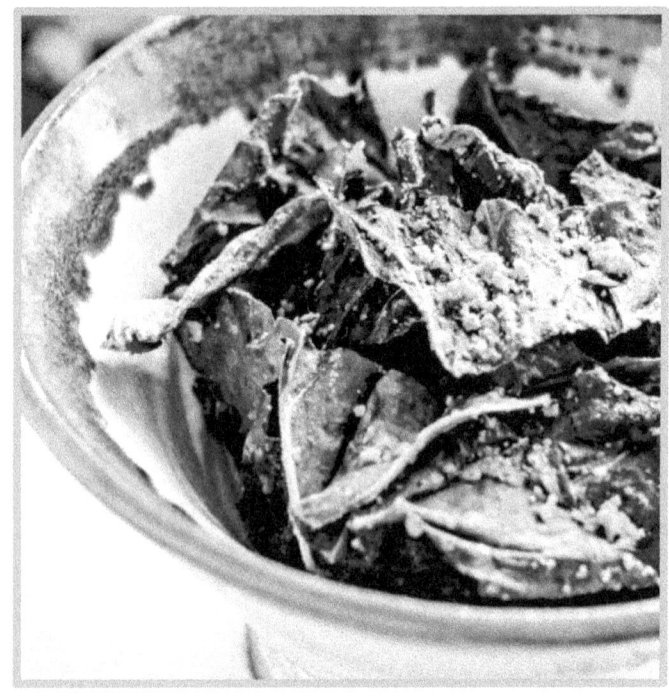

NUTRITION

Calories: 24
Total Fat: 1g
Saturated Fat: 0g
Cholesterol: 0mg
Carbohydrates: 3g
Fiber: 1g
Protein: 1g
Phosphorus: 6mg
Potassium: 72mg
Sodium: 8mg

PREP TIME
5 min

COOK TIME
20 min

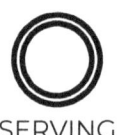
SERVING
4 people

DIRECTIONS

1. Preheat the oven to 350°F. Line a baking sheet with parchment paper.
2. Cut the collards into 2-by-2-inch squares and pat dry with paper towels.
3. Toss greens with the olive oil, lemon juice, garlic powder, and pepper in a large bowl. Use your hands to mix well, massaging the dressing into the greens until evenly coated.
4. Arrange the collards in a single layer on the baking sheet, and cook for 8 minutes. Flip the pieces and cook for an additional 8 minutes, until crisp. Remove from oven, let cool.

Substitution tip: If you prefer, use fresh garlic instead of dried. Mince 2 or 3 cloves, toss with the collards and proceed as directed.

INGREDIENTS

- 1 bunch of collard greens
- 1 teaspoon of extra-virgin olive oil
- Juice of ½ lemon
- ½ teaspoon of garlic powder
- ¼ teaspoon of freshly ground black pepper

41. Roasted Red Pepper Hummus

PREP TIME
10 min

COOK TIME
10 min

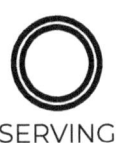

SERVING
8 people

NUTRITION

Calories: 103
Total Fat: 6g
Saturated Fat: 1g
Cholesterol: 0mg
Carbohydrates: 10g
Fiber: 3g
Protein: 3g
Phosphorus: 58mg
Potassium: 91mg
Sodium: 72mg

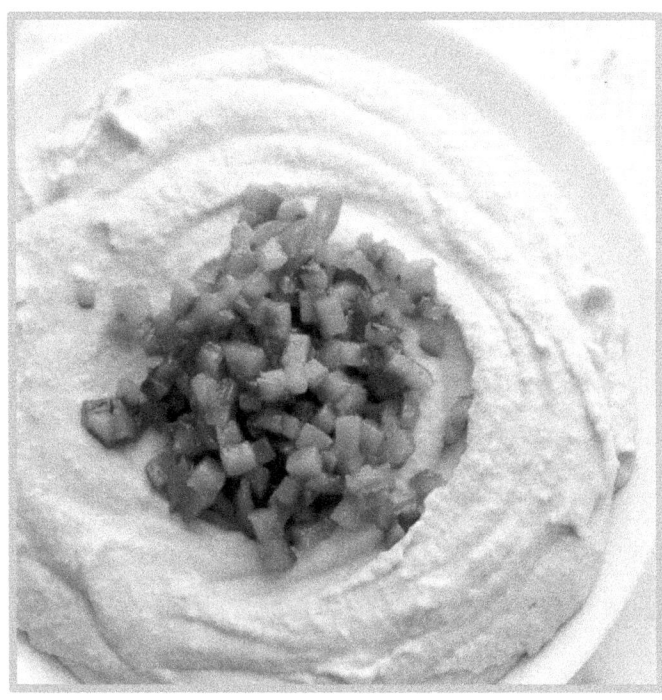

INGREDIENTS

- 1 red bell pepper
- 1 (15-ounce) can of chickpeas, drained and rinsed
- Juice of 1 lemon
- 2 tablespoons of tahini
- 2 garlic cloves
- 2 tablespoons of extra-virgin olive oil

DIRECTIONS

1. Move the rack of the oven to the highest position. Heat the broiler to high.
2. Core the pepper and cut it into three or four large pieces. Arrange them on a baking sheet, skin-side up.
3. Broil the peppers for 5 to 10 minutes, until the skins are charred. Remove from the oven then transfer the peppers to a small bowl. Cover with plastic wrap and let them steam for 10 to 15 minutes, until cool enough to handle.
4. Peel the charred skin off the peppers, and place the peppers in a blender.
5. Add the chickpeas, lemon juice, tahini, garlic, and olive oil. Wait until smooth, then add up to 1 tablespoon of water to adjust consistency as desired.

Substitution tip: This hummus can also be made without the red pepper if desired. To do this, simply follow Step 5. This will cut the potassium to 59mg per serving.

42. Thai-Style Eggplant Dip

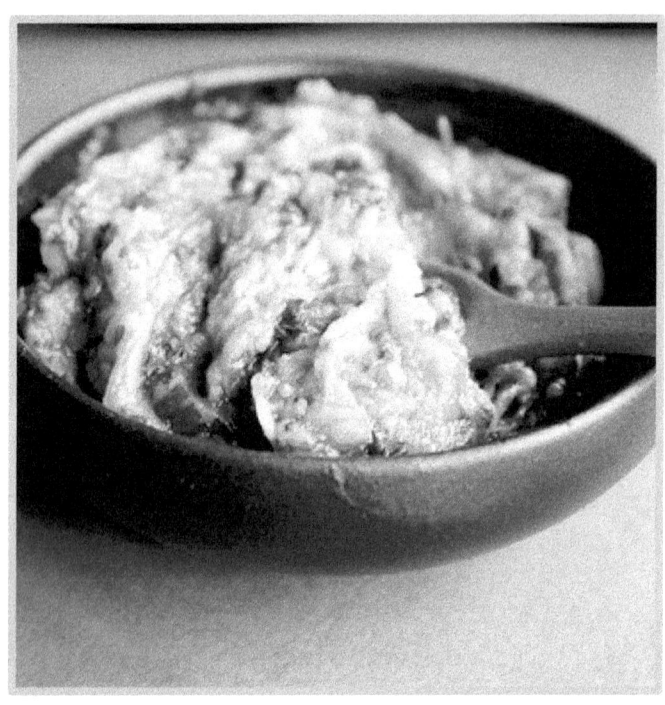

NUTRITION

Calories: 40
Total Fat: 0g
Saturated Fat: 0g
Cholesterol: 0mg
Carbohydrates: 10g
Fiber: 4g
Protein: 2g
Phosphorus: 34mg
Potassium: 284mg
Sodium: 47mg

PREP TIME
10 min

COOK TIME
30 min

SERVING
4 people

DIRECTIONS

1. Preheat the oven to 425°F to get it ready.
2. Pierce every eggplant with a skewer or knife. Place on a rimmed baking sheet and cook until soft, about 30 minutes. Let cool, cut in half, and scoop out the flesh of the eggplant into a blender.
3. Add the rice vinegar, sugar, soy sauce, jalapeño, garlic, and basil to the blender. Process until smooth. Serve with cut vegetables or crackers.

Lower-sodium tip: If you need to lower your sodium further, omit the soy sauce to lower the sodium to 3mg.

INGREDIENTS

- 1 pound of Thai eggplant (or Japanese or Chinese eggplant)
- 2 tablespoons of rice vinegar
- 2 teaspoons of sugar
- 1 teaspoon of low-sodium soy sauce
- 1 jalapeño pepper
- 2 garlic cloves
- ¼ cup of chopped basil
- Cut vegetables or crackers, for serving

43. Coconut Pancakes

PREP TIME
5 min

COOK TIME
10 min

SERVING
2 people

NUTRITION

Calories: 177

Fat: 13g

Carbohydrates: 12g

Phosphorus: 37mg

Potassium: 133mg

Sodium: 133mg

Protein: 5g

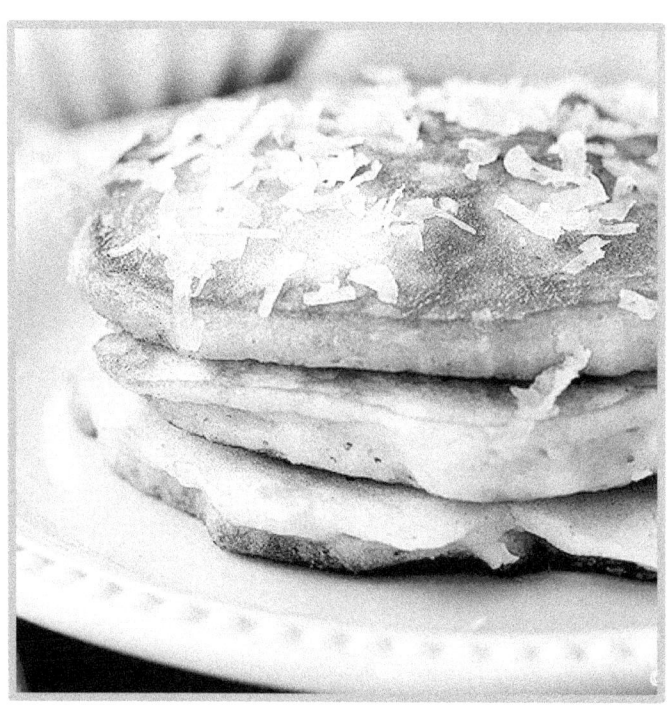

INGREDIENTS

- 2 free-range egg whites
- 2 tbsp. of all-purpose white flour
- 3 tbsp. of coconut shavings
- 2 tbsp. of coconut milk (optional)
- 1 tbsp. of coconut oil

DIRECTIONS

1. Get a bowl and combine all the ingredients.
2. Mix well until you get a thick batter.
3. Heat a skillet on medium heat and heat the coconut oil.
4. Pour half the mixture to the center of the pan, forming a pancake and cook through for 3-4 minutes on each side.
5. Serve with your choice of berries on the top.

Tip: Check with your doctor or dietitian as to whether you can still have coconut milk. Alternatively, use non-dairy milk, such as almond.

44. Spiced Peaches

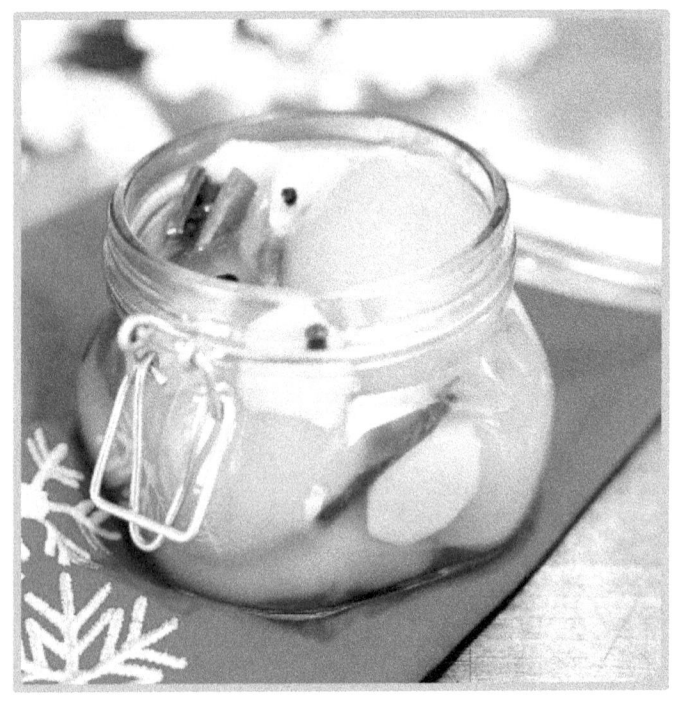

NUTRITION

Calories: 70
Fat: 1g
Carbohydrates: 18g
Phosphorus: 26mg
Potassium: 184mg
Sodium: 9mg
Protein: 1g

PREP TIME
5 min

COOK TIME
10 min

SERVING
2 people

DIRECTIONS

1. Drain peaches.
2. Combine water, cornstarch, cinnamon, nutmeg, ground cloves, and lemon zest in a pan on the stove.
3. Heat on medium heat and add peaches.
4. Bring to a boil, reduce the heat and simmer for 10 minutes.
5. Serve warm.

INGREDIENTS

- 1 cup of canned peaches in their own juices
- 1/2 tsp. of cornstarch
- 1 tsp. of ground cloves
- 1 tsp. of ground cinnamon
- 1 tsp. of ground nutmeg
- 1/2 lemon zest
- 1/2 cup of water

45. Pumpkin Cheesecake Bar

PREP TIME
10 min

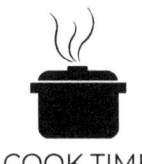

COOK TIME
50 min

SERVING
4 people

NUTRITION

Calories: 296

Fat: 17g

Carbohydrates: 30g

Phosphorus: 62mg

Potassium: 164g

Sodium: 159mg

Protein: 5g

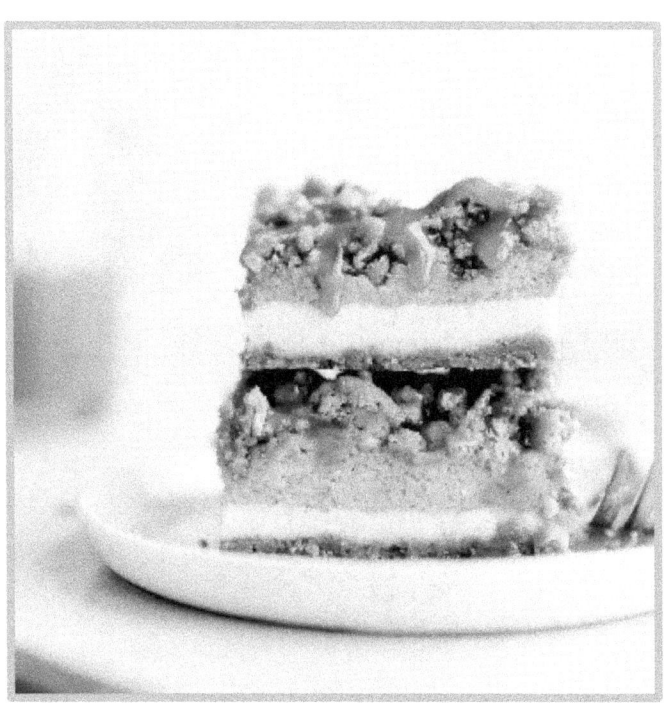

INGREDIENTS

- 2 ½ tbsp. of unsalted butter
- 4 oz. of cream cheese
- 1/2 cup of all-purpose white flour
- 3 tbsp. of golden brown sugar
- 1/4 cup of granulated sugar
- 1/2 cup of puréed pumpkin
- 2 egg whites
- 1 tsp. of ground cinnamon
- 1 tsp. of ground nutmeg
- 1 tsp. of vanilla extract

DIRECTIONS

1. Set the oven 350°F/170°C/Gas Mark 4 for Preheating.
2. Mix the flour and brown sugar in a mixing bowl.
3. Mix in the butter with your fingertips to form 'breadcrumbs.'
4. Place 3/4 of this mixture into the bottom of an ovenproof dish.
5. Bake in the oven for 15 minutes and remove to cool.
6. Lightly whisk the egg and fold in the cream cheese, sugar (or substitute stevia), pumpkin, cinnamon, nutmeg, and vanilla until smooth.
7. Pour this mixture over the oven-baked base and sprinkle with the rest of the breadcrumbs from earlier.
8. Place back in the oven and bake for a further 30–35 minutes.
9. Allow to cool and slice to serve.

46. Blueberry and Vanilla Mini Muffins

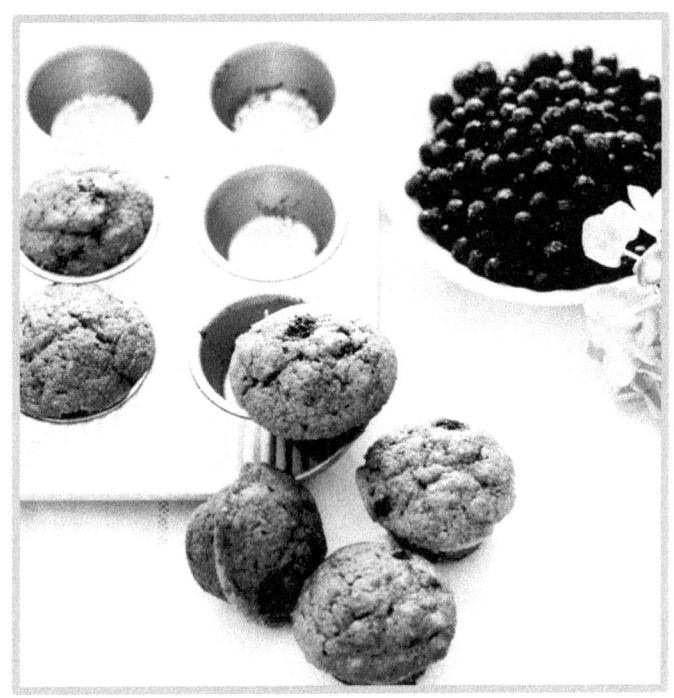

NUTRITION

Calories: 48
Fat: 1g
Carbohydrates: 8g
Phosphorus: 14mg
Potassium: 44mg
Sodium: 298mg
Protein: 2g

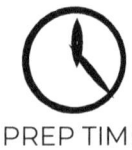
PREP TIME
10 min

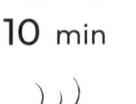
COOK TIME
35 min

SERVING
5 people

DIRECTIONS

1. Set the oven 325°F/170°C/Gas Mark 3 for Preheating.
2. Add all the ingredients in a bowl.
3. Divide the batter into 4 and spoon into a lightly oiled muffin tin.
4. Bake in the oven for 15–20 minutes or until cooked through.
5. Your knife should pull out clean from the middle of the muffin once done.
6. Allow to cool on a wired rack before serving.

INGREDIENTS

- 3 egg whites
- 1/4 cup of all-purpose white flour
- 1 tbsp. of coconut flour
- 1 tsp. of baking soda
- 1 tbsp. of nutmeg, grated
- 1 tsp. of vanilla extract
- 1 tsp. of stevia
- 1/4 cup of fresh blueberries

47. Puffy French Toast

PREP TIME
10 min

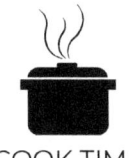
COOK TIME
8 min

SERVING
4 people

NUTRITION

Calories: 293.75

Carbohydrate: 25.3g

Protein: 9.27g

Sodium: 211g

Potassium: 97mg

Phosphorus: 165mg

Dietary Fiber: 12.3g

Fat: 16.50g

Kidney Disease Stage 2

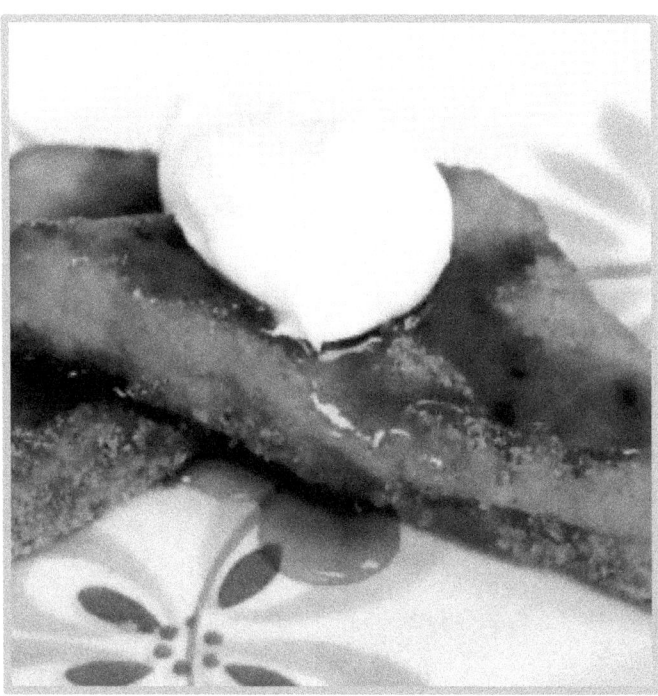

INGREDIENTS

- 4 slices of white bread, cut in half diagonally
- 3 whole eggs and 1 egg white
- 1 cup of plain almond milk
- 2 tbsp. of canola oil
- 1 tsp. of cinnamon

DIRECTIONS

1. Preheat your oven to 400F/180C
2. Beat the eggs and the almond milk.
3. Heat the oil in a pan.
4. Dip each bread slice/triangle into the egg and almond milk mixture.
5. Fry in the pan until golden brown on each side.
6. Place the toasts in a baking sheet and let cook in the oven for another 5 minutes.
7. Serve warm and drizzle with some honey, icing sugar, or cinnamon on top.

48. Puff Oven Pancakes

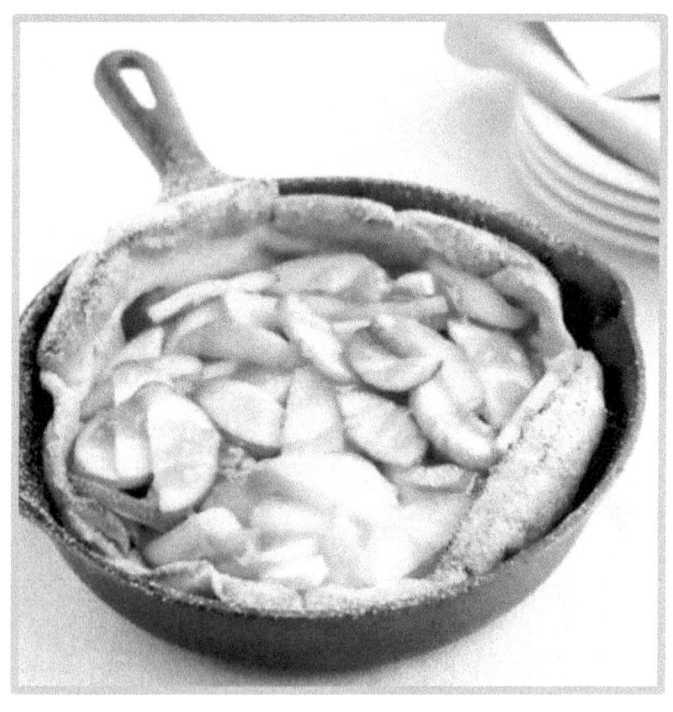

NUTRITION

Calories: 159.75

Carbohydrate: 17g

Protein: 5g

Sodium: 120g

Potassium: 52mg

Phosphorus: 66.25mg

Dietary Fiber: 0.5g

Fat: 9g

PREP TIME
5 min

COOK TIME
30 min

SERVING
4 people

DIRECTIONS

1. Preheat the oven at 400°F/190°C.
2. Grease a 10-inch skillet or Pyrex with the butter and heat in the oven until it melts.
3. Beat the eggs and whisk in the rice milk, flour and salt in a mixing bowl until smooth.
4. Take off the skillet or pie dish from the oven.
5. Transfer the batter directly into the skillet and put back in the oven for 25–30 minutes.
6. Place in a serving dish and cut into 4 portions.
7. Serve hot with honey or icing sugar on top.

INGREDIENTS

- 2 large eggs.
- ½ cup of rice flour
- ½ cup of rice milk
- 2 tbsp. of unsalted butter
- ⅛ tsp. of salt

49. Savory Muffins with Protein

PREP TIME
5 min

COOK TIME
35 min

SERVING
12 people

NUTRITION

Calories: 106.58

Carbohydrate: 8.20g

Protein: 4.77g

Sodium: 51.91mg

Potassium: 87.83 mg

Phosphorus: 49.41 mg

Dietary Fiber: 0.58 g

Fat: 5 g

Kidney Disease Stage 2

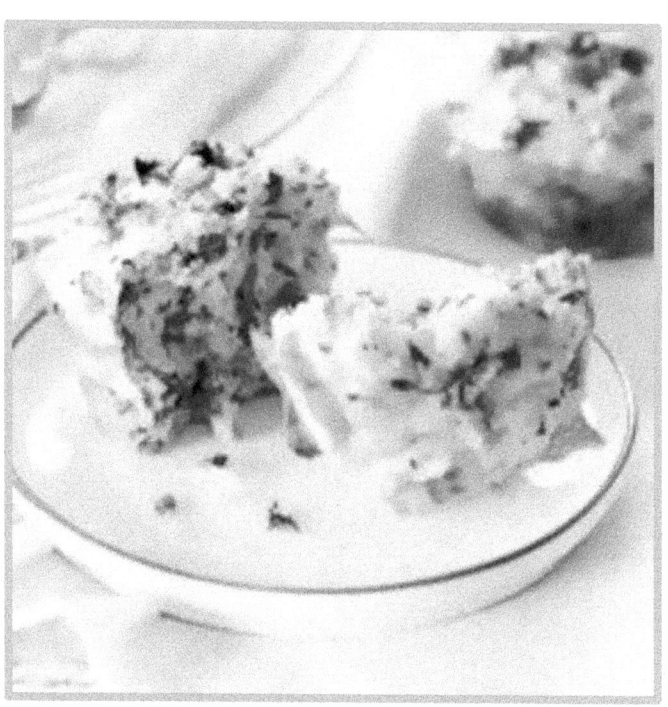

INGREDIENTS

- 2 cups of corn flakes
- ½ cup of unfortified almond milk
- 4 large eggs
- 2 tbsp. of olive oil
- 1/2 cup of almond milk
- 1 medium white onion, sliced
- 1 cup of plain Greek yogurt
- ¼ cup of pecans, chopped
- 1 tbsp. of mixed seasoning blend, e.g., Mrs. dash

DIRECTIONS

1. Preheat the oven at 350°F/180°C.
2. Heat the olive oil in the pan. Saute the onions with the pecans and seasoning blend for a couple of minutes.
3. Add the rest of the ingredients and toss well.
4. Split the mixture into 12 small muffin cups (lightly greased) and bake for 30–35 minutes or until an inserted knife or toothpick is coming out clean.
5. Serve warm or keep at room temperature for a couple of days.

50. European Pancakes

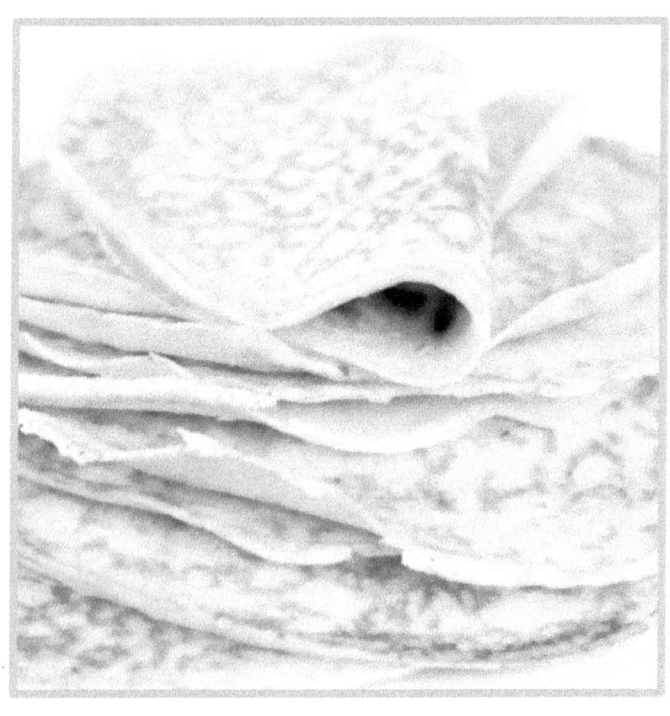

NUTRITION

Calories: 74
Carbohydrate: 10g
Protein: 4g
Sodium: 39mg
Potassium: 73mg
Phosphorus: 73mg
Dietary Fiber: 0.2g
Fat: 2g
Kidney Disease Stage 4

PREP TIME
5 min

COOK TIME
20 min

SERVING
10 people

DIRECTIONS

1. Mix flour and sugar, then whisk in the eggs and combine well in a medium.
2. Put then the milk, vanilla, and lemon zest to the mix and whisk well.
3. Spray a small 8–10-inch pan with cooking spray and pour around 4 tbsp. of the mixture and distribute evenly by tilting the pan from one side to another.
4. Cook until the batter is solid and light golden brown (around 50 seconds on each side). Flip.
5. Repeat the above two steps until all the batter has finished.

INGREDIENTS

- 2/3 cups of all-purpose flour
- 4 large eggs
- 2 tbsp. of sugar
- ½ tsp. of lemon zest
- 1 cup of low-fat milk
- ¼ tsp. of vanilla extract

51. Easy and Fast Mac-n-Cheese

PREP TIME
5 min

COOK TIME
8-10 min

SERVING
4 people

NUTRITION

Calories: 231.68
Carbohydrate: 32.65g
Protein: 9.74g
Sodium: 107.25mg
Potassium: 29.52mg
Phosphorus: 159.93mg
Dietary Fiber: 0.12g
Fat: 7.2g
Kidney Disease Stage 2

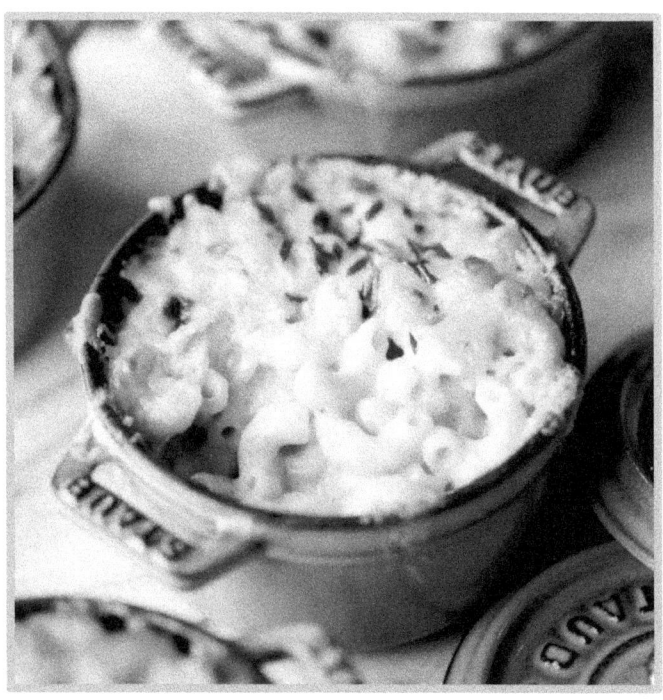

INGREDIENTS

- 1 cup of dry elbow macaroni pasta
- ½ cup of mild cheddar cheese
- 3 cups of water
- 1 tsp. of unsalted butter
- ½ tsp. of dry mustard powder
- ½ tsp. of paprika

DIRECTIONS

1. Boil the elbow macaroni in boiling water for 7–8 minutes (or until soft).
2. Drain all the water out and transfer it in the bowl.
3. Add the butter cheese, mustard, and paprika while the pasta is still hot, toss and serve.

52. Sandwich with Chicken Salad

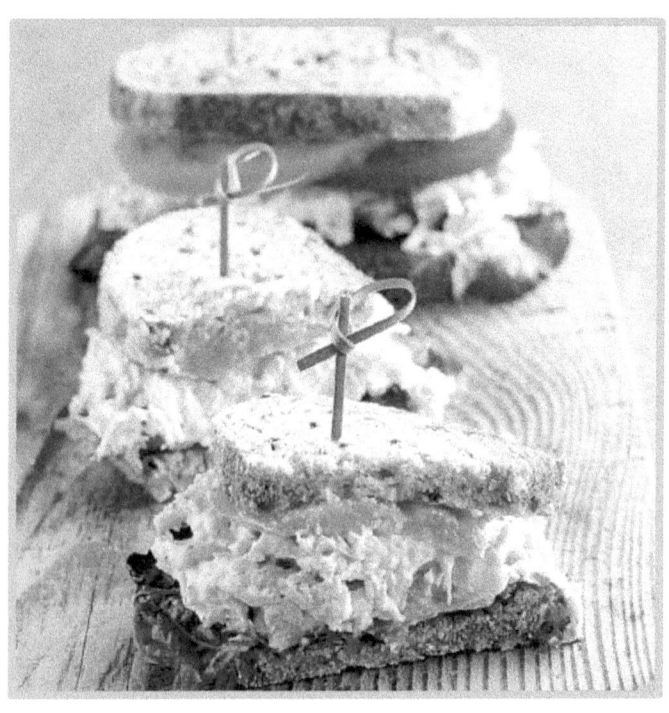

NUTRITION

Calories: 345

Protein: 22g

Sodium: 395mg

Potassium: 330mg

Phosphorus: 165mg

PREP TIME

10 min

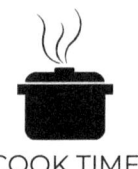

COOK TIME

10 min

SERVING

2 people

DIRECTIONS

1. Prepare aside the diced chicken and drain pineapple, adding green bell pepper, black pepper, and carrots.
2. Combine all in a bowl and refrigerate until chilled.
3. Later on, serve the chicken salad on the flatbread. Enjoy!

INGREDIENTS

- 2 bowls of cooked chicken
- 1/2 cup of low-fat mayonnaise
- 1/2 cup of green bell pepper
- 1 cup of pieces pineapple
- 1/3 cup of carrots
- 4 slices of flatbread
- 1/2 tsp. of black pepper

53. Celery and Arugula Salad

PREP TIME
10 min

COOK TIME
0 min

SERVING
4 people

NUTRITION

Calories: 45

Fat: 4g

Carbs: 1g

Protein: 1g

Phosphorus: 23mg

Potassium: 47mg

Sodium: 47mg

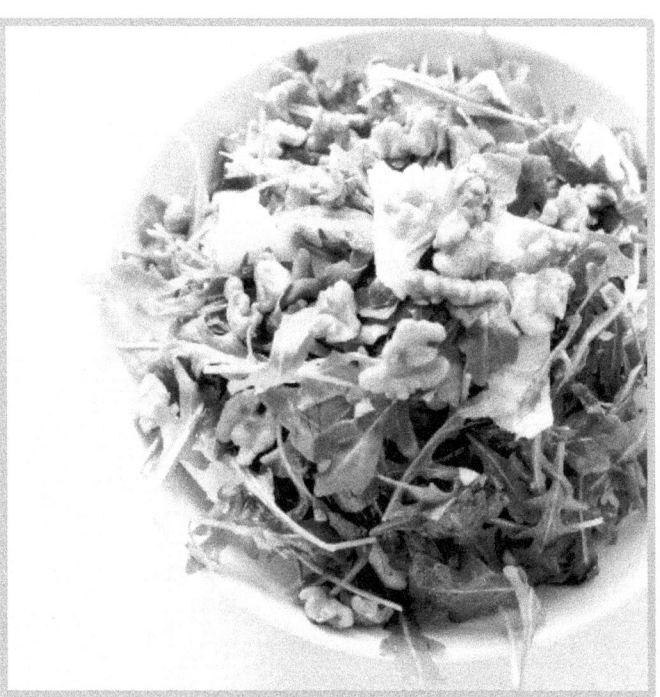

INGREDIENTS

- 1 shallot, thinly sliced
- 3 celery stalks, cut into 1-inch pieces about ¼ inch thick
- 2 cups of loosely packed arugula
- 1 tablespoon of extra-virgin olive oil
- 2 tablespoons of white wine vinegar
- Freshly ground black pepper
- 2 tablespoons of grated Parmesan cheese

DIRECTIONS

1. In a medium bowl, toss the shallot, celery stalks, and arugula.
2. In a small bowl, whisk the olive oil, vinegar, and pepper.
3. Toss your salad with your dressing.
4. Top with Parmesan cheese and serve.

54. Chicken, Charred Tomato, and Broccoli Salad

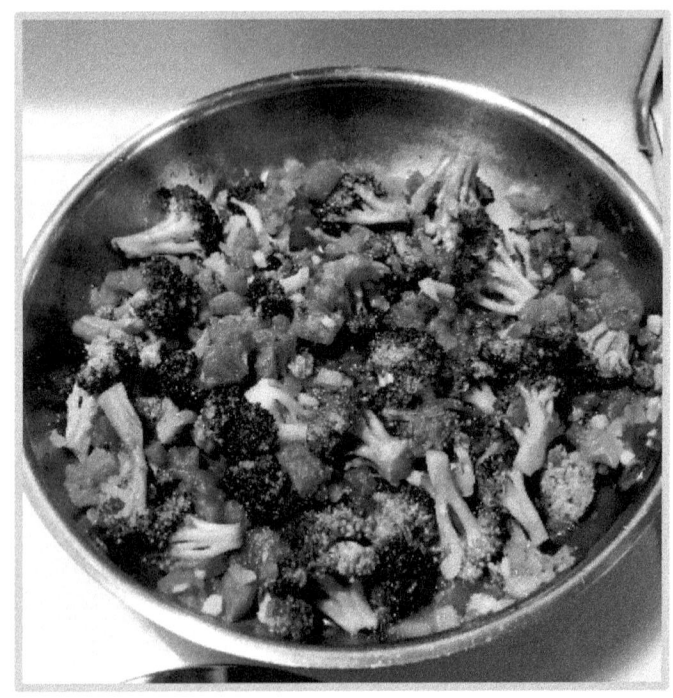

NUTRITION

Calories: 277

Carbs: 6g

Protein: 28g

Fat: 9g

Phosphorus: 292mg

Potassium: 719mg

Sodium: 560mg

PREP TIME
10 min

COOK TIME
30 min

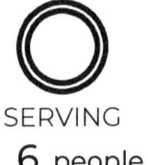
SERVING
6 people

DIRECTIONS

1. Place the chicken in a skillet and add just enough water to cover the chicken.
2. Bring to a simmer over high heat. Reduce the heat once the liquid boils and cook the chicken thoroughly for 12 minutes. Once cooked, shred the chicken into bite-sized pieces.
3. On a large pot, bring water to a boil and add the broccoli. Cook for 5 minutes until slightly tender.
4. Drain and rinse the broccoli with cold water. Set aside. Core the tomatoes and cut them crosswise.
5. Discard the seeds and set the tomatoes cut-side down on paper towels. Pat them dry.
6. In a heavy skillet, heat the pan over high heat until very hot. Brush the cut sides of the tomatoes with olive oil and place them on the pan. Cook the tomatoes until the sides are charred. Set aside.
7. In the same pan, heat the remaining 3 tablespoon olive oil over medium heat. Stir the salt, chili powder, and pepper and stir for 45 seconds. Pour over the lemon juice and remove the pan from the heat. Plate the broccoli, shredded chicken, and chili powder mixture dressing.

INGREDIENTS

- ¼ cup of lemon juice
- ½ tsp. of chili powder
- 1 ½ lb. of boneless chicken breast
- 1 ½ lb. of a medium tomato
- 1 tsp. of freshly ground pepper
- 1 tsp. of sea salt
- 4 cups of broccoli florets
- 5 tbsp. of extra virgin olive oil, divided to 2 and 3 tablespoons

55. Easy Baked Shepherd's Pie

PREP TIME
10 min

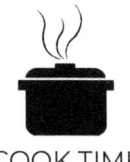
COOK TIME
25 min

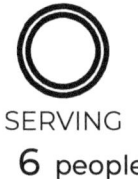
SERVING
6 people

NUTRITION

Calories: 1639

Carbs: 27g

Protein: 31g

Fat: 163g

Phosphorus: 425mg

Potassium: 896mg

Sodium: 419mg

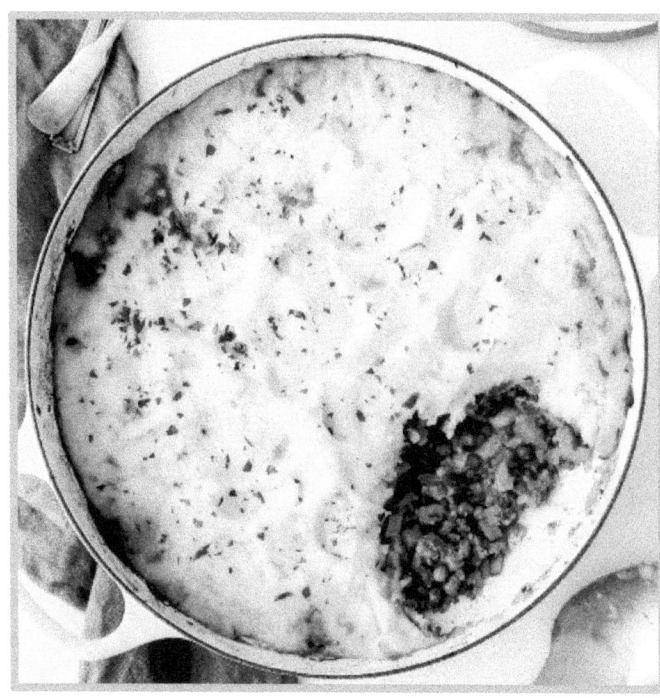

INGREDIENTS

- ½ cup of shredded cheddar cheese
- ¾ cup of reduced-sodium chicken broth
- 4 cups of frozen mixed vegetables
- 2 tbsps. of flour
- 1 garlic clove, minced
- 1 medium onion, chopped
- 1 lb. of lean ground chicken
- ½ cup of low-fat milk
- 2 large baked potatoes, peeled and diced

DIRECTIONS

1. In a saucepan, bring to boil potatoes with water barely covering it.
2. Once boiling, reduce fire to a simmer and cook for 15 minutes or until soft while covered. Once soft, drain potatoes, transfer to a bowl, and mash. Add milk and mix well.
3. Preheat oven to 375°F. In a large skillet, grease with cooking spray and sauté garlic and onions for a minute. Add ground chicken and sauté until brown around 8 to 10 minutes. Add flour and sauté for another minute.
4. Add broth and mixed vegetables. Sauté until bubbly, around 5 minutes—transfer mixture into an 8-inch square baking sheet.
5. Cover the top with mashed potato mixture and sprinkle cheese on top. Pop into the oven and bake until bubbly around 25 minutes. Serve and enjoy.

56. Crunchy Potato Croquettes

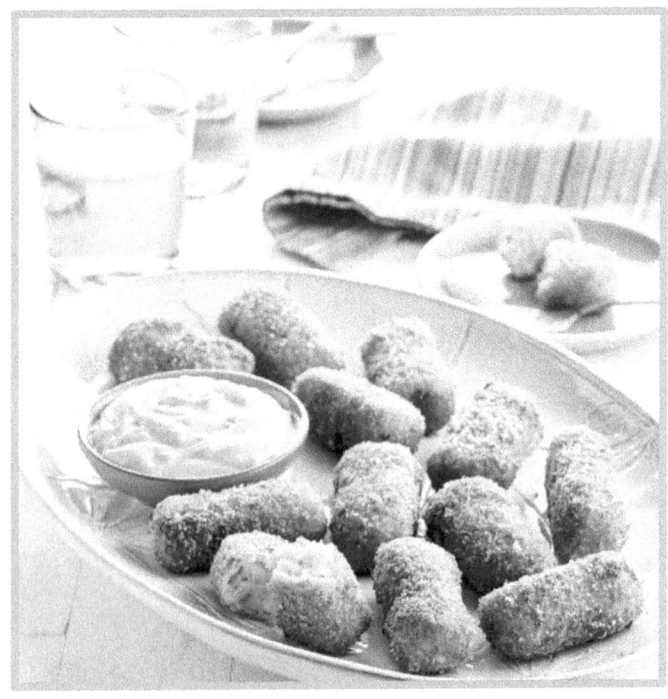

NUTRITION

Calories: 322.1

Protein: 7.5g

Sodium: 399.7mg

Phosphorus: 13.5mg

Potassium: 233.5mg

PREP TIME
15 min

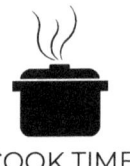

COOK TIME
20 min

SERVING
4 people

DIRECTIONS

1. Mash potatoes with milk, butter, and pepper.
2. Form cooled potatoes into balls with your hands.
3. Dip balls in beaten egg.
4. Next, roll balls in bread crumbs.
5. Then place balls in a hot oiled skillet and fry until golden brown.

INGREDIENTS

- 4 medium "leached" potato, cooked and peeled
- 1 tbsp. of butter
- 1 tbsp. of rice milk
- 1 tsp. of pepper
- 1 beaten egg
- 1 cup of white bread crumbs
- 2 tbsp. of canola oil

57. Vegetarian Summer Rolls

PREP TIME
3 min

COOK TIME
0 min

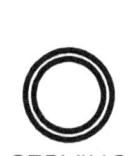
SERVING
24 people

NUTRITION

Calories: 94.5

Protein: 0.2g

Sodium: 562.6mg

Phosphorus: 0.5mg

Potassium: 34.0mg

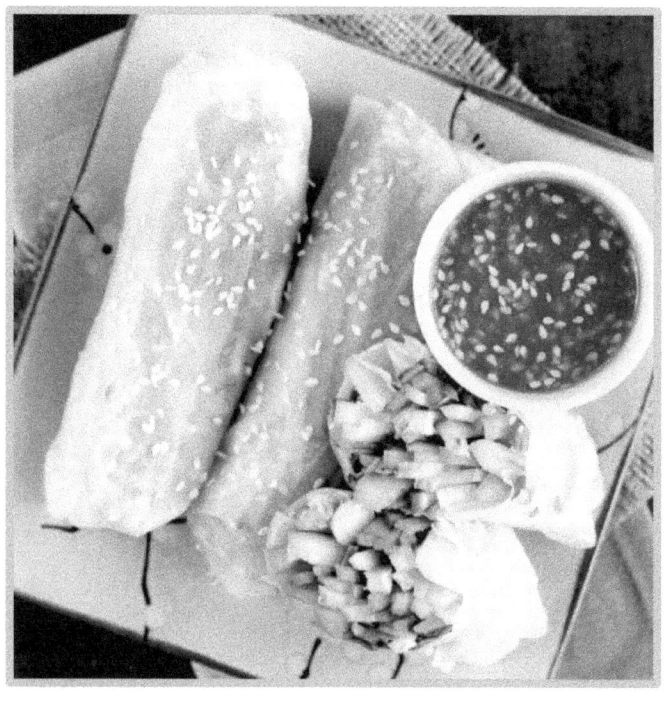

INGREDIENTS

- 1 ounce of rice vermicelli noodles
- 2 zucchinis shredded
- 2 carrots shredded
- 2 shallots finely chopped
- 2 small cucumbers peeled and diced
- 1/3 cup of fresh basil chopped
- ½ cup of fresh cilantro chopped
- 24 spring roll wrappers

Dipping Sauce:
- 1/4 cup of sugar
- 1/4 cup of rice vinegar
- 2 fresh red chilies

DIRECTIONS

1. Place sugar, vinegar, and 2 tbsp. of water in a saucepan and boil gently.
2. Remove from heat, add chilies, and set aside.
3. In a large bowl, combine all rest of the ingredients (except wrappers).
4. Place a moistened wrapper on a work surface.
5. Put a spoonful of filling in the center and fold to encase, bringing corner to corner.
6. Fold in sides and roll up tightly. Brush end with water to seal.
7. Repeat until all filling is used.
8. Serve with dipping sauce.

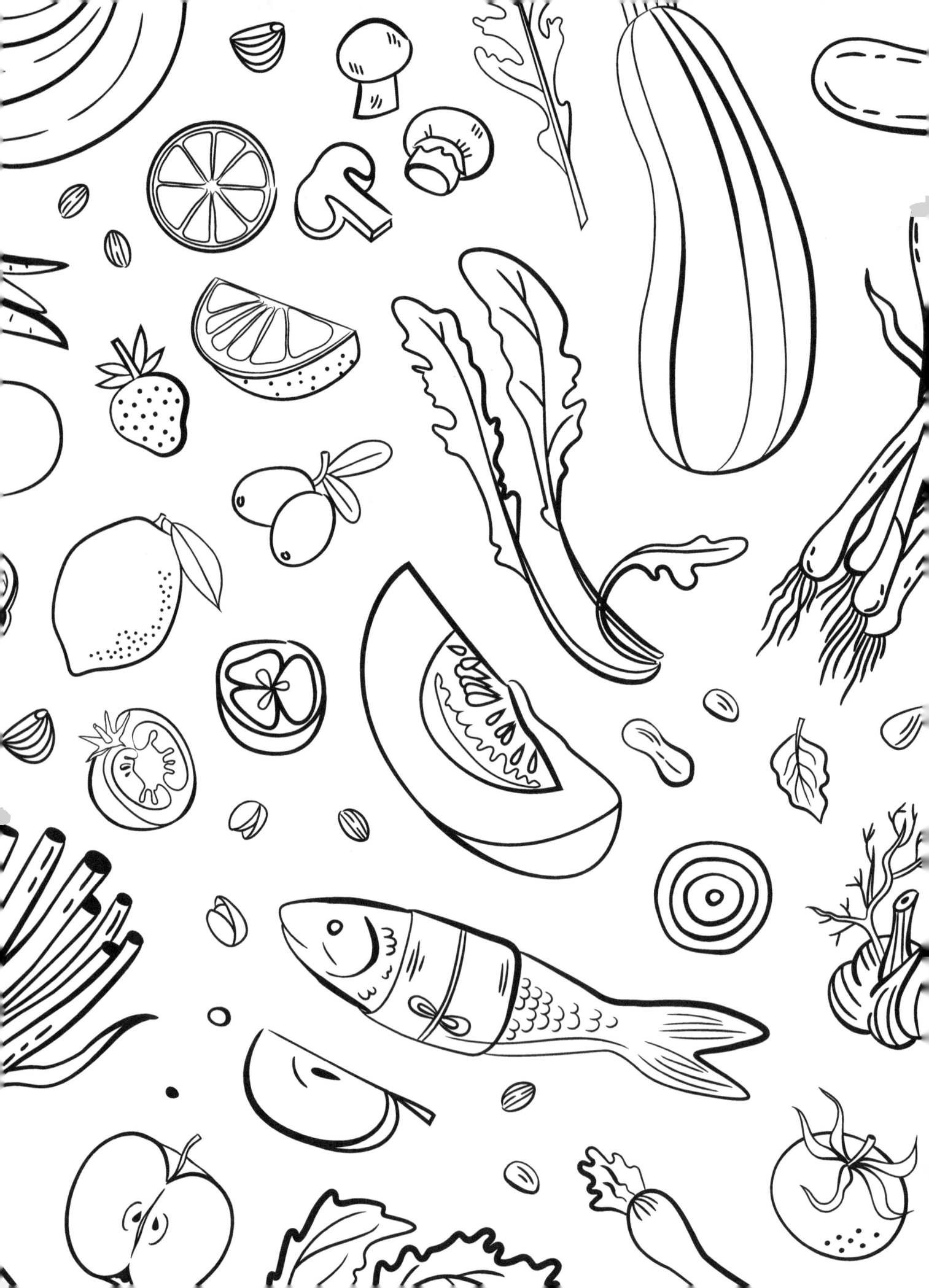

Chapter 9

SOUPS

58. Tofu Soup

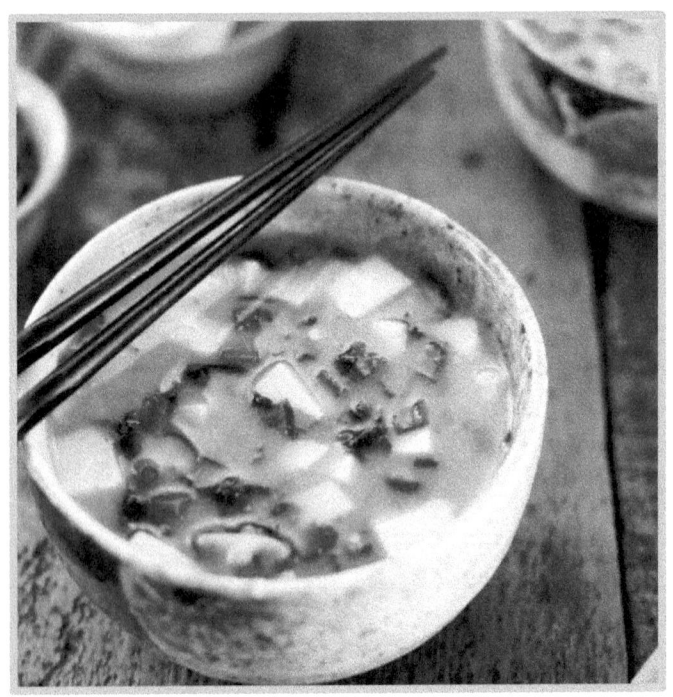

NUTRITION

Calories: 129

Fat: 7.8g

Sodium: 484mg

Potassium: 435mg

Protein: 11g

Carbs: 5.5g

Phosphorus: 73.2mg

PREP TIME
5 min

COOK TIME
10 min

SERVING
2 people

DIRECTIONS

1. Take a saucepan, pour the stock into this pan and let it boil on high heat.
2. Reduce heat to medium and let this stock simmer. Add mushrooms in this stock and cook for almost 3 minutes.
3. Take a bowl and mix soy sauce (reduced salt) and miso paste together in this bowl.
4. Add this mixture and tofu in stock. Simmer for nearly 5 minutes and serve with chopped green onion.

INGREDIENTS

- 1 tbsp. of miso paste
- 1/8 cup of cubed soft tofu
- 1 chopped green onion
- ¼ cup of sliced Shiitake mushrooms
- 3 cups of Renali stock
- 1 tbsp. of soy sauce

59. Onion Soup

PREP TIME
15 min

COOK TIME
45 min

SERVING
6 people

NUTRITION

Calories: 22

Fat: 0g

Sodium: 602.3mg

Potassium: 54.1mg

Carbs: 4.9g

Protein: 0.6g

Phosphorus: 15.8mg

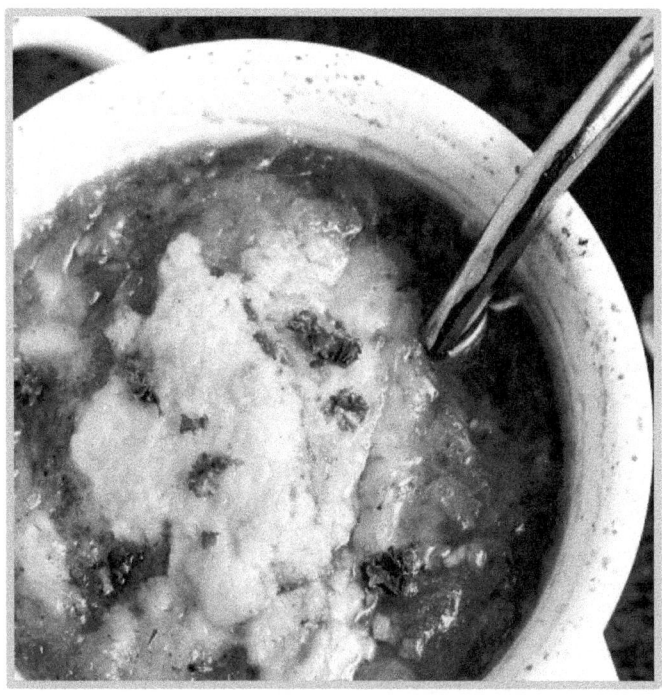

INGREDIENTS

- 2 tbsps. of chicken stock
- 1 cup of chopped Shiitake mushrooms
- 1 tbsp. of minced chives
- 3 tsps. of beef bouillon
- 1 tsp. of grated ginger root
- ½ chopped carrot
- 1 cup of sliced Portobello mushrooms
- 1 chopped onion
- ½ chopped celery stalk
- 2 quarts of water
- ¼ tsp. of minced garlic

DIRECTIONS

1. Take a saucepan and combine carrot, onion, celery, garlic, mushrooms (some mushrooms), and ginger in this pan. Add water, beef bouillon, and chicken stock in this pan.
2. Put this pot on high heat and let it boil. Decrease flame to medium and cover this pan to cook for almost 45 minutes.
3. Put all remaining mushrooms in one separate pot.
4. Once the boiling mixture is completely done, put one strainer over this new bowl with mushrooms and strain cooked soup in this pot over mushrooms. Discard solid-strained materials.
5. Serve delicious broth with yummy mushrooms in small bowls and sprinkle chives over each bowl.

60. Roasted Carrot Soup

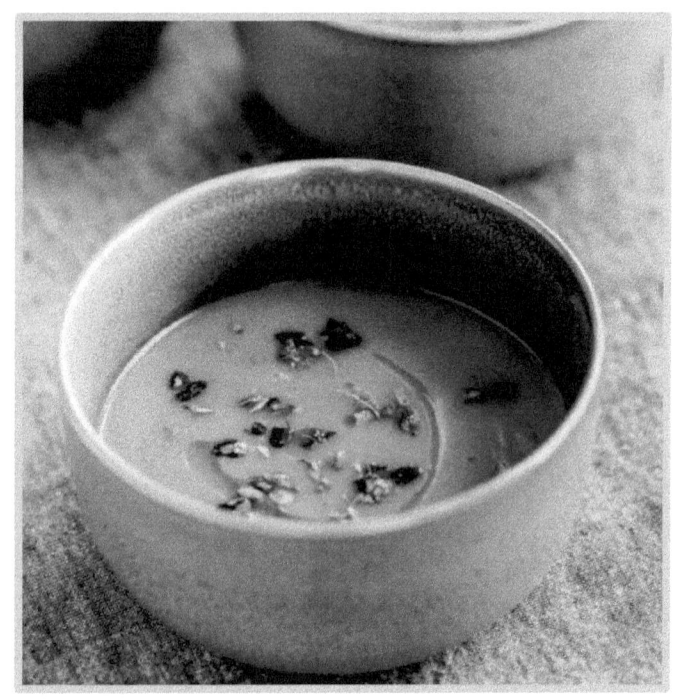

NUTRITION

Calories: 222

Fat: 18g

Net Carbohydrates: 7g

Protein: 5g

PREP TIME
10 min

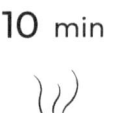

COOK TIME
50 min

SERVING
4 people

DIRECTIONS

1. Preheat your oven to 425°F.
2. Take a baking sheet and add carrots, drizzle olive oil, and roast for 30–45 minutes.
3. Put roasted carrots into a blender and add the broth, puree.
4. Pour into saucepan and heat soup.
5. Season with salt, pepper, and cayenne.
6. Drizzle olive oil.
7. Serve and enjoy!

INGREDIENTS

- 8 large carrots, washed and peeled
- 6 tablespoons of olive oil
- 1-quart of broth
- Cayenne pepper to taste
- Salt and pepper to taste

61. Mushroom Cream Soup

PREP TIME 5 min

COOK TIME 30 min

SERVING 4 people

NUTRITION

Calories: 200

Fat: 17g

Carbohydrates: 5g

Protein: 4g

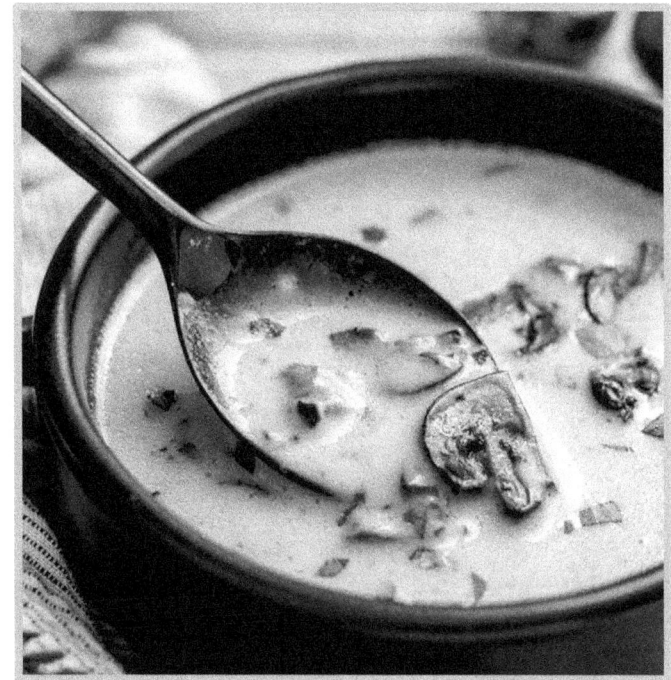

INGREDIENTS

- 1 tablespoon of olive oil
- ½ large onion, diced
- 20 ounces of mushrooms, sliced
- 6 garlic cloves, minced
- 2 cups of vegetable broth
- 1 cup of coconut cream
- ¾ teaspoon of salt
- ¼ teaspoon of black pepper

DIRECTIONS

1. Using a large-sized pot, heat it over medium heat.
2. Add onion and mushrooms in olive oil and Sauté for 10–15 minutes.
3. Make sure to keep stirring it from time to time until browned evenly.
4. Add garlic and Sauté for 10 minutes more.
5. Add vegetable broth, coconut cream, coconut milk, black pepper, and salt.
6. Bring to a boil then reduce the temperature to low.
7. Simmer for 15 minutes.
8. Use a blender to puree the mixture.
9. Enjoy

62. Garlic Soup

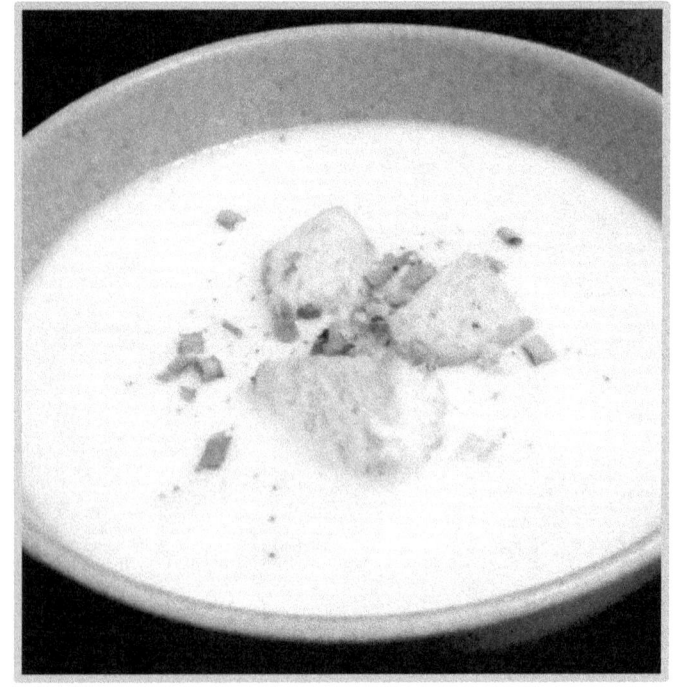

NUTRITION

Calories: 142
Fat: 8g
Carbohydrates: 3.4g
Protein: 4g

PREP TIME
10 min

COOK TIME
60 min

SERVING
10 people

DIRECTIONS

1. Preheat your oven to 400°F.
2. Slice ¼ inch top off the garlic bulb and place it in aluminum foil.
3. Grease with olive oil and roast in the oven for 35 minutes.
4. Squeeze the flesh out of the roasted garlic.
5. Heat oil in a saucepan and add shallots; sauté for 6 minutes.
6. Add the garlic and remaining ingredients.
7. Cover the pan and then reduce to low heat.
8. Let it cook for 15–20 minutes.
9. Use an immersion blender to puree the mixture.
10. Season soup with salt and pepper.
11. Serve and enjoy!

INGREDIENTS

- 1 tablespoon of olive oil
- 2 bulbs of garlic, peeled
- 3 shallots, chopped
- 1 large head cauliflower, chopped
- 6 cups of vegetable broth
- Salt and pepper to taste

63. Pesto Green Vegetable Soup

PREP TIME
10 min

COOK TIME
15 min

SERVING
6 people

NUTRITION

Calories: 170
Total fat: 13g
Saturated fat: 3g
Cholesterol: 2g
Sodium: 333mg
Carbohydrates: 8g
Fiber: 1g
Phosphorus: 42mg
Potassium: 200mg
Protein: 3g

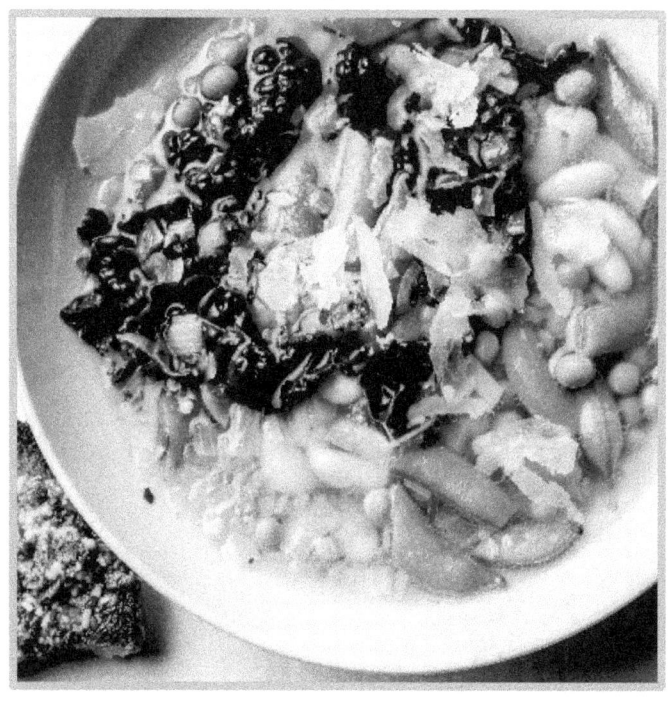

INGREDIENTS

- 2 teaspoons of olive oil
- 1 leek, white and light green parts, sliced and washed thoroughly
- 2 celery stalks, diced
- 1 teaspoon of minced garlic
- 2 cups of sodium-free chicken stock
- 1 cup of chopped snow peas
- 1 cup of shredded spinach
- 1 tablespoon of chopped fresh thyme
- Juice and zest of ½ lemon
- ¼ teaspoon of freshly ground black pepper
- 1 tablespoon of Basil Pesto

DIRECTIONS

1. In a large saucepan over medium-high heat, heat the olive oil.
2. Add the leek, celery, and garlic, and sauté until tender, about 3 minutes.
3. Stir in the stock, and bring to a boil.
4. Stir in the snow peas, spinach, and thyme, and simmer for about 5 minutes.
5. Remove the pan from the heat, and stir in the lemon juice, lemon zest, pepper, and pesto.
6. Serve immediately.

64. Cucumber Soup

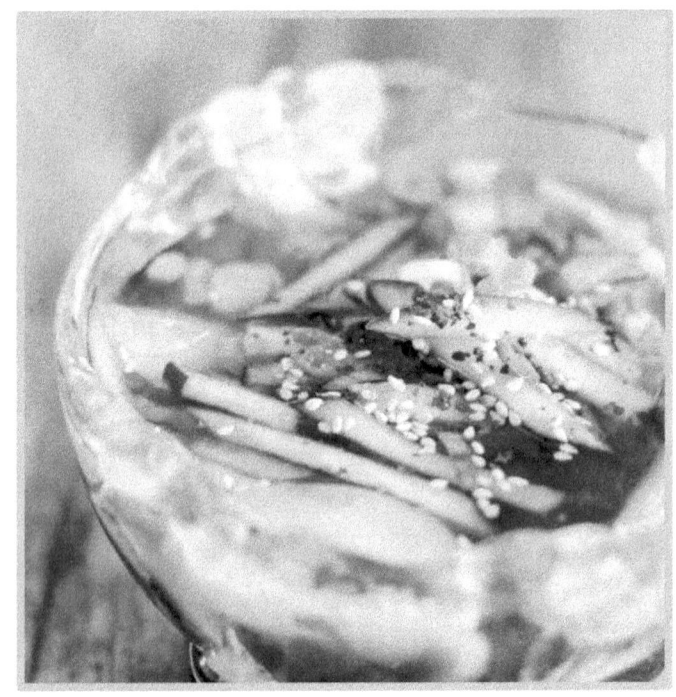

NUTRITION

Calories: 371

Fat: 36g

Carbohydrates: 8g

Protein: 4g

PREP TIME
14 min

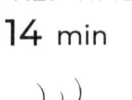

COOK TIME
0 min

SERVING
4 people

DIRECTIONS

1. Pour the ingredients to a blender and emulsify by blending them (except ½ cup of chopped cucumbers)
2. Blend until smooth
3. Divide the soup amongst 4 servings and top with extra cucumbers
4. Enjoy chilled!

INGREDIENTS

- 2 tablespoons of garlic, minced
- 4 cups of English cucumbers, peeled and diced
- ½ cup of onions, diced
- 1 tablespoon of lemon juice
- 1 ½ cups of vegetable broth
- ½ teaspoon of salt
- ¼ teaspoon of red pepper flakes
- ¼ cup of parsley, diced
- ½ cup of Greek yogurt, plain

65. Tangy Orange Shrimp

PREP TIME
15 min

COOK TIME
15 min

SERVING
4 people

NUTRITION

Calories: 140

Total fat: 3g

Saturated fat: 1g

Cholesterol: 130g

Sodium: 132mg

Carbohydrates: 8g

Fiber: 1g

Phosphorus: 196mg

Potassium: 329mg

Protein: 18g

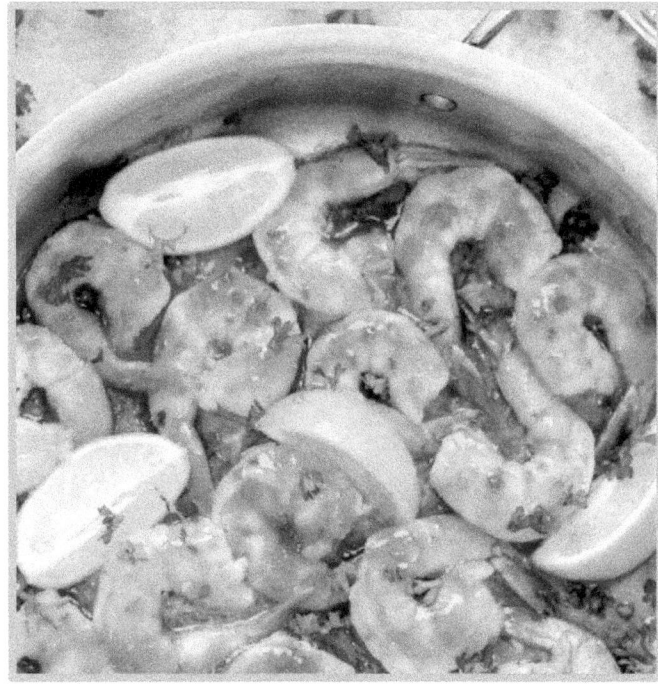

INGREDIENTS

- ½ cup of freshly squeezed orange juice
- ½ teaspoon of cornstarch
- ¼ teaspoon of freshly grated orange zest
- 1 teaspoon of olive oil
- 12 ounces (26/30 count) of shrimp, peeled and deveined, tails left on
- 1 cup of broccoli florets
- 1 teaspoon of unsalted butter
- ½ cup of orange segments
- Freshly ground black pepper

DIRECTIONS

1. In a small bowl, whisk together the orange juice, cornstarch, and orange zest and set aside.
2. In a large skillet over medium-high heat, heat the olive oil.
3. Add the shrimp and sauté until just cooked through and opaque, about 5 minutes. Transfer the cooked shrimp to a plate. Add the broccoli and sauté until tender, about 4 minutes. Transfer to the plate with the shrimp.
4. Pour the orange juice mixture into the skillet, and whisk until the sauce has thickened and is glossy about 3 minutes.
5. Whisk in the butter, and add the orange segments, shrimp, and broccoli to the skillet.
6. Toss to combine and season with pepper. Serve immediately.

66. Shrimp and Greens

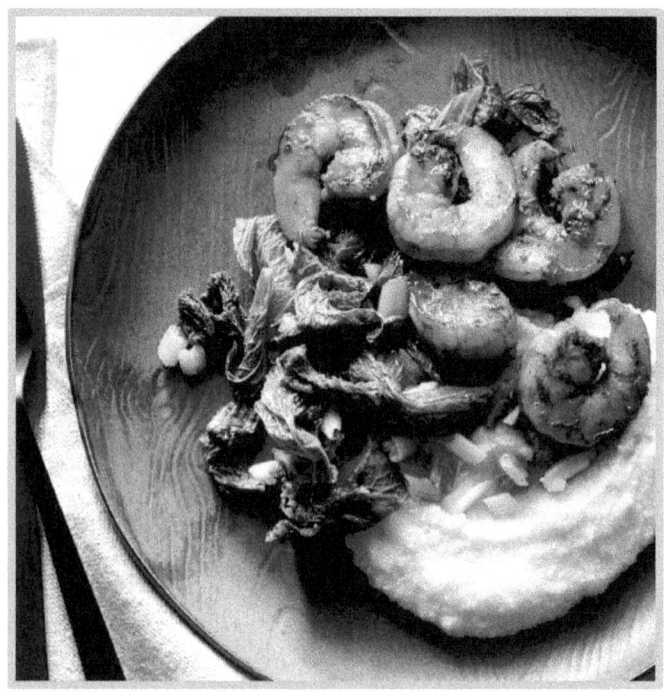

NUTRITION

Calories: 127
Total fat: 8g
Saturated fat: 1g
Cholesterol: 85mg
Sodium: 96mg
Carbohydrates: 2g
Fiber: 1g
Phosphorus: 178mg
Potassium: 287mg
Protein: 18g

PREP TIME
10 min

COOK TIME
15 min

SERVING
4 people

DIRECTIONS

1. In a large skillet over medium-high heat, heat the olive oil.
2. Add the shrimp and sauté until opaque and pink, about 6 minutes.
3. With a slotted spoon, remove the shrimp to a plate.
4. In the skillet, sauté the garlic until softened, about 3 minutes.
5. Stir in the spinach and tomatoes, and sauté until the spinach has wilted and the tomatoes are cooked, about 5 minutes.
6. Stir in the shrimp, sprinkle in the nutmeg, and toss to combine.
7. Season with pepper, and serve.

INGREDIENTS

- 1 tablespoon of olive oil
- 12 ounces (26/30 count) of shrimp, peeled, deveined, tails removed
- 2 teaspoons of minced garlic
- 2 cups of fresh spinach
- ½ cup of halved cherry tomatoes
- ½ teaspoon of ground nutmeg
- Freshly ground black pepper

67. Seared Herbed Scallops

PREP TIME
10 min

COOK TIME
5 min

SERVING
4 people

NUTRITION

Calories: 131
Total fat: 5g
Saturated fat: 1g
Cholesterol: 35mg
Sodium: 136mg
Carbohydrates: 2g
Fiber: 0g
Phosphorus: 176mg
Potassium: 268mg
Protein: 14g

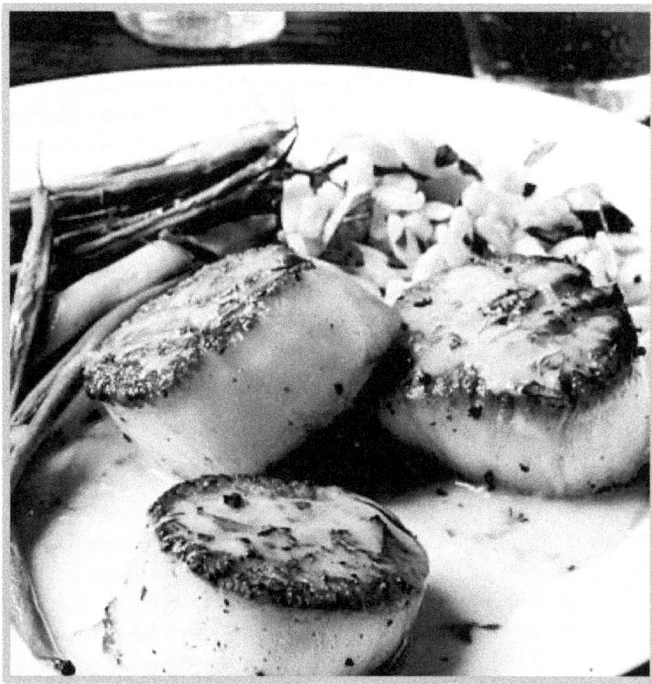

INGREDIENTS

- 1 tablespoon of olive oil
- 12 ounces of sea scallops, rinsed and patted dry
- Freshly ground black pepper
- 2 tablespoons of freshly squeezed lemon juice
- 1 teaspoon of chopped fresh parsley
- 1 teaspoon of chopped fresh thyme
- 1 teaspoon of chopped fresh chives

DIRECTIONS

1. In a large skillet over medium-high heat, heat the olive oil.
2. Lightly season the scallops with pepper. Add them to the skillet.
3. Sear the scallops, turning once, until just cooked through and browned, about 4 minutes total.
4. Stir in the lemon juice, parsley, thyme, and chives.
5. Turn the scallops to coat in the herb sauce.
6. Serve hot.

68. Almond-Crusted Sole

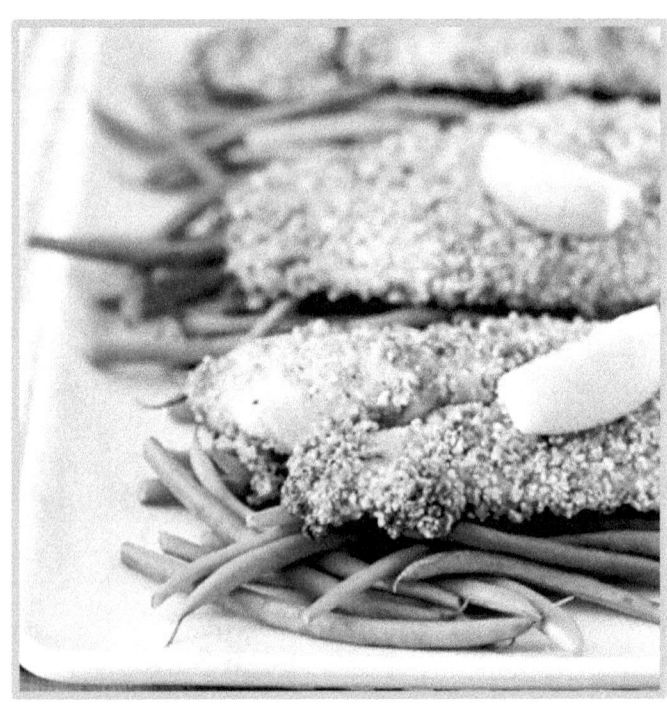

NUTRITION

Calories: 113

Total fat: 3g

Saturated fat: 1g

Cholesterol: 41mg

Sodium: 70mg

Carbohydrates: 1g

Fiber: 0g

Phosphorus: 168mg

Potassium: 327mg

Protein: 17g

PREP TIME
15 min

COOK TIME
15 min

SERVING
4 people

DIRECTIONS

1. Preheat the oven to 350°F.
2. Line a baking sheet with parchment paper.
3. Lightly season the sole fillets with pepper.
4. In a shallow bowl, mix together the almond flour, parsley, and thyme until blended.
5. Lightly brush the fish with the olive oil, and dredge in the almond flour mixture.
6. Place the sole fillets on the prepared baking sheet, and bake until the fish is opaque, about 15 minutes.
7. Serve immediately.

Ingredient tip: Black pepper is something most people are used to seeing in shakers on the table, and the taste is very familiar. However, pepper can go stale and lose potency, so the best way to enjoy it is to fill your pepper grinder with black peppercorns and freshly grind your own pepper as needed.

INGREDIENTS

- 4 (3-ounce) sole fillets, patted dry
- Freshly ground black pepper
- 3 tablespoons of almond flour
- 1 tablespoon of chopped fresh parsley
- 1 teaspoon of chopped fresh thyme
- 1 teaspoon of olive oil

69. Breaded Baked Sole

PREP TIME 10 min

COOK TIME 10 min

SERVING 4 people

NUTRITION

Calories: 103
Total fat: 3g
Saturated fat: 2g
Cholesterol: 35mg
Sodium: 96mg
Carbohydrates: 5g
Fiber: 0g
Phosphorus: 116mg
Potassium: 200mg
Protein: 8g

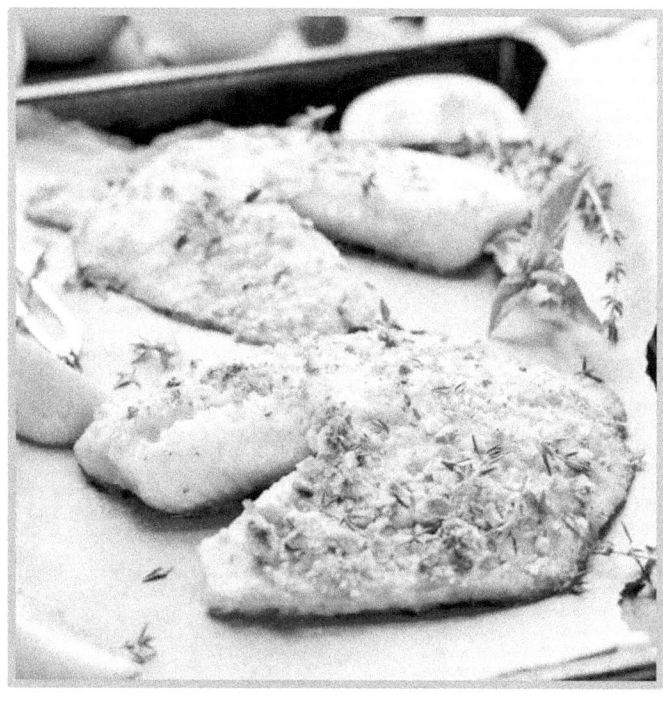

INGREDIENTS

- ¼ cup of bread crumbs
- 1 tablespoon of unsalted butter, at room temperature
- 2 teaspoons of chopped fresh parsley
- 2 teaspoons of chopped fresh thyme
- 2 teaspoons of freshly grated lemon zest
- 4 (2-ounce) sole fillets, skinless, patted dry
- Freshly ground black pepper

DIRECTIONS

1. Preheat the oven to 400°F.
2. In a small bowl, stir together the bread crumbs, butter, parsley, thyme, and lemon zest.
3. Lightly season the fish fillets with pepper, and place them on a baking sheet.
4. Divide the bread crumb mixture evenly among the fillets, pressing it down lightly to adhere.
5. Bake until the fish is just cooked through and the bread crumbs are golden, about 10 minutes.

70. Roasted Tilapia with Garlic Butter

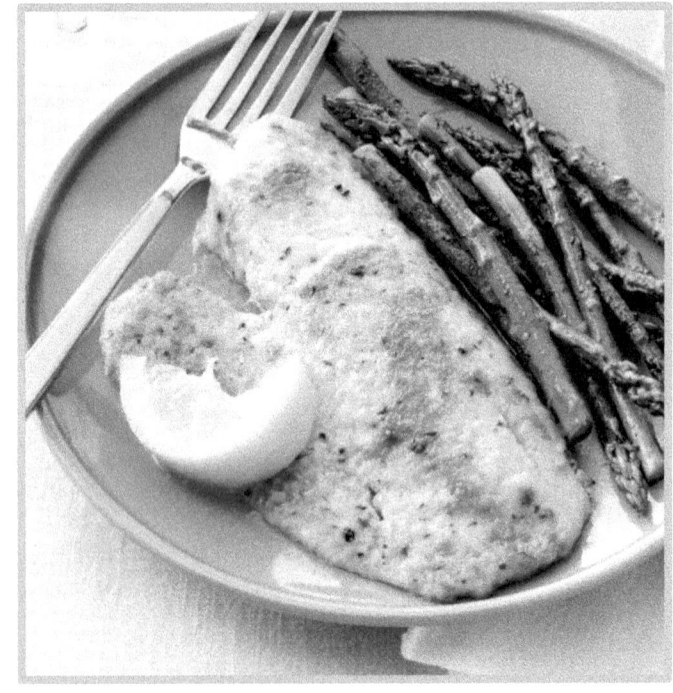

NUTRITION

Calories: 219
Total fat: 16g
Saturated fat: 8g
Cholesterol: 72mg
Sodium: 45mg
Carbohydrates: 2g
Fiber: 0g
Phosphorus: 149mg
Potassium: 252mg
Protein: 17g

PREP TIME
10 min

COOK TIME
10 min

SERVING
4 people

DIRECTIONS

1. Preheat the oven to 400°F.
2. In a small bowl, stir together the butter, shallot, garlic, lemon juice, lemon zest, parsley, and flour and set aside.
3. In a large ovenproof skillet over medium-high heat, heat the oil. Season the fillets with pepper and set them in the skillet. Brown the fish, turning once, about 4 minutes total.
4. Pour the butter mixture over the fish, and place the skillet, uncovered, in the oven. Roast the fish until just cooked through and opaque in the center, about 4 minutes.
5. Serve immediately with a spoonful of sauce from the skillet.

Substitution tip: Onion or scallion can be substituted for the shallot in the sauce. Shallot has a lighter, sweeter flavor.

INGREDIENTS

- ¼ cup of melted unsalted butter
- 1 shallot, minced
- 1 teaspoon of minced garlic
- Juice and zest of ½ lemon
- 2 tablespoons of chopped fresh parsley
- 1 tablespoon of all-purpose flour
- 1 tablespoon of olive oil
- 4 (3-ounce) tilapia fillets, patted dry
- Freshly ground black pepper

71. Pesto-Crusted Tilapia

PREP TIME
10 min

COOK TIME
15 min

SERVING
4 people

NUTRITION

Calories: 159
Total fat: 5g
Saturated fat: 1g
Cholesterol: 43mg
Sodium: 162mg
Carbohydrates: 10g
Fiber: 1g
Phosphorus: 164mg
Potassium: 272mg
Protein: 19g

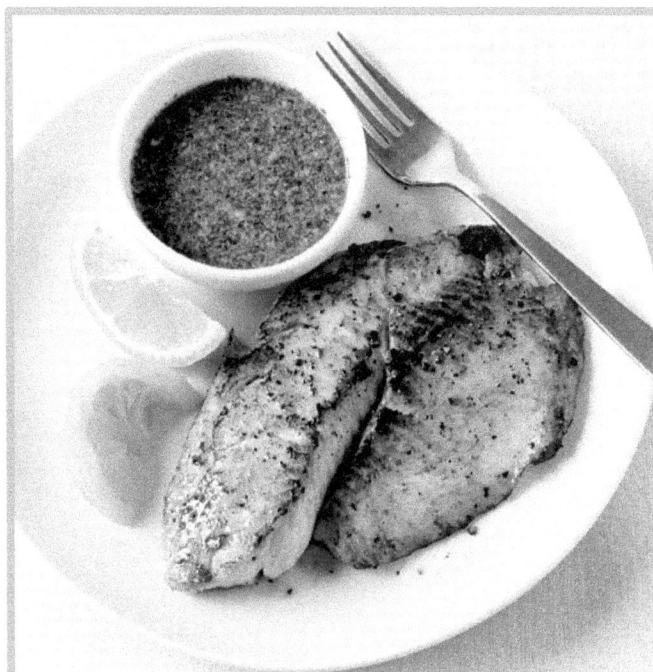

INGREDIENTS

- Olive oil, for the baking sheet
- ½ cup of bread crumbs
- 1 tablespoon of grated Parmesan cheese
- 1 tablespoon of Basil Pesto (here)
- 4 (3-ounce) tilapia fillets, patted dry

DIRECTIONS

1. Preheat the oven to 400°F.
2. Lightly coat a 9-by-9-inch baking sheet with olive oil, and set it aside.
3. In a small bowl, add the bread crumbs, Parmesan cheese, and pesto and stir until blended.
4. Place the fish in the baking sheet, and spoon the pesto mixture over the fish, so each piece is evenly coated.
5. Bake until just cooked through, about 15 minutes.
6. Serve hot.

Cooking tip: If you have a barbecue, this recipe is perfect for cooking outdoors on a balmy summer evening. Turn one side of your barbecue on high, and leave the other side off. Place the fish in a foil package instead of a baking sheet, on the cool side of the barbecue, for about 25 minutes.

72. Lime Baked Haddock

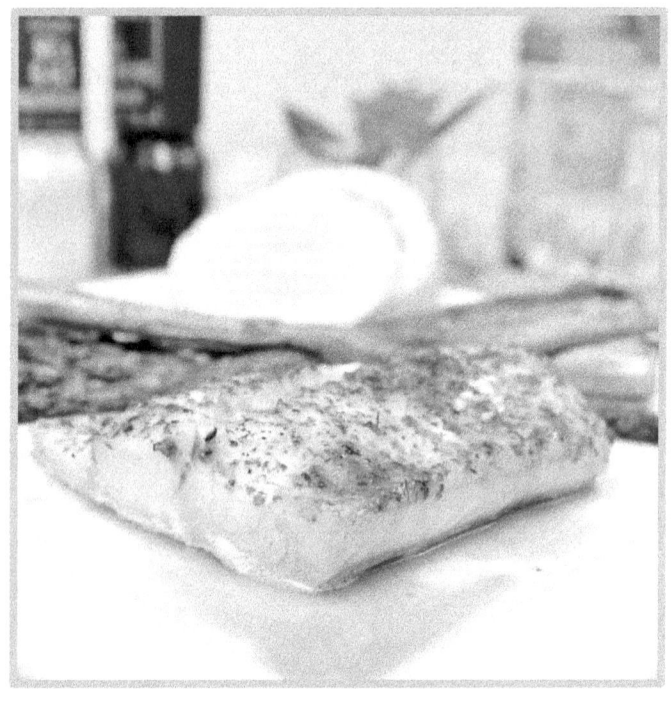

NUTRITION

Calories: 124
Total fat: 6g
Saturated fat: 0g
Cholesterol: 55mg
Sodium: 59mg
Carbohydrates: 1g
Fiber: 0g
Phosphorus: 176mg
Potassium: 283mg
Protein: 17g

PREP TIME
10 min

COOK TIME
10 min

SERVING
4 people

DIRECTIONS

1. Preheat the oven to 400°F.
2. Lightly season the fish with pepper.
3. Lightly coat a 9-by-9-inch baking sheet with cooking spray.
4. Lay the lime slices in the bottom of the baking sheet, and arrange the fish fillets on top.
5. Brush the fish with the olive oil, and sprinkle them with the almonds.
6. Bake the fish until just cooked through, and the almonds are golden, about 10 minutes.
7. Serve with the chopped dill.

INGREDIENTS

- 4 (3-ounce) haddock fillets, patted dry
- Freshly ground black pepper
- Olive oil cooking spray
- 3 limes, thinly sliced
- 1 tablespoon of olive oil
- 3 tablespoons of crushed almonds
- 2 teaspoons of chopped fresh dill

73. Fish Tacos with Vegetable Slaw

PREP TIME 20 min

COOK TIME 0 min

SERVING 4 people

NUTRITION

Calories: 131
Total fat: 3g
Saturated fat: 1g
Cholesterol: 32mg
Sodium: 57mg
Carbohydrates: 13g
Fiber: 2g
Phosphorus: 144mg
Potassium: 307mg
Protein: 12g

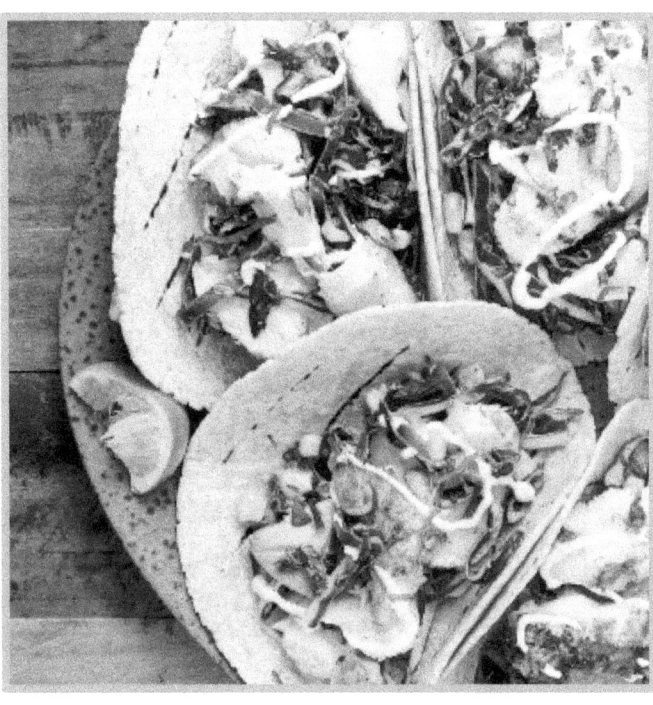

INGREDIENTS

- 2 cups of finely shredded red cabbage
- 1 carrot, shredded
- 3 radishes, grated
- 2 tablespoons of apple cider vinegar
- Juice of 1 lime
- 1 teaspoon of honey
- 1 teaspoon of chopped fresh cilantro

For the tacos:
- 4 (6-inch) flour tortillas
- 8 ounces of halibut fillet, cooked

DIRECTIONS

To make the slaw:
1. In a medium bowl, toss together the cabbage, carrot, radishes, vinegar, lime juice, honey, and cilantro until well mixed.
2. Place the bowl in the refrigerator for 1 hour to let the flavors mellow.
3.

To make the tacos:
1. Place the tortillas on a clean work surface. Divide the fish evenly among them, then top with the slaw.
2. Fold the tortillas over the fish and serve.

74. Eggplant and Red Pepper Soup

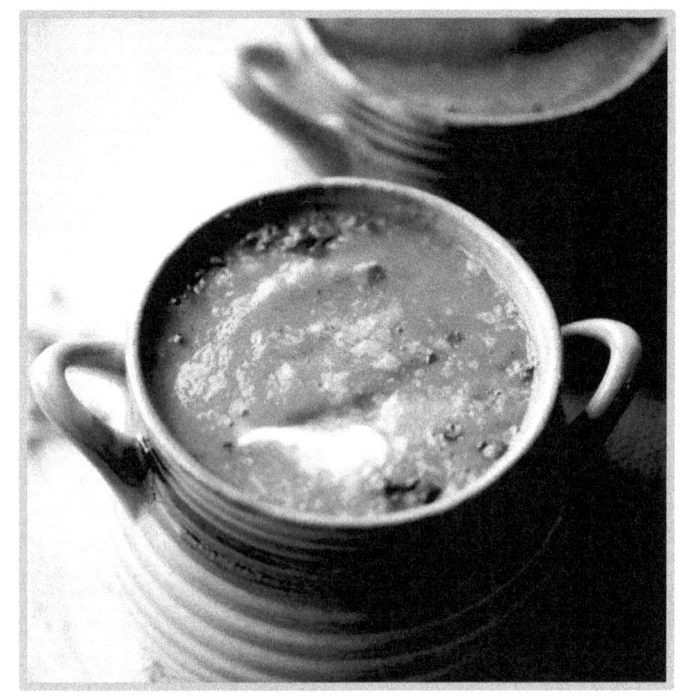

NUTRITION

Calories: 61
Fat: 2g
Carb: 9g
Phosphorus: 33mg
Potassium: 198mg
Sodium: 98mg
Protein: 2g

PREP TIME
20 min

COOK TIME
40 min

SERVING
4 people

DIRECTIONS

1. Preheat the oven to 350°F.
2. Put the onions, red peppers, eggplant, and garlic in a baking sheet.
3. Drizzle the vegetables with the olive oil.
4. Roast the vegetables for 30 minutes or until they are slightly charred and soft.
5. Cool the vegetables slightly and remove the skin from the peppers.
6. Puree the vegetables with a hand mixer (with the chicken stock).
7. Transfer the soup to a medium pot and add enough water to reach the desired thickness.
8. Heat the soup to a simmer and add the basil.
9. Season with pepper and serve.

INGREDIENTS

- 1 small, cut into quarters sweet onion
- 2 halves red bell peppers
- 2 cups of eggplant, cubed
- 2 garlic cloves, crushed
- 1 tbsp. of olive oil
- 1 cup of chicken stock
- Water
- ¼ cup of chopped fresh basil
- Ground black pepper

75. Chicken Pho

PREP TIME
10 min

COOK TIME
15 min

SERVING
4 people

NUTRITION

Calories: 325

Fat: 3g

Carbs: 55g

Protein: 21g

Phosphorus: 205mg

Potassium: 389mg

Sodium: 313mg

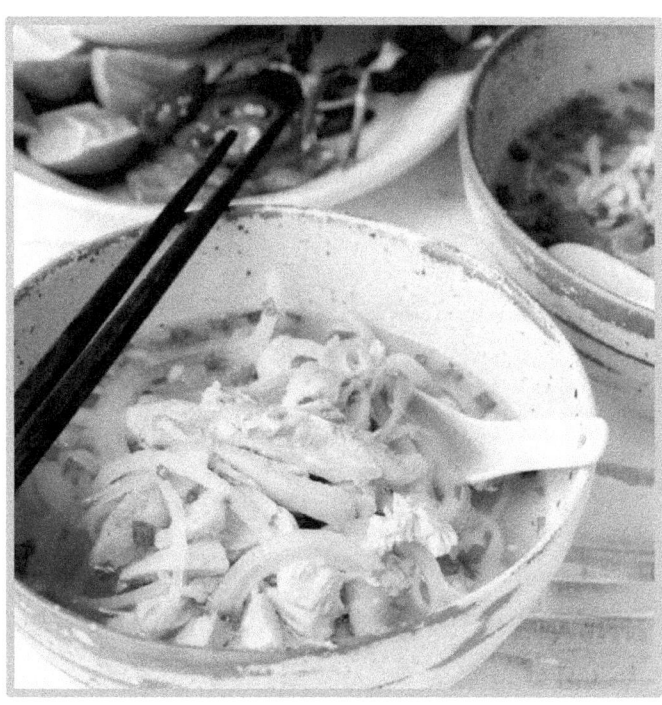

INGREDIENTS

- 5 cups of Simple Chicken Broth or low-sodium, store-bought chicken stock
- 1-inch piece of ginger, cut lengthwise into 2 or 3 strips
- 1 cup of cooked chicken breast, diced
- Several fresh Thai basil sprigs
- 1 cup of mung bean sprouts
- 1 lime, cut into wedges
- 1 jalapeño pepper, stemmed, seeded, and thinly sliced
- 1 (16-ounce) package of dried rice vermicelli noodles, cooked according to package
- 4 tablespoons (¼ cup) of sliced scallions
- 4 tablespoons (¼ cup) of chopped cilantro leaves

DIRECTIONS

1. In a medium stockpot over medium-high heat, add the broth and ginger, and bring to a simmer. Add the chicken and simmer for 5 minutes. Remove the ginger from the pot and discard it.

2. On a plate, arrange the Thai basil, bean sprouts, lime wedges, and jalapeño slices. Distribute the noodles among four bowls. Add 1¼ cups of broth to each bowl. Top with 1 tablespoon each of the scallions and cilantro. Serve immediately alongside the plate of garnishes.

76. Herbed Cabbage Stew

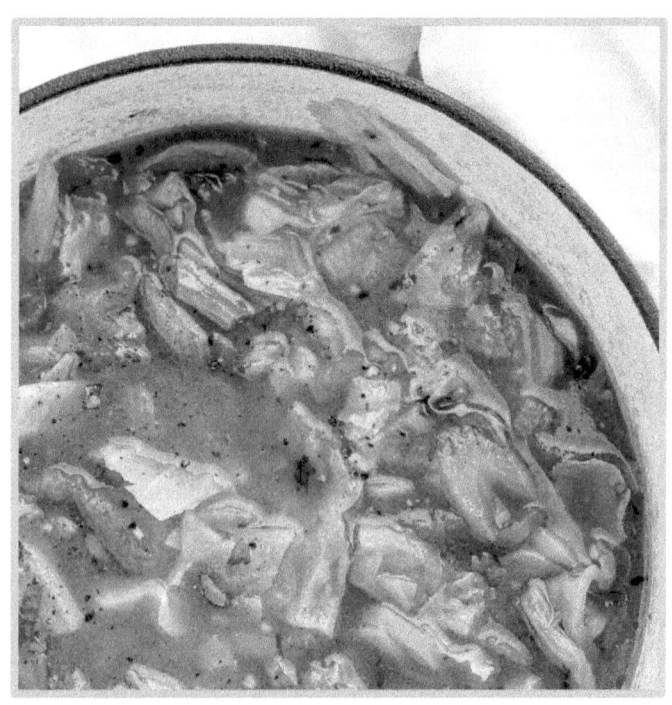

NUTRITION

Calories: 33
Fat: 1g
Carbs: 6g
Phosphorus: 29mg
Potassium: 187mg
Sodium: 20mg
Protein: 1g

PREP TIME
20 min

COOK TIME
35 min

SERVING
6 people

DIRECTIONS

1. In a medium stockpot over medium-high heat, melt the butter.
2. Sauté the onion and garlic in the melted butter for about 3 minutes or until the vegetables are softened.
3. Add the cabbage, celery, scallion, parsley, lemon juice, thyme, savory herb, and oregano to the pot, and add enough water to cover the vegetables by about 4 inches.
4. Bring the soup to a boil, reduce the heat to low, and simmer the soup for about 25 minutes or until the vegetables are tender. Add the green beans and simmer 3 minutes—season with pepper.

INGREDIENTS

- 1 teaspoon of unsalted butter
- ½ large sweet onion, chopped
- 1 teaspoon of minced garlic
- 6 cups of shredded green cabbage
- 3 celery stalks, chopped with the leafy tops
- 1 scallion, both green and white parts, chopped
- 2 tablespoons of chopped fresh parsley
- 2 tablespoons of freshly squeezed lemon juice
- 1 tablespoon of chopped fresh thyme
- 1 teaspoon of chopped savory herb
- 1 teaspoon of chopped fresh oregano
- Water
- Green beans, 1 cup, chopped
- Freshly ground black pepper

77. Vegetable Lentil Soup

PREP TIME
10 min

COOK TIME
25 min

SERVING
4 people

NUTRITION

Calories: 195

Fat: 6g

Carbs: 25g

Protein: 13g

Phosphorus: 228mg

Potassium: 707mg

Sodium: 157mg

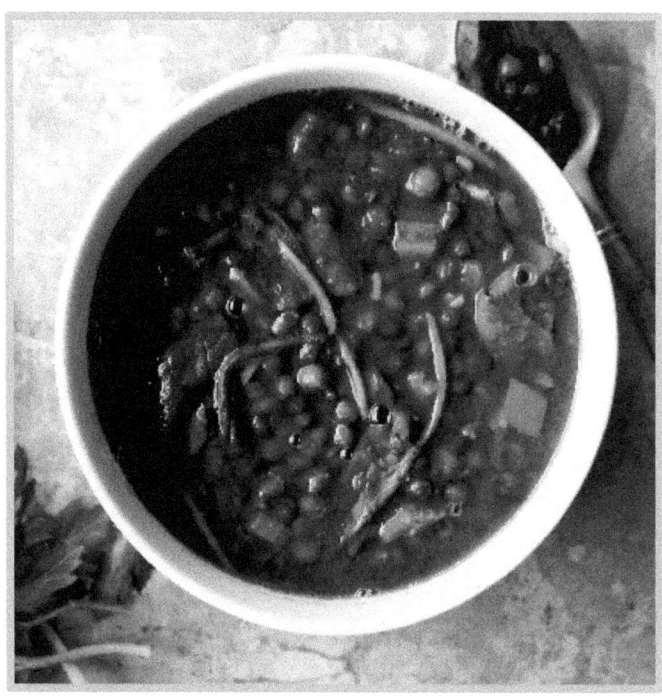

INGREDIENTS

- 1 tablespoon of extra-virgin olive oil
- ½ sweet onion, diced
- 2 carrots, diced
- 2 celery stalks, diced
- ½ cup of lentils
- 5 cups of Simple Chicken Broth or low-sodium store-bought chicken stock
- 2 cups of sliced chard leaves
- Freshly ground black pepper
- 1 lemon

DIRECTIONS

1. In a medium stockpot over medium-high heat, heat the olive oil.
2. Add the onion and stir until softened, about 3 to 5 minutes.
3. Add the carrots, celery, lentils, and broth.
4. Bring to a boil, reduce the heat, and simmer, uncovered, for 15 minutes, until the lentils are tender.
5. Add the chard and cook for 3 additional minutes, until wilted—season with the pepper and lemon juice.
6. Serve.

78. French Onion Soup

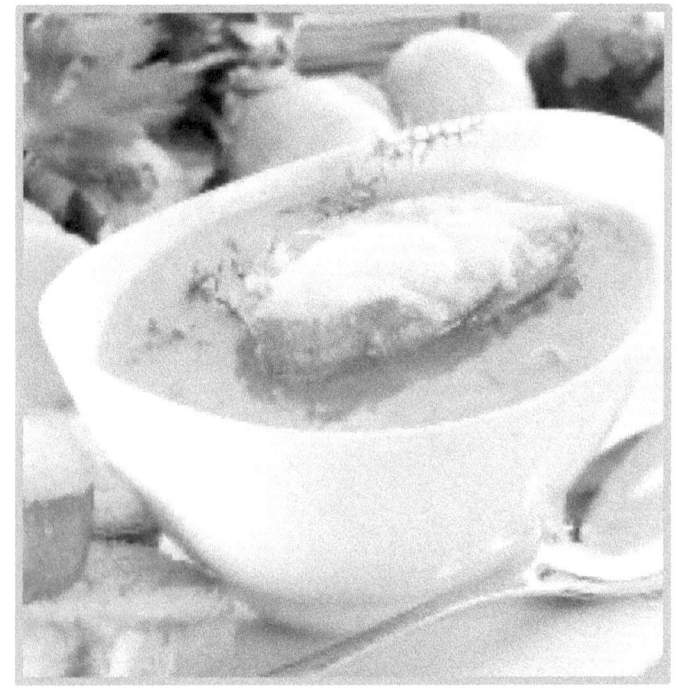

NUTRITION

Calories: 90
Fat: 6g
Carbs: 7g
Phosphorus: 22mg
Potassium: 192mg
Sodium: 57mg
Protein: 2g

PREP TIME
20 min

COOK TIME
50 min

SERVING
4 people

DIRECTIONS

1. Set your butter on to melt in a saucepan on medium heat. Add the onions to the saucepan and cook them slowly, frequently stirring, for about 30 minutes or until the onions are caramelized and tender.
2. Add the chicken stock and water and bring the soup to a boil. Switch to low heat to simmer for 15 minutes. Stir in the thyme and season the soup with pepper. Serve piping hot.

INGREDIENTS

- 2 tablespoons of unsalted butter
- 4 Vidalia onions, sliced thin
- 2 cups of Easy Chicken Stock
- 2 cups of water
- 1 tablespoon of chopped fresh thyme
- Freshly ground black pepper

79. Creamy Broccoli Soup

PREP TIME
10 min

COOK TIME
15 min

SERVING
4 people

NUTRITION

Calories: 88
Fat: 3g
Carbs: 12g
Protein: 4g
Phosphorus: 87mg
Potassium: 201mg
Sodium: 281mg

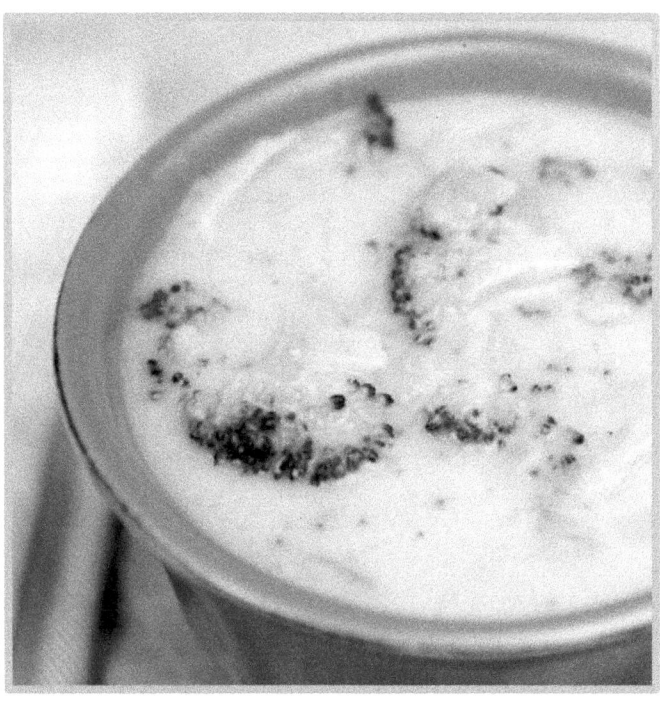

INGREDIENTS

- 1 teaspoon of extra-virgin olive oil
- ½ sweet onion, roughly chopped
- 2 cups of chopped broccoli
- 4 cups of low-sodium vegetable broth
- Freshly ground black pepper
- 1 cup of Homemade Rice Milk or unsweetened store-bought rice milk
- ¼ cup of grated Parmesan cheese

DIRECTIONS

1. In a medium saucepan over medium-high heat, heat the olive oil.
2. Add the onion and cook for 3 to 5 minutes, until it begins to soften. Add the broccoli and broth, and season with pepper.
3. Bring to a boil, reduce the heat, and simmer uncovered for 10 minutes, until the broccoli is just tender but still bright green.
4. Transfer the soup mixture to a blender. Add the rice milk, and process until smooth.
5. Return to the saucepan, stir in the Parmesan cheese, and serve.

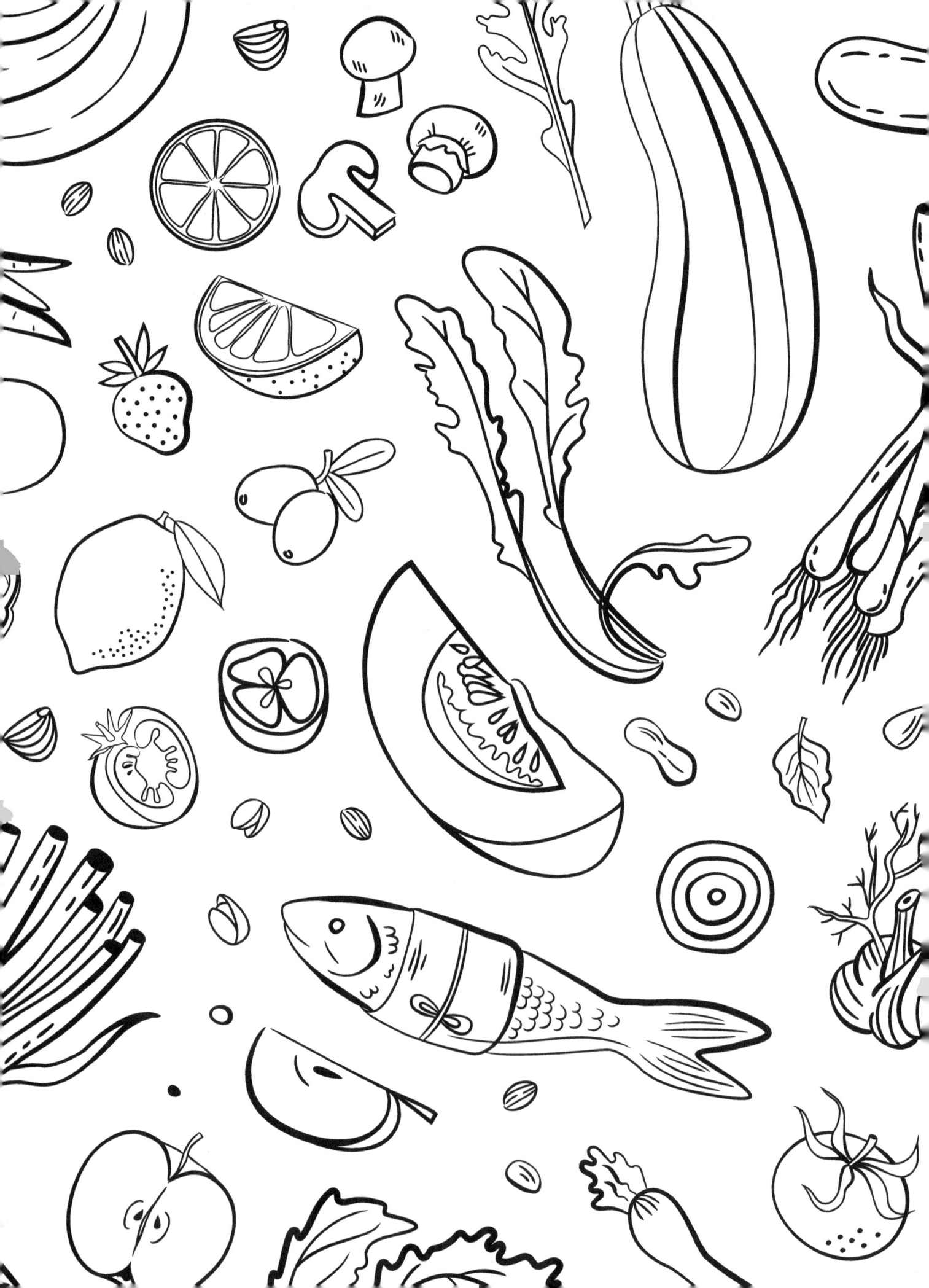

Chapter 10

SALAD

80. Cucumber Salad

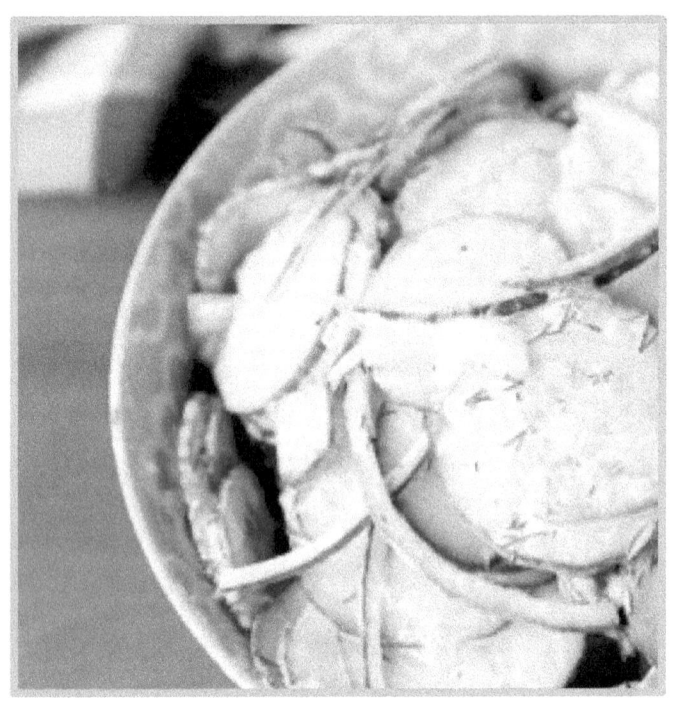

NUTRITION

Calories: 49
Fat: 0.1g
Sodium: 341mg
Potassium: 171mg
Protein: 0.8g
Carbs: 11g
Phosphorus: 24mg

PREP TIME
5 min

COOK TIME
0 min

SERVING
4 people

DIRECTIONS

1. Mix all the ingredients in a bowl.
2. Serve with dressing

INGREDIENTS

- 1 tbsp. of dried dill
- 1 onion
- ¼ cup of water
- 1 cup of vinegar
- 3 cucumbers
- ¾ cup of white sugar

81. Thai Cucumber Salad

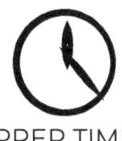

PREP TIME
5 min

COOK TIME
5 min

SERVING
2 people

NUTRITION

Calories: 20

Fat: 0g

Sodium: 85mg

Carbs: 5g

Protein: 1g

Potassium: 190.4mg

Phosphorus: 46.8mg

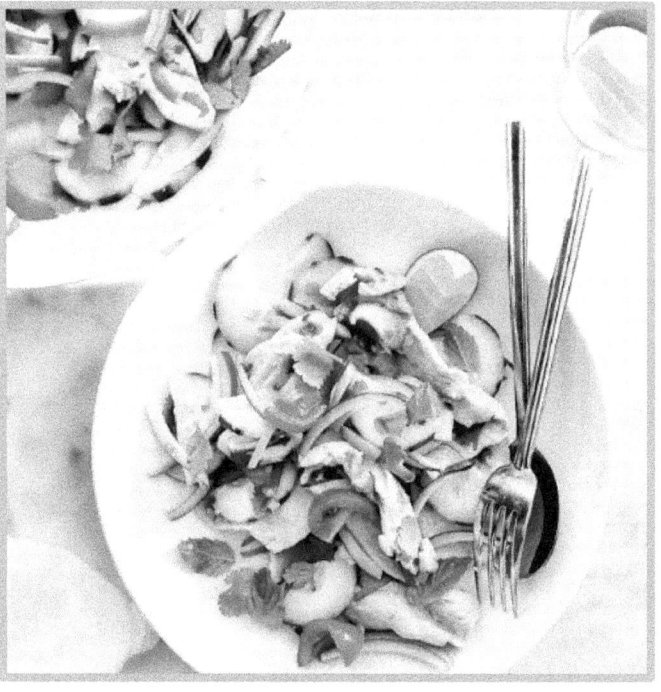

INGREDIENTS

- ¼ cup chopped peanuts
- ¼ cup white sugar
- ½ cup cilantro
- ¼ cup rice wine vinegar
- 3 cucumbers
- 2 jalapeno peppers

DIRECTIONS

1. Mix all the ingredients in a bowl.
2. Serve with dressing

82. Red Potato Salad

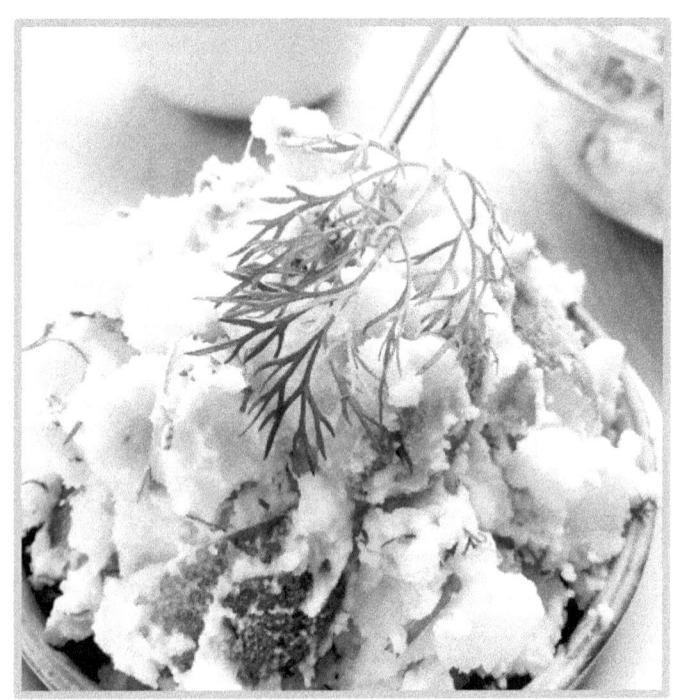

NUTRITION

Calories: 280
Fat: 20.0g
Sodium: 180.0mg
Potassium: 0.0mg
Carbs: 26.0g
Protein: 2.0g
Phosphorus: 130mg

PREP TIME
5 min

COOK TIME
5 min

SERVING
2 people

DIRECTIONS

1. In a pot, add water, potatoes, and cook until tender.
2. Remove, drain, and set aside.
3. Place eggs in a saucepan, add water and bring to a boil.
4. Cover and let eggs stand for 10–15 minutes.
5. When ready, remove, meanwhile in a deep skillet, cook bacon on low heat.
6. Mix all the ingredients in a bowl.
7. Serve with dressing.

INGREDIENTS

- 2 cups of mayonnaise
- 1 lb. of bacon
- 1 stalk celery
- 4 eggs
- Pepper
- 2 lbs. of red potatoes
- 1 onion

83. Broccoli-Cauliflower Salad

PREP TIME
5 min

COOK TIME
5 min

SERVING
4 people

NUTRITION

Calories: 89.8
Fat: 4.5g
Sodium: 51.2mg
Potassium: 257.6mg
Carbs: 11.5g
Protein: 3.0g
Phosphorus: 47mg

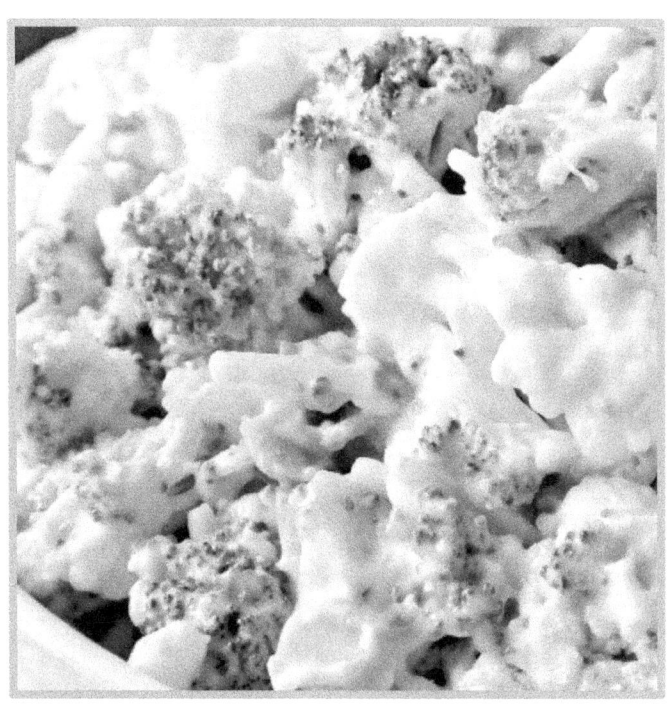

INGREDIENTS

- 1 tbsp. of wine vinegar
- 1 cup of cauliflower florets
- ¼ cup of white sugar
- 2 cups of hard-cooked eggs
- 5 slices of bacon
- 1 cup of broccoli florets
- 1 cup of cheddar cheese
- 1 cup of mayonnaise

DIRECTIONS

1. Boil the cauliflower florets for 5 minutes.
2. Mix all the ingredients in a bowl.
3. Serve with dressing.

84. Macaroni Salad

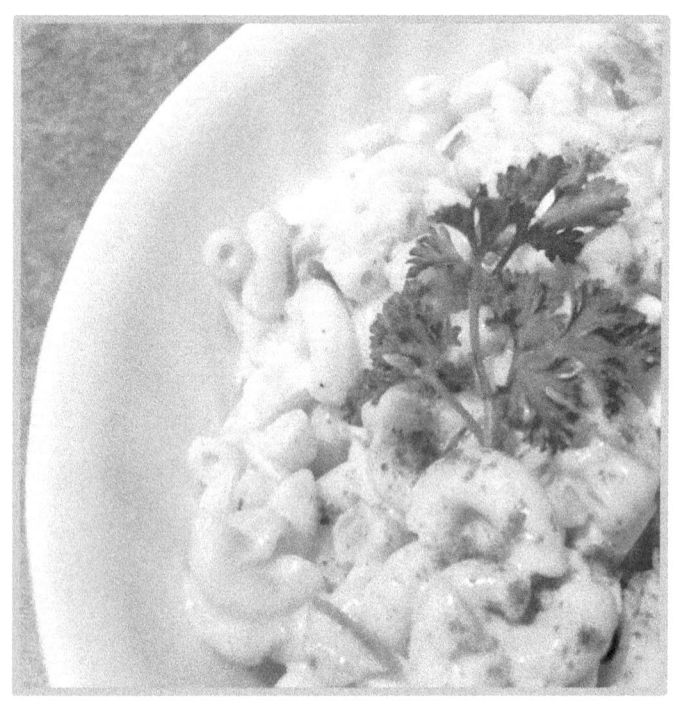

NUTRITION

Calories: 360
Fat: 21g
Sodium: 400mg
Carbs: 36g
Protein: 6g
Potassium: 68mg
Phosphorus: 36mg

PREP TIME
5 min

COOK TIME
0 min

SERVING
4 people

DIRECTIONS

1. Mix all the ingredients in a bowl.
2. Serve with dressing.

INGREDIENTS

- ¼ tsp. of celery seed
- 2 hard-boiled eggs
- 2 cups of salad dressing
- 1 onion
- 2 tsps. of white vinegar
- 2 stalks of celery
- 2 cups of cooked macaroni
- 1 red bell pepper
- 2 tbsps. of mustard

85. Green Bean and Potato Salad

PREP TIME
5 min

COOK TIME
5 min

SERVING
4 people

NUTRITION

Calories: 153.2

Fat: 2.0g

Sodium: 77.6mg

Potassium: 759.0mg

Carbs: 29.0g

Protein: 6.9g

Phosphorus: 49mg

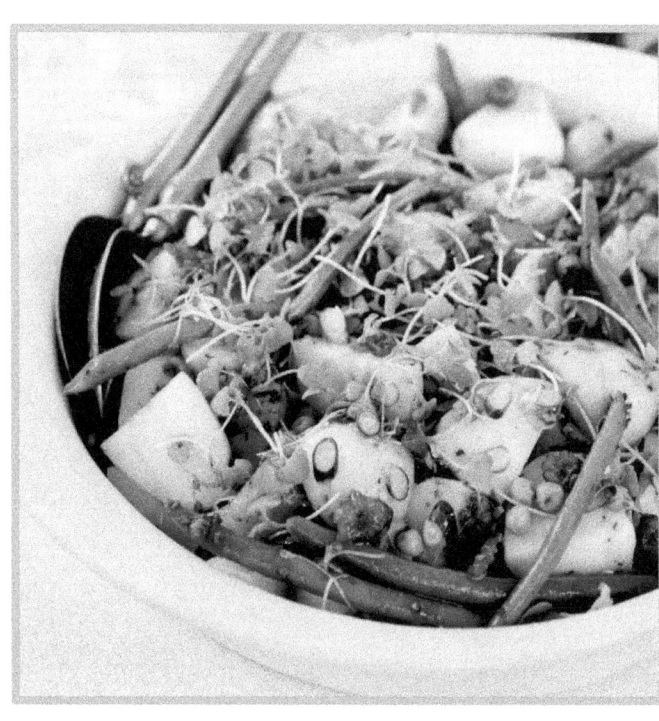

INGREDIENTS

- ½ cup of basil
- ¼ cup of olive oil
- 1 tbsp. of mustard
- ¾ lb. of green beans
- 1 tbsp. of lemon juice
- ½ cup of balsamic vinegar
- 1 red onion
- 1 lb. of red potatoes
- 1 garlic clove

DIRECTIONS

1. Boil potatoes using a pot for 15–18 minutes or until tender.
2. Throw in the green beans after 5–6 minutes.
3. Drain and cut into cubes.
4. In a bowl, add all ingredients and mix well.
5. Serve with dressing.

86. Eggplant Salad

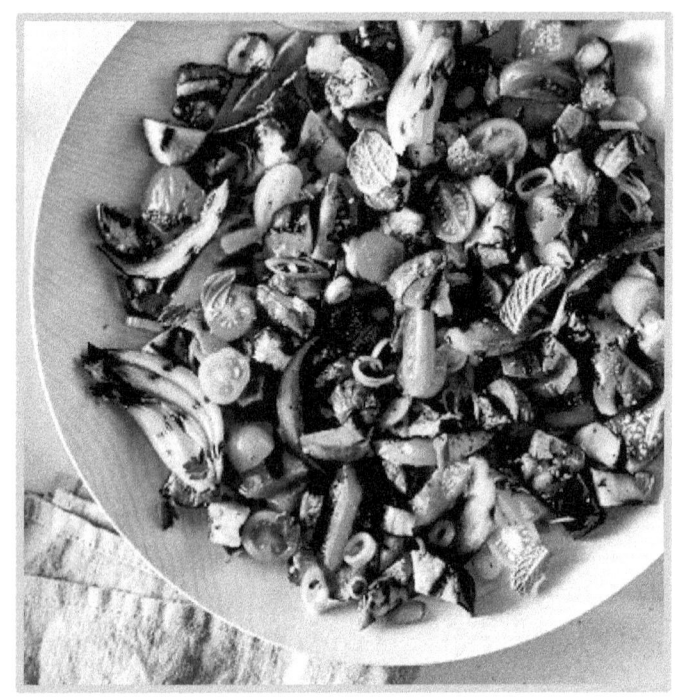

NUTRITION

Calories: 196
Fat: 108.g
Carbohydrates: 13.4g
Protein: 14.6g

PREP TIME
10 min

COOK TIME
30 min

SERVING
3 people

DIRECTIONS

1. Preheat your oven to 480°F.
2. Take a baking pan and add the eggplants and black pepper.
3. Bake for about 30 minutes.
4. Flip the vegetables after 20 minutes.
5. Then, take a bowl and add baked vegetables and all the remaining ingredients.
6. Mix well.
7. Serve and enjoy!

INGREDIENTS

- 2 eggplants, peeled and sliced
- 2 garlic cloves
- 2 green bell paper, sliced, seeds removed
- ½ cup of fresh parsley
- ½ cup of egg-free mayonnaise
- Salt and black pepper

87. Spinach Salad with Orange Vinaigrette

PREP TIME
5 min

COOK TIME
0 min

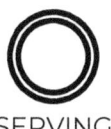
SERVING
4 people

NUTRITION

Calories: 73
Total fat: 4g
Saturated fat: 1g
Cholesterol: 0mg
Carbohydrates: 10g
Fiber: 2g
Protein: 2g
Phosphorus 33mg
Potassium: 353mg
Sodium: 35mg
Kidney Disease Stage 3

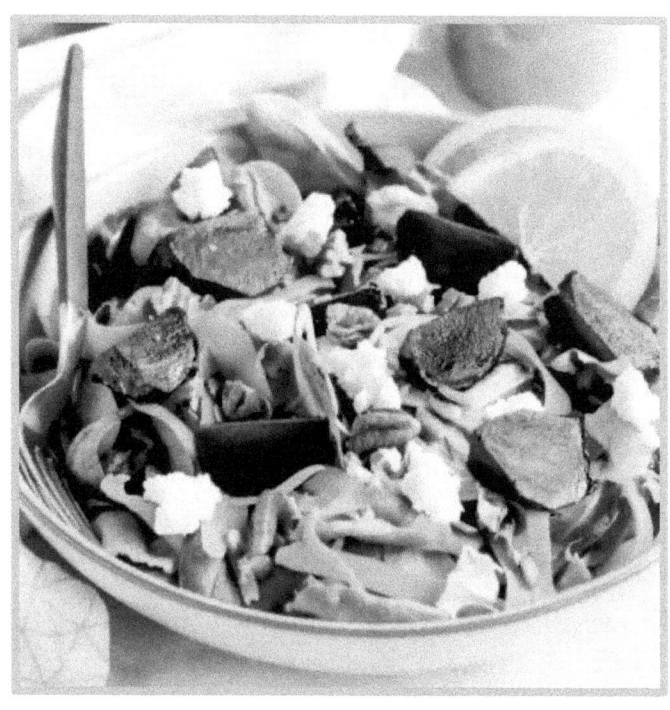

INGREDIENTS

- Zest and juice of 1 mandarin orange
- 1 tablespoon of extra-virgin olive oil
- Freshly ground black pepper
- 6 ounces of baby spinach
- 2 mandarin oranges, peeled, membranes removed

DIRECTIONS

1. In a small bowl, whisk the orange zest, orange juice, and olive oil. Season with pepper.
2. In a medium bowl, toss the spinach and pieces of orange. Drizzle the dressing over the salad, and toss to coat.
3. Serve.

Substitution tip: To make a heartier and stand-alone salad as a meal, add 1 cup of diced avocado. This will increase the fat content to 9g, the phosphorus to 53mg, and the potassium to 535mg.

88. Mixed Green Leaf and Citrus Salad

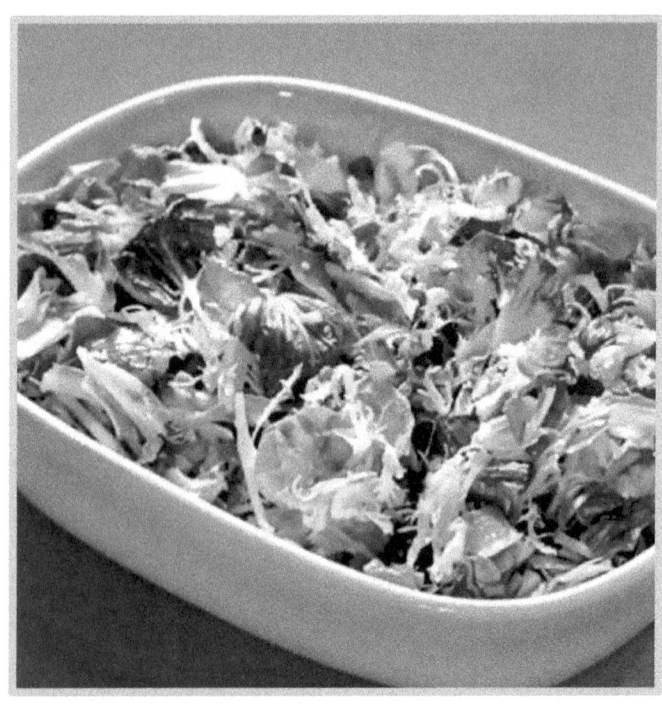

NUTRITION

Calories: 142
Total fat: 9g
Saturated fat: 1g
Cholesterol: 0mg
Carbohydrates: 15g
Fiber: 2g
Protein: 3g
Phosphorus 116mg
Potassium: 219mg
Sodium: 137mg
Kidney Disease Stage 4

PREP TIME
10 min

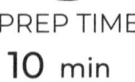

COOK TIME
0 min

SERVING
4 people

DIRECTIONS

1. In a large bowl, toss the greens, pepitas, lemon juice, and olive oil. Season with pepper.
2. Arrange the greens on four plates, and top each with 2 slices of orange and lemon.
3. Add 1 tablespoon each of cranberries and Kalamata olives to each plate.
4. Serve.

Ingredient tip: Toasted pepitas are delicious in this salad. To toast them, Preheat the oven to 25°F. Toss the pepitas with ½ teaspoon of olive oil, then spread them on a baking sheet. Roast for about 15 minutes, until golden. Let cool before adding to the salad.

Substitution tip: Use any combination of citrus in this salad for different effects. Sliced grapefruit, limes, and different types of oranges can all be used based on your preference.

INGREDIENTS

- 4 cups of mixed salad greens
- ¼ cup of pepitas
- Juice of 1 lemon
- 2 teaspoons of extra-virgin olive oil
- Freshly ground black pepper
- 1 orange, peeled and thinly sliced
- ½ lemon, peeled and thinly sliced
- 4 tablespoons of (¼ cup) dried cranberries
- 4 tablespoons of (¼ cup) pitted Kalamata olives

89. Roasted Beet Salad

PREP TIME
10 min

COOK TIME
30 min

SERVING
4 people

NUTRITION

Calories: 170
Total fat: 9g
Saturated fat: 2g
Cholesterol: 4mg
Carbohydrates: 20g
Fiber: 5g
Protein: 4g
Phosphorus 93mg
Potassium: 585mg
Sodium: 217mg
Kidney Disease Stage 3

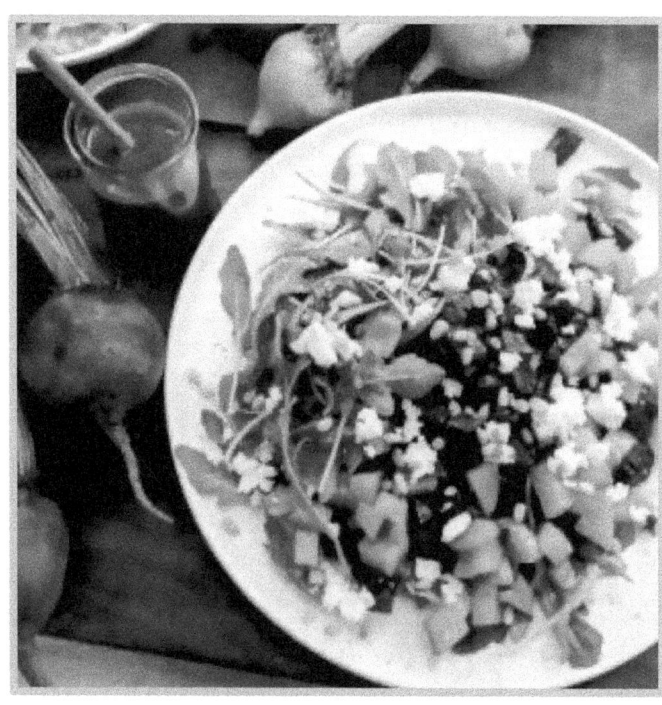

INGREDIENTS

- 8 small beets, trimmed
- 2 tablespoons of plus 1 teaspoon extra-virgin olive oil, divided
- 1 tablespoon of white wine vinegar
- 1 teaspoon of Dijon mustard
- Freshly ground black pepper
- 4 cups of baby salad greens
- ½ sweet onion, sliced
- 2 tablespoons of crumbled feta cheese
- 2 tablespoons of walnut pieces

DIRECTIONS

1. Preheat the oven to 400°F.
2. Toss the beets with 1 teaspoon of olive oil, wrap them in aluminum foil, and cook for 30 minutes, until fork-tender.
3. In a small bowl, whisk the remaining 2 tablespoons of olive oil, vinegar, and mustard—season with pepper.
4. In a medium bowl, mix the salad greens, onion, feta cheese, and walnuts. Toss with about half of the vinaigrette. Arrange on four plates.
5. Slice the beets into wedges and top the salads. Serve with the remaining dressing.

Cooking tip: To make this salad in advance, just assemble the salad greens, onion, feta, and walnuts in a bowl—hold off on tossing it with the vinaigrette until ready to serve, to prevent wilting. Store refrigerated up to three days before serving.

90. Appealing Green Salad

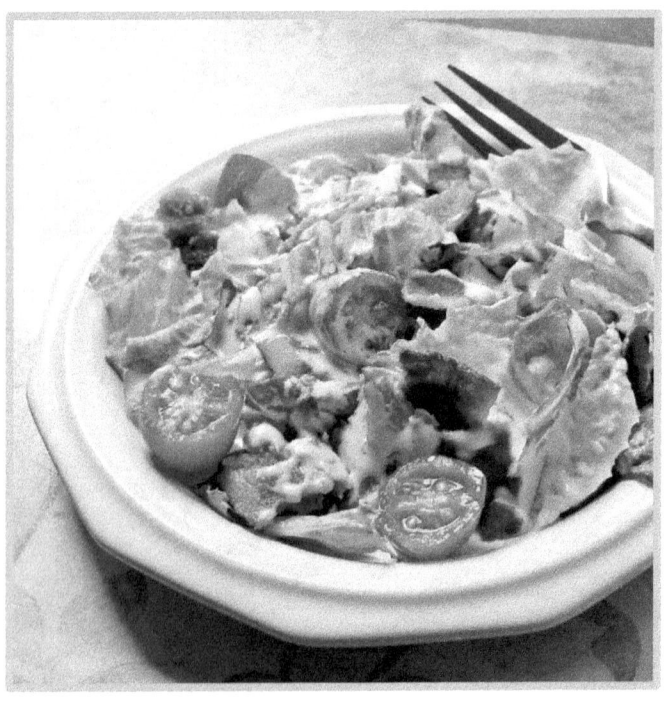

NUTRITION

Calories: 179
Fat: 17.1g
Carbs: 7.5g
Protein: 1.7g
Fiber: 1.9g
Potassium: 249mg
Sodium: 21mg

PREP TIME
10 min

COOK TIME
0 min

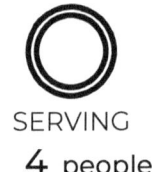

SERVING
4 people

DIRECTIONS

1. In a bowl, add all dressing ingredients and beat till well combined. Keep aside.
2. In another large bowl, mix all salad ingredients.
3. Add dressing and gently toss to coat well.
4. Serve immediately.

INGREDIENTS

For Dressing:
- 1 tbsp. of shallot, minced
- 1/3 cup of olive oil
- 2 tbsp. of fresh lemon juice
- 1 tsp. of honey
- Freshly ground black pepper, to taste

For Salad:
- 1½ cups of chopped broccoli florets
- 1½ cups of shredded cabbage
- 4 cups of chopped lettuce

91. Mango with Avocado Salad

NUTRITION

PREP TIME 10 min

COOK TIME 0 min

SERVING 4 people

Calories: 259.3
Carbohydrates: 19.59g
Proteins: 4.15g
Fiber: 5.77g
Fat: 16.98g

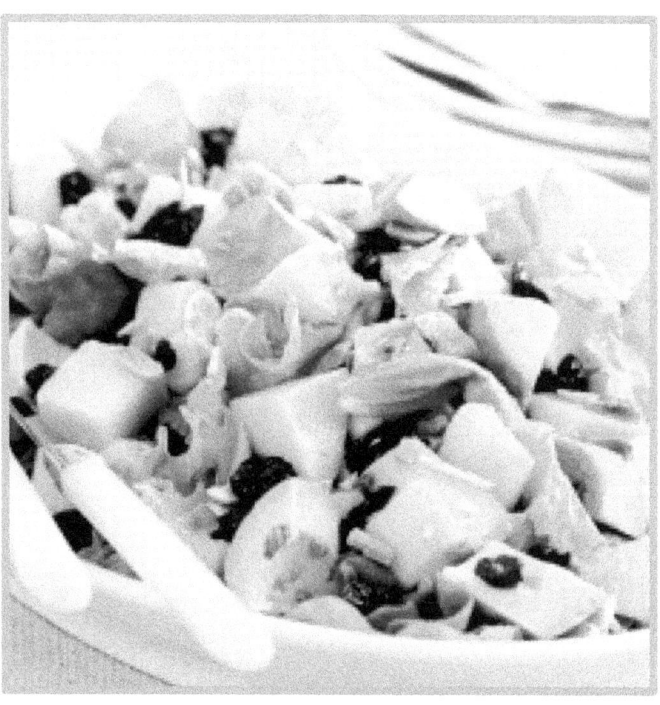

INGREDIENTS

- 1 chopped Lettuce
- 1 pinch of Pepper
- 1 Avocado
- 1 Mango
- 1 tablespoon of White wine vinegar
- 1 tablespoon of olive oil
- 2 tablespoon of chopped toasted almonds
- 2 tablespoon of dried cranberries

DIRECTIONS

1. Peel and chop the vegetables.
2. Put the lettuce, mango, avocado, almonds, and cranberries in a bowl.
3. On the other hand, mix the oil with the vinegar and add pepper.
4. Pour over the salad and mix.
5. Serve on plates and enjoy.

92. Avocado and Lettuce Salad

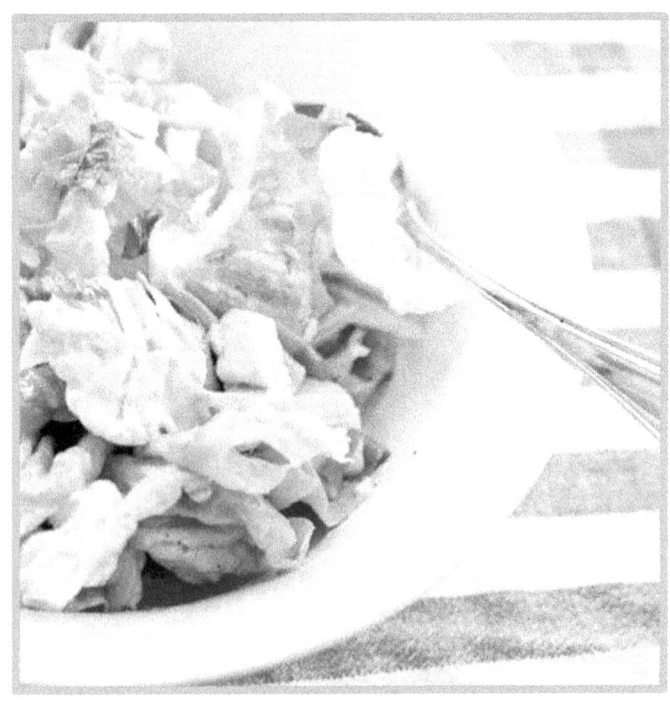

NUTRITION

Calories: 315.53

Carbohydrates: 10.8g

Proteins: 6.55g

Fiber: 7.55g

Fat: 25.88g

PREP TIME

10 min

COOK TIME

0 min

SERVING

2 people

DIRECTIONS

1. Wash the lettuce well and chop it.
2. Wash and chop the remaining ingredients such as the Tomato, red pepper or diced julienne, Avocado, Nuez chopped, Modena balsamic vinegar.
3. Mix the lemon juice, vinegar, virgin oil, and pepper. Then toss on the salad.
4. Remove and add the nuts (optional) to garnish.

INGREDIENTS

- 1 tomato
- 1 lettuce
- ½ red pepper, diced julienne
- 1 pinch of Pepper
- 1 Avocado
- 2 tablespoon of Nuez chopped (walnut crepes)
- 2 tablespoon of Modena balsamic vinegar
- 2 tablespoon of lemon juice
- 1 pinch of extra virgin olive oil

93. Rocket Salad with Mango, Avocado, and Cherry Tomatoes

PREP TIME
10 min

COOK TIME
0 min

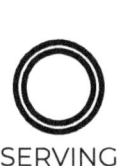
SERVING
2 people

NUTRITION

Calories: 306

Protein: 16.0g

Fiber: 6.8g

Sugar: 5.0g

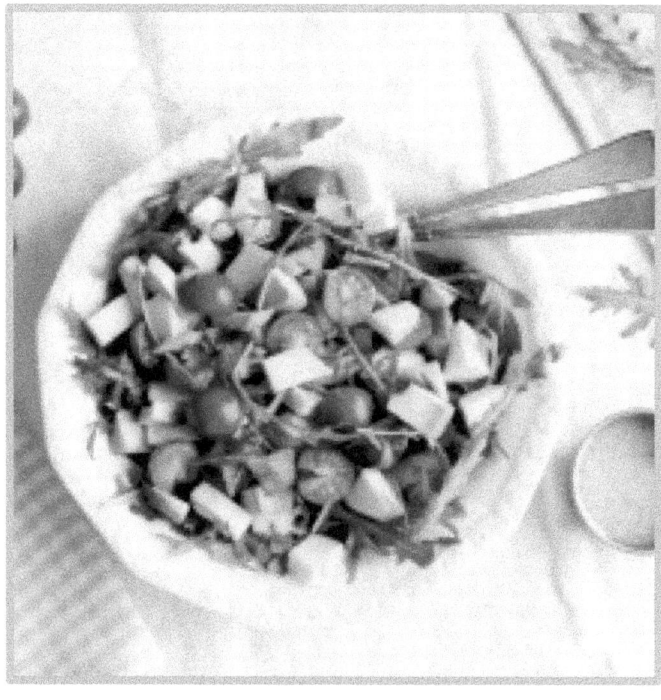

INGREDIENTS

- 1 tbsp. of lime juice
- 2 tbsps. of white balsamic vinegar
- 2 tbsps. of rapeseed oil
- 2 tbsps. of olive oil
- 1 tsp. of honey
- 1 tsp. of medium-hot mustard
- Pepper
- 3 handful of rocket (120g)
- 200g of cherry tomatoes
- 1 ripe mango
- 2 avocados

DIRECTIONS

1. For the vinaigrette, whip lime juice with balsamic vinegar, rapeseed, and olive oils.
2. Whisk in honey and mustard and then season with pepper.
3. Wash the rocket and spin dry.
4. Wash tomatoes and halve.
5. Peel the mango, slice the pulp from the core, and dice it.
6. Halve the avocados, core them, remove the pulp from the skin and dice them as well.
7. Add cherry tomatoes, ripe mango, avocados—all the salad ingredients inside a bowl with the vinaigrette, and spread on four plates.

94. Chickpea Salad

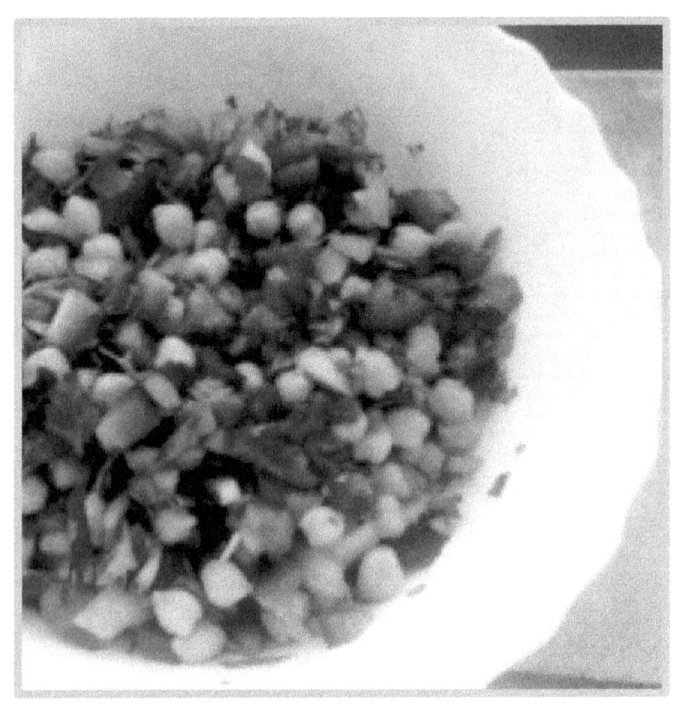

NUTRITION

Calories: 511.42
Carbohydrates: 37.33g
Proteins: 16.66g
Fiber: 11.54g
Fat: 31.84g

PREP TIME
5 min

COOK TIME
10 min

SERVING
2 people

DIRECTIONS

1. Chop the all the red peppers, Green pepper, onion, and parsley and mix them with the chickpeas.
2. In a separate bowl, mix an abundant stream of oil, another stream of vinegar, lemon juice, a teaspoon of paprika (sweet), a pinch of pepper, a clove of garlic, chopped into small pieces, and a little salt (optional).
3. Add the canned Garbanzo
4. Then add the dressing to the vegetables.

INGREDIENTS

- 1 garlic (one clove)
- 1 unit of chickpeas
- 1 onion, medium
- 1 red pepper
- Pinch of paprika
- Pinch of pepper
- Parsley (one bunch)
- 1 pinch of salt (optional)
- 1 glass of vinegar
- 1 glass of olive oil
- 1 unit (s) of green pepper
- 400 grams of canned garbanzo
- 1 tablespoon of lemon juice

95. Bulgur and Broccoli Salad

PREP TIME
10 min

COOK TIME
15 min

SERVING
4 people

NUTRITION

Calories: 156

Fat: 6g

Carbs: 24g

Protein: 6g

Phosphorus: 101mg

Potassium: 315mg

Sodium: 21mg

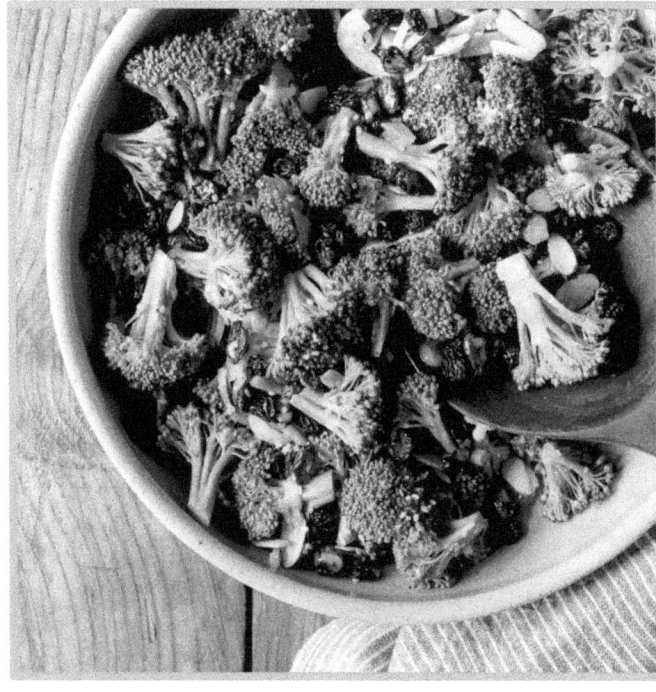

INGREDIENTS

- 3 cups of broccoli florets
- 1 cup of bulgur
- ½ cup of halved cherry tomatoes
- ¼ cup of raw sunflower seeds
- ¼ cup of chopped mint leaves
- Juice of 1 lemon
- 1 tablespoon of extra-virgin olive oil

DIRECTIONS

1. In a medium bowl, prepare an ice-water bath by filling the bowl with ice and water.
2. Set a pot of water on to boil. Add the broccoli and blanch for 3 minutes.
3. With a slotted spoon, remove the broccoli and transfer it to the ice bath, retaining the cooking water over the heat.
4. Once cool, after about 3 minutes, drain the ice and water. Set the broccoli aside.
5. Add the bulgur to the hot water, remove from the heat, cover, and let sit for 15 minutes.
6. Drain, pressing the bulgur with the back of a spoon to remove excess moisture.
7. In a medium bowl, toss the broccoli, bulgur, tomatoes, sunflower seeds, mint, lemon juice, and olive oil.
8. Serve immediately.

96. Pear and Watercress Salad

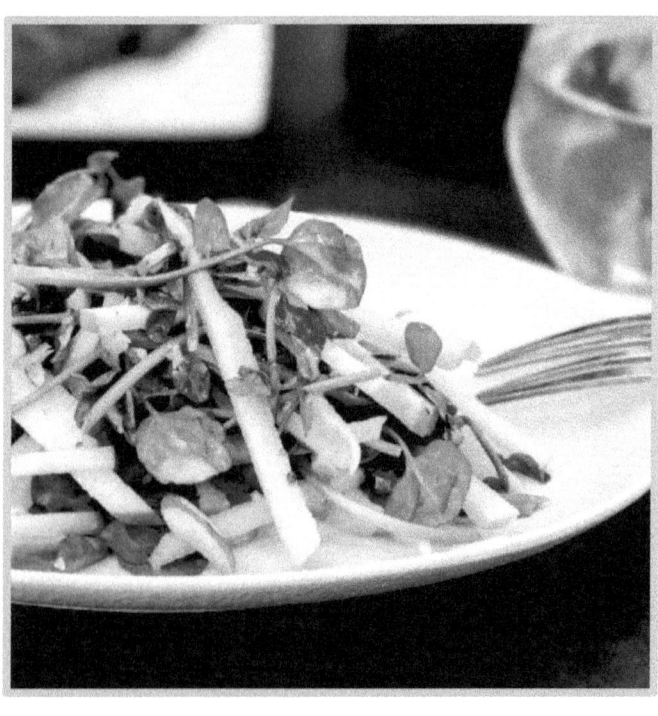

NUTRITION

Calories: 144
Fat: 8g
Carbs: 17g
Protein: 3g
Phosphorus: 70mg
Potassium: 310mg
Sodium: 134mg

PREP TIME
10 min

COOK TIME
0 min

SERVING
4 people

DIRECTIONS

1. In a food processor or blender, combine the onion, mustard, olive oil, vinegar, and honey.
2. Process until smooth.
3. In a medium bowl, toss the watercress with the dressing.
4. Arrange on four plates.
5. Top each with pear slices and crumbled feta cheese.

INGREDIENTS

- ¼ cup of sweet onion, coarsely chopped
- 1 teaspoon of Dijon mustard
- 2 tablespoons of extra-virgin olive oil
- 1 tablespoon of white wine vinegar
- 1 teaspoon of honey
- 1 bunch of watercress, thick stems removed, washed well
- 2 ripe pears, cored and cut into wedges
- 1 ounce of crumbled feta cheese

97. Tropical Chicken Salad

PREP TIME
20 min

COOK TIME
0 min

SERVING
4 people

NUTRITION

Calories: 443.8

Protein: 33.1g

Sodium: 245.5mg

Phosphorus: 30.2mg

Potassium: 563.5mg

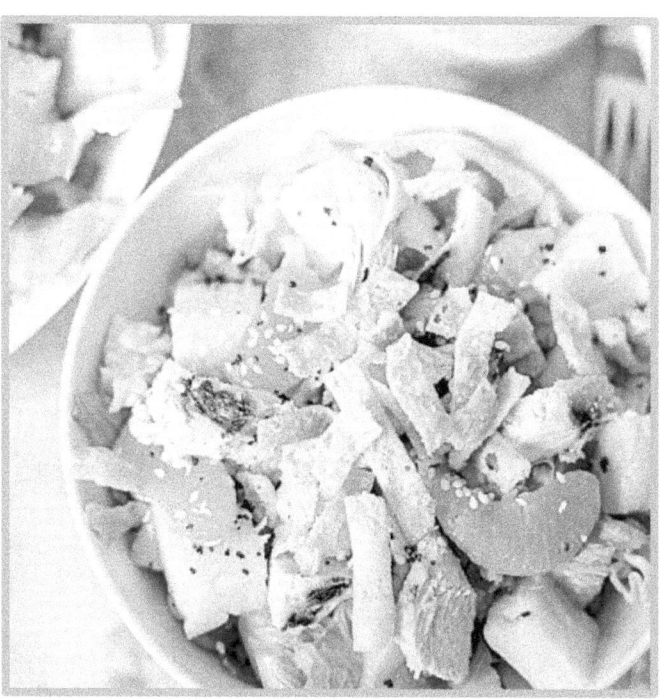

INGREDIENTS

- 1/2 cup of diced celery
- 1 1/2 cup of shredded cooked chicken
- 1 cup of peeled and diced apples
- 1 cup of drained unsweetened pineapple chunks
- 1/2 cup of seedless grapes
- 1 cup of diced pears
- 1/2 tsp. of sugar
- 2 tbsp. of lemon juice
- 1/2 cup of mayonnaise
- Dash hot sauce
- 1 tsp. of pepper
- Paprika for garnish

DIRECTIONS

1. Mix sugar, juice, mayo, hot sauce, and pepper.
2. In a large bowl, mix together the rest of the ingredients.
3. Add dressing to fruit and chicken and combine well.
4. Serve on a bed of lettuce and sprinkle with paprika.

98. Chicken and Grape Salad

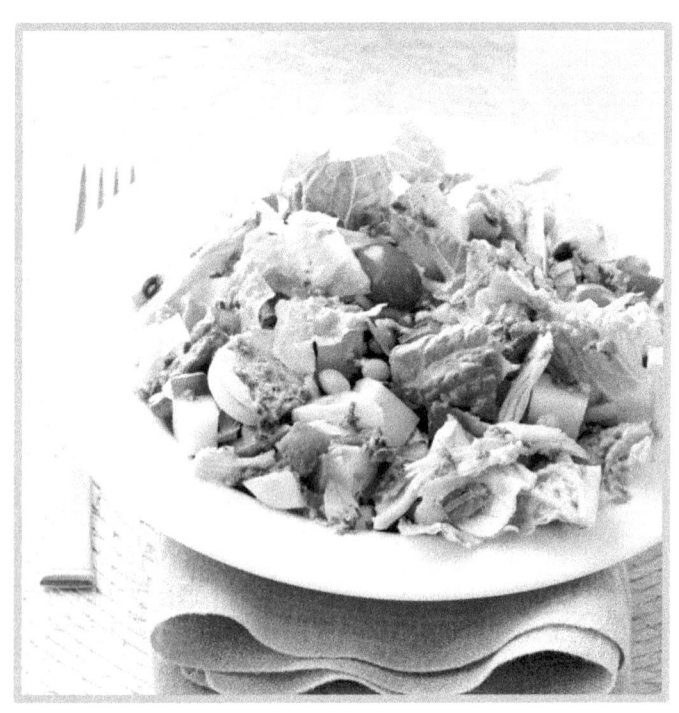

NUTRITION

Calories: 290.7

Protein: 8.3g

Sodium: 112.3mg

Phosphorus: 7.1mg

Potassium: 91.8mg

PREP TIME
20 min

COOK TIME
0 min

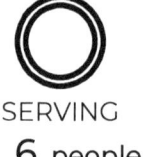

SERVING
6 people

DIRECTIONS

1. Combine dressing ingredients in a large bowl and mix well.
2. Add cooked pasta and mix well.
3. Add grapes and apples and mix well.
4. Transfer to serving plates and top with sliced chicken.

INGREDIENTS

- 1 diced apple
- 1 lb. of rotelle pasta cooked (according to package directions)
- 1/2 cup of seedless grapes
- 1 cup of sliced cooked chicken

Dressing:

- 1/2 cup of mayonnaise
- 2 tbsp. of sriracha hot sauce
- 1/4 cup of light sour cream

99. Fresh Berry Salad

PREP TIME
15 min

COOK TIME
0 min

SERVING
4 people

NUTRITION

Calories: 142.4

Protein: 1.0g

Sodium: 51.5mg

Phosphorus: 3.7mg

Potassium: 394.0mg

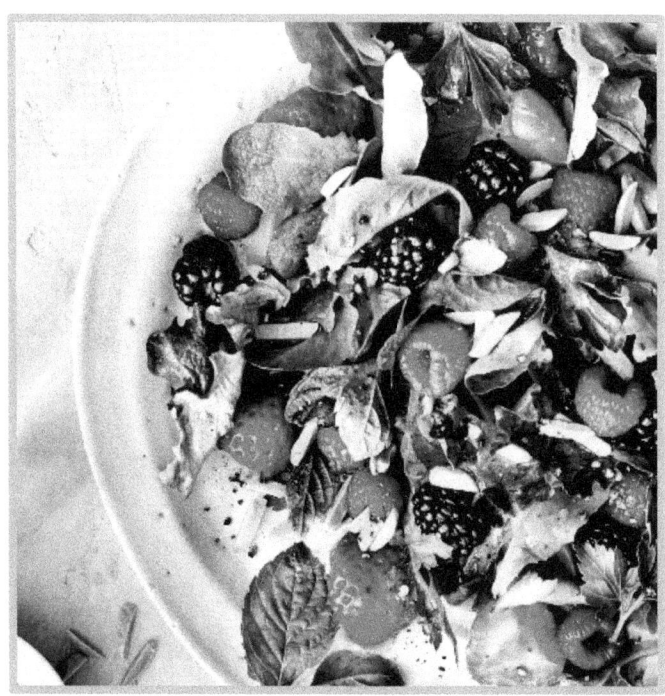

INGREDIENTS

- 3 tbsp. of balsamic vinegar
- 2 tbsp. of honey
- Dash of ground cardamom
- Ground pepper
- 1 lb. of hulled and quartered strawberries
- 1 pint of blueberries
- 1 sprig mint leaves roughly torn

DIRECTIONS

1. Whisk together in a large bowl the vinegar, honey, pepper, and cardamom.
2. Tumble in the berries and mint leaves.

100. Cauliflower Mash

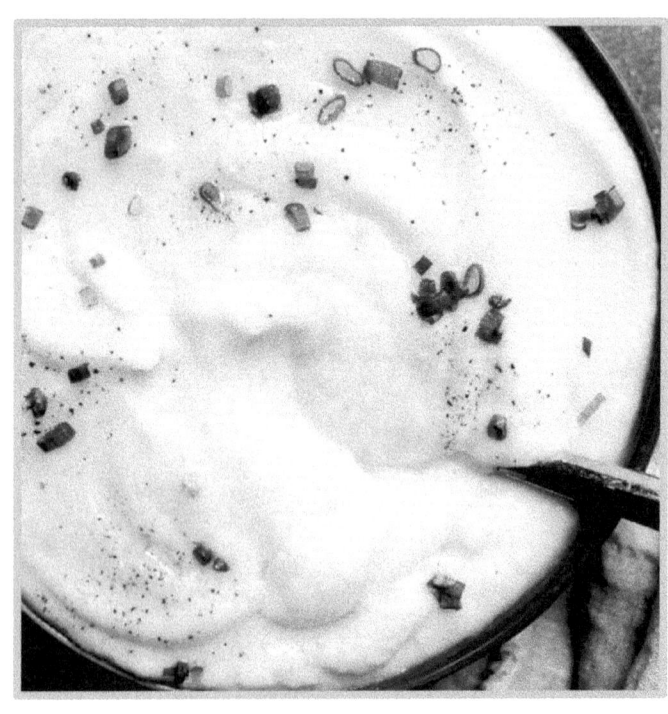

NUTRITION

Calories: 158.4

Protein: 5.2g

Sodium: 384.7mg

Phosphorus: 13.7mg

Potassium: 414.2mg

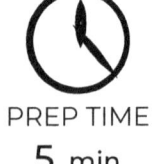

PREP TIME
5 min

COOK TIME
10 min

SERVING
4 people

DIRECTIONS

1. Cut potatoes into quarters.
2. Break apart cauliflower.
3. Add veggies to a large pot of boiling water.
4. Cook until veggies are tender, about 10 minutes.
5. Remove from heat, and drain.
6. Add milk, butter, and pepper.
7. With an immersion blender, cream veggies.
8. Serve hot.

INGREDIENTS

- 2 cups of "leached" potatoes
- 2 cups of cauliflower florets
- 2 tbsp. of softened butter
- 3/4 cup of tepid milk
- 1 tsp. of ground black pepper

101. Asian Cucumber Salad

PREP TIME 15 min

COOK TIME 0 min

SERVING 4 people

NUTRITION

Calories: 34.0

Protein: 0.9g

Sodium: 50.0mg

Phosphorus: 28.3mg

Potassium: 198.0mg

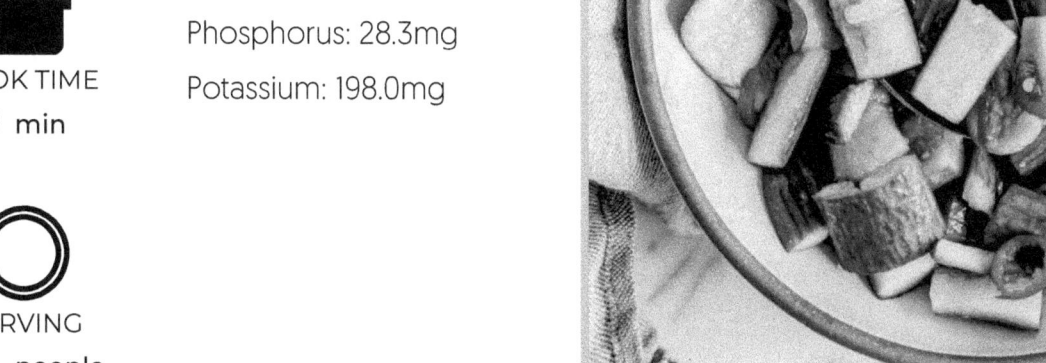

INGREDIENTS

- 2 sliced banana peppers
- 1/2 cup of diced radishes
- 4 tsp. of red diced onion
- 4 tsp. of mirin
- 1 tsp. of sesame oil
- 1/2 tsp. of fresh ginger minced
- 2 tsp. of rice wine vinegar
- 4 cups of cucumbers partially peeled cut into thin slices
- 1 green onion sliced thin
- 1 tsp. of pepper

DIRECTIONS

1. In a large bowl, toss together peppers, radishes, and red onions.
2. In a separate bowl, whisk together Mirin, sesame oil, ginger, vinegar, and pepper.
3. Pour dressing over cucumber medley and refrigerate for 2 hours or overnight.
4. Serve with a sprinkling of green onions.

102. Garden Fresh Salad

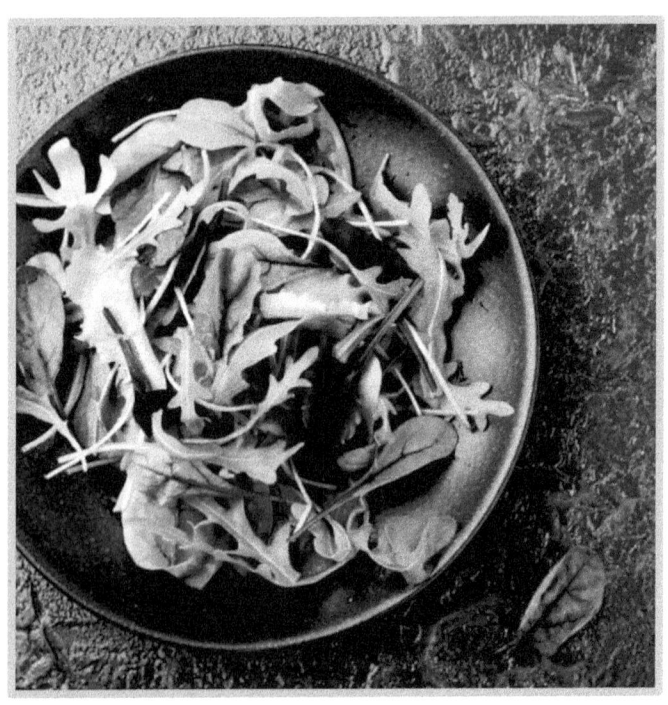

NUTRITION

Calories: 71
Fat: 17.1g
Carbs: 7.2g
Protein: 1.1g
Fiber: 2.2g
Potassium: 247mg
Sodium: 63mg

PREP TIME
15 min

COOK TIME
0 min

SERVING
6 people

DIRECTIONS

1. In a large serving bowl, add all salad ingredients
2. In another bowl, all dressing ingredients and mix till well combined.
3. Pour dressing over salad and toss to coat well.
4. Serve immediately.

INGREDIENTS

For Salad:
- 2 cups of peeled and shredded carrots
- 1½ cups of shredded green cabbage
- 1½ cups of shredded purple cabbage
- 1 cup of chopped cucumber
- 2 chopped large scallions
- ¼ cup of chopped fresh parsley leaves

For Dressing:
- 2 tbsp. of olive oil
- 2 tbsp. of fresh lemon juice
- 1 tsp. of finely grated fresh lemon zest
- Pinch of salt
- Freshly ground black pepper, to taste

103. Avocado Boats with Shrimp Salad and Crostinis

PREP TIME
25 min

COOK TIME
15 min

SERVING
4 people

NUTRITION

Calories: 250
Total Fat: 20.4g
Cholesterol: 75.9mg
Sodium: 411.7mg
Total Carbohydrate: 9.9g
Dietary Fiber: 6.9g
Sugars: 0.9g
Protein: 10g
Phosphorus: 29g

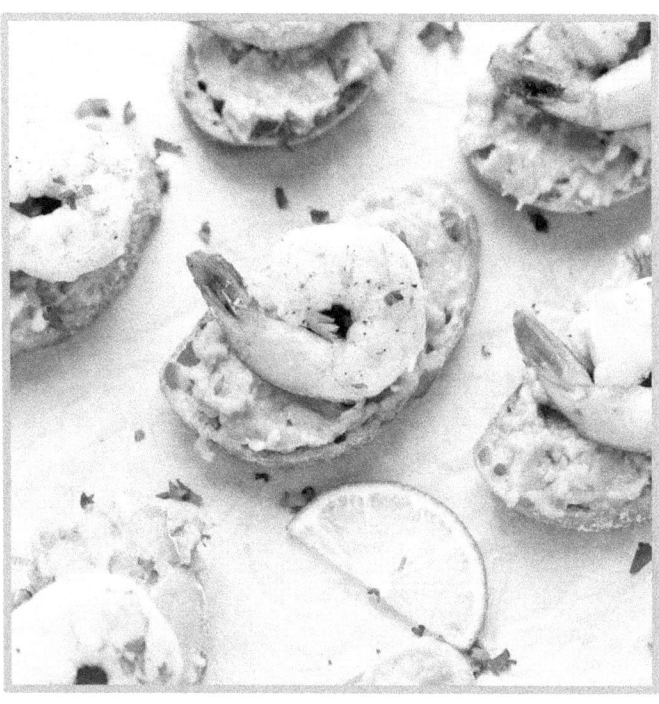

INGREDIENTS

- 2 ripe avocados
- 100g of shrimp
- 1/2 red onion—chopped
- 2 tbsp. of mayo
- 1 small apple—cubes
- 1/4 lemon juice
- A handful of fresh chives—finely sliced
- Few sprigs of fresh dill as a garnish

For the crostini:
- 1 pistoled—cut into 8 slices
- Dash of olive oil
- Clove of garlic

DIRECTIONS

1. Preheat the oven to 200° and rub the sandwiches with olive oil, garlic, and a pinch of salt. Roast them crispy in 10 to 15 minutes.
2. Halve the avocados and remove the seed. Try to halve them in equal parts so that you get nice boats. Cut the flesh into cubes with the convex side of a knife and spoon it out.
3. Mix the avocado with the shrimp, chives, lemon juice, mayo, apple, and red onion in a bowl. Taste for a moment and add a pinch of salt and pepper to taste.
4. Place the scooped boats on plates and fill them with shrimp salad. Finish with fresh dill and crostinis.

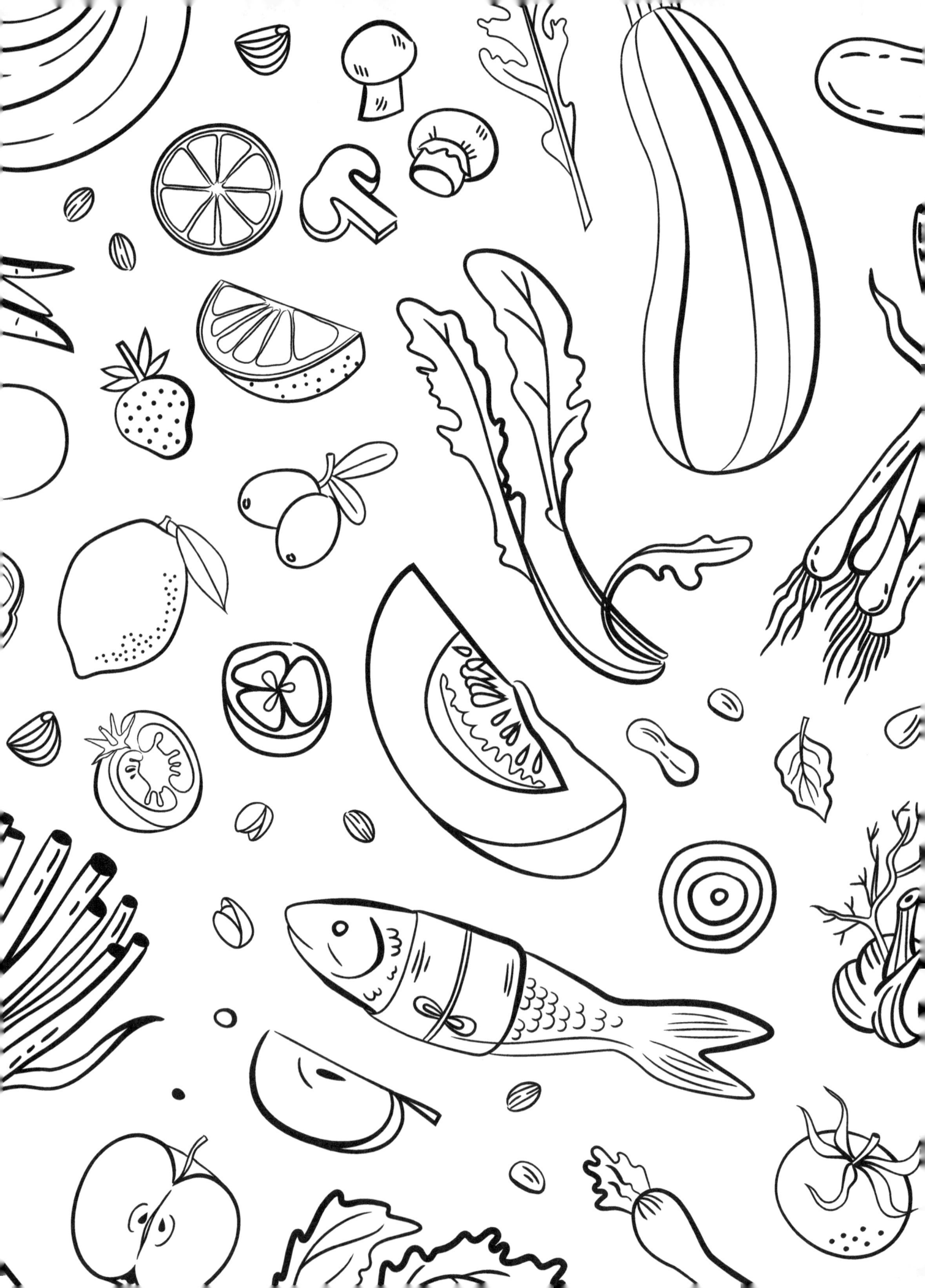

Chapter 11

VEGETABLES

104. Curried Veggie Stir-Fry

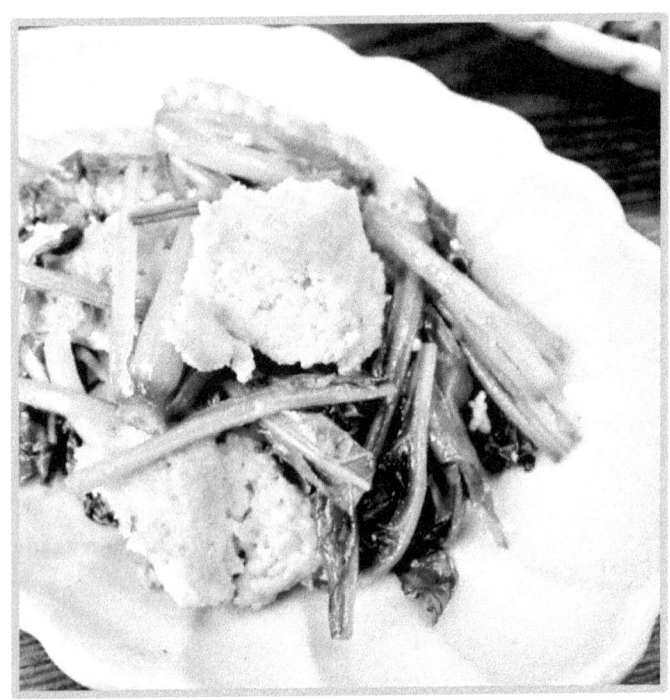

NUTRITION

Calories: 293
Total fat: 18g
Saturated fat: 10g
Sodium: 247mg
Phosphorus: 138mg
Potassium: 531mg
Carbohydrates: 28g
Fiber: 7g
Protein: 7g
Sugar: 4g

PREP TIME
20 min

COOK TIME
10 min

SERVING
6 people

DIRECTIONS

1. In a wok or non-stick, heat the olive oil over medium-high heat. Stir-fry the onion and garlic for 2 to 3 minutes, until fragrant.
2. Add the frozen stir-fry vegetables and continue to cook for 3 to 4 minutes longer, or until the vegetables are hot.
3. Meanwhile, in a small bowl, combine coconut milk, water, and curry paste. Stir until the paste dissolves.
4. Add the broth mixture to the wok and cook for another 2 to 3 minutes, or until the sauce has reduced slightly and all the vegetables are crisp-tender.
5. Serve over couscous or hot cooked rice.

Ingredient Tip: When you buy frozen stir-fry vegetables, make sure you purchase a variety that doesn't include seasonings or sauce, which would increase the sodium content. You could also use separate veggies; try a combination of broccoli with carrots or asparagus with zucchini.

INGREDIENTS

- 2 tablespoons of extra-virgin olive oil
- 1 onion, chopped
- 4 garlic cloves, minced
- 4 cups of frozen stir-fry vegetables
- 1 cup of canned unsweetened full-fat coconut milk
- 1 cup of water
- 2 tablespoons of green curry paste

105. Chilaquiles

PREP TIME
20 min

COOK TIME
20 min

SERVING
4 people

NUTRITION

Calories: 312

Total fat: 20g

Saturated fat: 8g

Sodium: 345mg

Phosphorus: 280mg

Potassium: 453mg

Carbohydrates: 19g

Fiber: 3g

Protein: 15g

Sugar: 5g

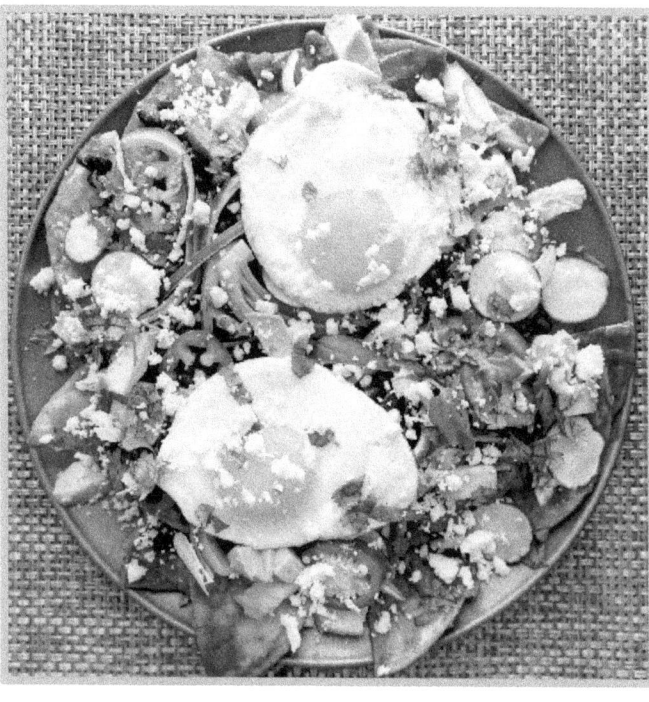

INGREDIENTS

- 3 (8-inch) corn tortillas, cut into strips
- 2 tablespoons of extra-virgin olive oil
- 12 tomatillos, papery covering removed, chopped
- 3 tablespoons fof reshly squeezed lime juice
- ⅛ teaspoon of salt
- ⅛ teaspoon of freshly ground black pepper
- 4 large egg whites
- 2 large eggs
- 2 tablespoons of water
- 1 cup of shredded pepper jack cheese

DIRECTIONS

1. In a dry nonstick skillet, toast the tortilla strips over medium heat until they are crisp, tossing the pan and stirring occasionally. This should take 4 to 6 minutes. Remove the strips from the pan and set aside.
2. In the same skillet, heat the olive oil over medium heat and add the tomatillos, lime juice, salt, and pepper. Cook and frequently stir for about 8 to 10 minutes until the tomatillos start to break down and form a sauce. Transfer the sauce to a bowl and set aside.
3. In a small bowl, beat the egg whites, eggs, and water and add to the skillet. Cook the eggs for 3 to 4 minutes, stirring occasionally until they are set and cooked to 160°F.
4. Preheat the oven to 400°F.
5. Toss the tortilla strips in the tomatillo sauce and place in a casserole dish. Top with the scrambled eggs and cheese.
6. Bake for 10 to 15 minutes, or until the cheese starts to brown. Serve.

106. Roasted Veggie Sandwiches

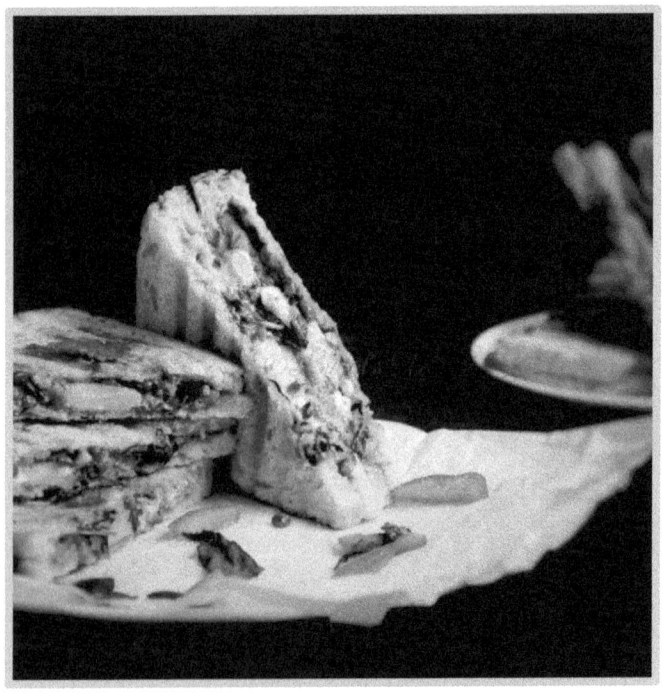

NUTRITION

Calories: 182
Total fat: 5g
Saturated fat: 1g
Sodium: 234mg
Phosphorus: 106mg
Potassium: 289mg
Carbohydrates: 31g
Fiber: 4g
Protein: 5g
Sugar: 6g

PREP TIME 20 min

COOK TIME 35 min

SERVING 6 people

DIRECTIONS

1. Preheat the oven to 400°F.
2. Prepare a parchment paper and line it in a rimmed baking sheet.
3. Spread the bell peppers, squash, and onion on the prepared baking sheet. Sprinkle with the olive oil, vinegar, salt, and pepper.
4. Roast for 30 to 40 minutes, turning the vegetables with a spatula once during cooking, until they are tender and light golden brown.
5. Pile the vegetables into the pita breads and serve.

Ingredient Tip: Pita breads are puffed rounds that have a natural pocket in the center that holds a filling. To prepare them, cut in half crosswise and gently separate the two halves, cutting the pocket if necessary. You can find pita breads in most supermarkets.

INGREDIENTS

- 3 bell peppers, assorted colors, sliced
- 1 cup of sliced yellow summer squash
- 1 red onion, sliced
- 2 tablespoons of extra-virgin olive oil
- 2 tablespoons of balsamic vinegar
- ⅛ teaspoon of salt
- ⅛ teaspoon of freshly ground black pepper
- 3 large whole-wheat pita breads, halved

107. Roasted Peach Open-Face Sandwich

PREP TIME
5 min

COOK TIME
15 min

SERVING
4 people

NUTRITION

Calories: 250
Total fat: 13g
Saturated fat: 6g
Sodium: 376mg
Phosphorus: 163mg
Potassium: 260mg
Carbohydrates: 28g
Fiber: 3g
Protein: 6g
Sugar: 8g

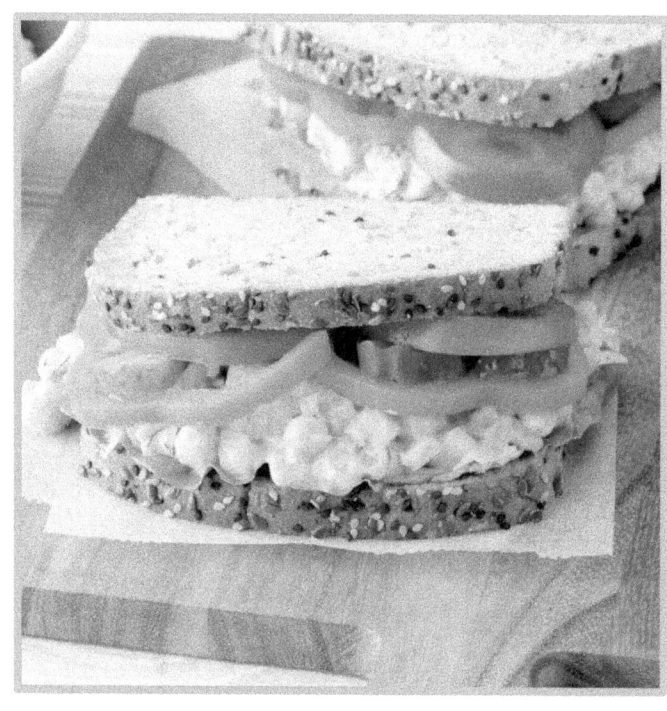

INGREDIENTS

- 2 fresh peaches, peeled and sliced
- 1 tablespoon of extra-virgin olive oil
- 1 tablespoon of freshly squeezed lemon juice
- ⅛ teaspoon of salt
- ⅛ teaspoon of freshly ground black pepper
- 4 ounces of cream cheese, at room temperature
- 2 teaspoons of fresh thyme leaves
- 4 whole-wheat sourdough bread slices

DIRECTIONS

1. Preheat the oven to 400°F.
2. Arrange the peaches on a rimmed baking sheet. Brush them with olive oil on both sides.
3. Roast the peaches for 10 to 15 minutes, until they are lightly golden brown around the edges. Sprinkle with lemon juice, salt, and pepper.
4. In a small bowl, combine the cream cheese and thyme and mix well.
5. Toast the bread. Get the toasted bread and spread it with the cream cheese mixture. Top with the peaches and serve.

108. Pasta Fagioli

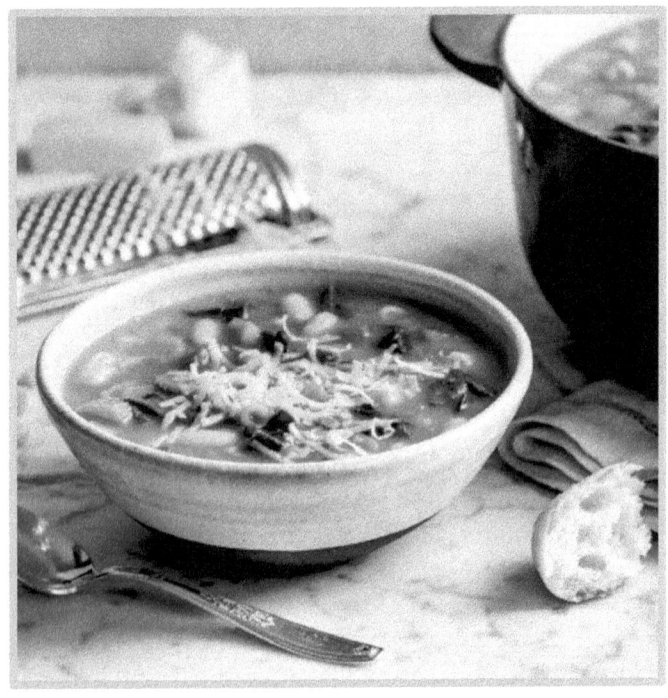

NUTRITION

Calories: 245
Total fat: 7g
Saturated fat: 2g
Sodium: 269mg
Phosphorus: 188mg
Potassium: 592mg
Carbohydrates: 36g
Fiber: 7g
Protein: 12g
Sugar: 4g

PREP TIME
25 min

COOK TIME
25 min

SERVING
6 people

DIRECTIONS

1. In a large saucepan, place the beans and cover with water. Bring to a boil over high heat and boil for 10 minutes. Drain the beans.
2. In a food processor or blender, combine ⅓ cup of beans and ⅓ cup of thawed peppers and onions. Process until smooth.
3. In the same saucepan, combine the pureed mixture, the remaining 1⅔ cups of peppers and onions, the remaining beans, the broth, and the salt and pepper and bring to a simmer.
4. Add the pasta to the saucepan. Make sure to stir it and bring it to boil, reduce the heat to low, and simmer for 8 to 10 minutes, or until the pasta is tender.
5. Serve drizzled with olive oil and topped with Parmesan cheese.

INGREDIENTS

- 1 (15-ounce) can low-sodium great northern beans, drained and rinsed, divided
- 2 cups frozen peppers and onions, thawed, divided
- 5 cups low-sodium vegetable broth
- ⅛ teaspoon salt
- ⅛ teaspoon freshly ground black pepper
- 1 cup whole-grain orecchiette pasta
- 2 tablespoons extra-virgin olive oil
- ⅓ cup grated Parmesan cheese

109. Spinach Alfredo Lasagna Rolls

PREP TIME
25 min

COOK TIME
50 min

SERVING
4 people

NUTRITION

Calories: 388

Total fat: 24g

Saturated fat: 7g

Sodium: 411mg

Phosphorus: 119mg

Potassium: 378mg

Carbohydrates: 34g

Fiber: 9g

Protein: 13g

Sugar: 5g

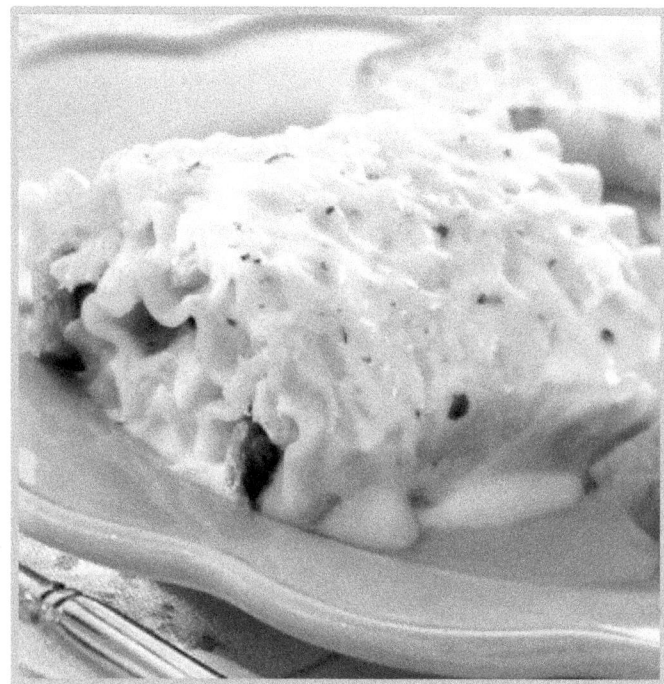

INGREDIENTS

- 4 whole-grain lasagna noodles
- 2 tablespoons of extra-virgin olive oil
- 1 large onion, chopped
- 2 cups of frozen whole-leaf spinach, thawed (measure while frozen)
- 1 (8-ounce) cream cheese, divided
- ⅓ cup of shredded Parmesan cheese

DIRECTIONS

1. Bring a large pot of water to a boil over high heat and add the lasagna noodles. Simmer for 8 to 9 minutes or until the pasta is almost al dente but still has a thin white line in the center. Drain, reserving ¼ cup of the pasta water, and set aside.
2. Meanwhile, in a saucepan, heat the olive oil over medium heat. Add the onions and cook for 6 to 8 minutes, stirring, until the onions are tender and starting to turn brown.
3. While the onions are cooking, drain the spinach and put the leaves into some paper towels. Squeeze well to remove most of the water from the spinach.
4. Add the spinach to the onions, stir, and turn off the heat. Add 6 ounces of cream cheese to the vegetables and stir until combined. Set aside.
5. In a small saucepan, combine the remaining 2 ounces of cream cheese with the reserved pasta water. Heat over low heat, often stirring with a wire whisk, until smooth.
6. In a 9-inch baking sheet, place 2 tablespoons of the cream cheese sauce.
7. On a work surface, place the lasagna noodles. Divide the spinach mixture among them and roll them up.
8. Place the rolls, seam-side down, on the sauce in the casserole. Top with the remaining sauce.
9. Sprinkle the lasagna rolls with the Parmesan cheese. Bake for 25 to 35 minutes, or until the lasagna is bubbling and the top starts to brown.

110. Spicy Corn and Rice Burritos

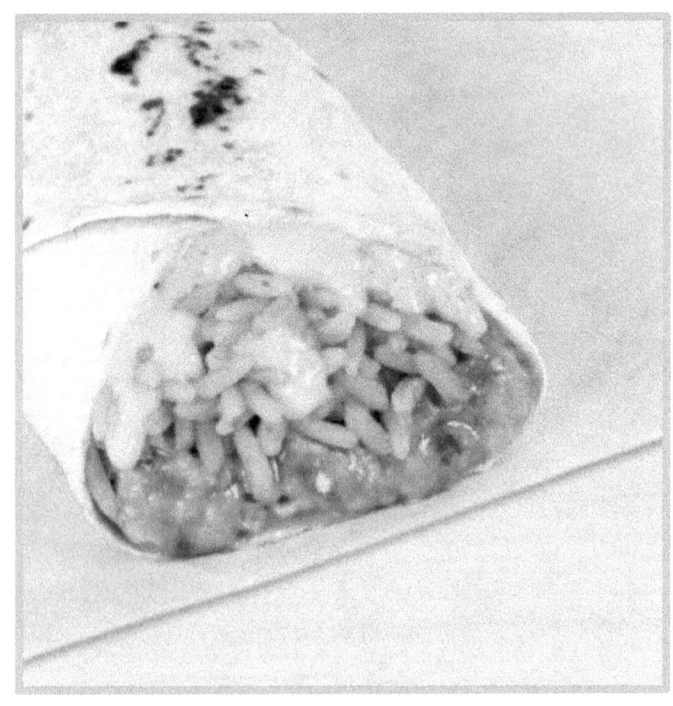

NUTRITION

Calories: 386
Total fat: 21g
Saturated fat: 7g
Sodium: 510mg
Phosphorus: 304mg
Potassium: 282mg
Carbohydrates: 41g
Fiber: 4g
Protein: 11g
Sugar: 2g

PREP TIME
10 min

COOK TIME
20 min

SERVING
4 people

DIRECTIONS

1. Put the skillet in over medium heat and put 2 tablespoons of olive oil. Add the rice, corn, and chili powder and cook for 4 to 6 minutes, or until the ingredients are hot.
2. Transfer the ingredients from the pan into a medium bowl. Let cool for 15 minutes.
3. Stir the cheese into the rice mixture.
4. Heat the tortillas using the directions from the package to make them pliable. Fill the corn tortillas with the rice mixture, then roll them up.
5. At this point, you can serve them as is, or you can fry them first. Heat the remaining tablespoon of olive oil in a large skillet. Fry the burritos, seam-side down at first, turning once, until they are brown and crisp, about 4 to 6 minutes per side, then serve.

INGREDIENTS

- 3 tablespoons of extra-virgin olive oil, divided
- 1 (10-ounce) package of frozen cooked brown rice
- 1½ cups of frozen yellow corn
- 1 tablespoon of chili powder
- 1 cup of shredded pepper jack cheese
- 4 large or 6 small corn tortillas

111. Crustless Cabbage Quiche

PREP TIME: 10 min
COOK TIME: 40 min
SERVING: 6 people

NUTRITION

Calories: 203
Total fat: 16g
Saturated fat: 6g
Sodium: 321mg
Phosphorus: 169mg
Potassium: 155mg
Carbohydrates: 5g
Fiber: 1g
Protein: 11g
Sugar: 4g

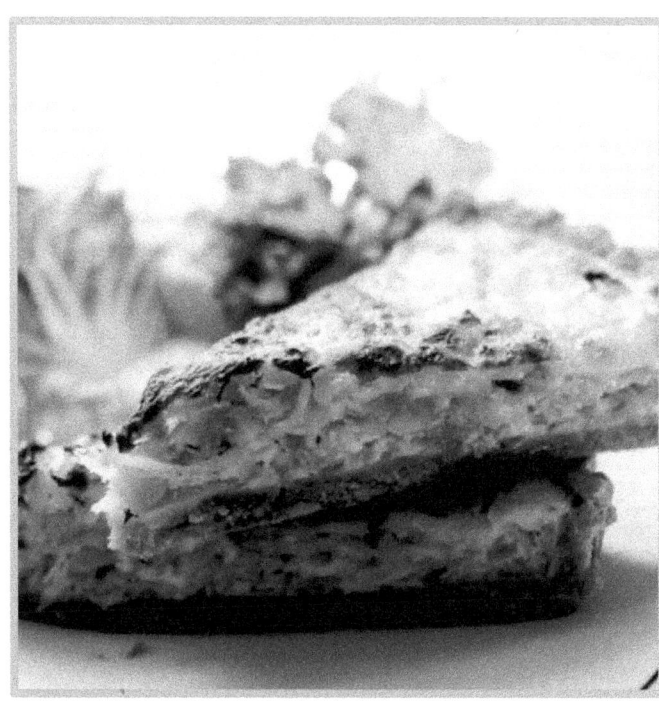

INGREDIENTS

- Olive oil cooking spray
- 2 tablespoons of extra-virgin olive oil
- 3 cups of coleslaw blend with carrots
- 3 large eggs, beaten
- 3 large egg whites, beaten
- ½ cup of half-and-half
- 1 teaspoon of dried dill weed
- ⅛ teaspoon of salt
- ⅛ teaspoon of freshly ground black pepper
- 1 cup of grated Swiss cheese

DIRECTIONS

1. Preheat the oven to 350°F. Spray pie plate (9-inch) with cooking spray and set aside.
2. In a skillet, put an oil and put it in medium heat. Add the coleslaw mix and cook for 4 to 6 minutes, stirring, until the cabbage is tender. Transfer the vegetables from the pan to a medium bowl to cool.
3. Meanwhile, in another medium bowl, combine the eggs and egg whites, half-and-half, dill, salt, and pepper and beat to combine.
4. Stir the cabbage mixture into the egg mixture and pour into the prepared pie plate.
5. Sprinkle with the cheese.
6. Bake for 30 to 35 minutes, or until the mixture is puffed, set, and light golden brown. Let stand for 5 minutes, then slice to serve.

112. Creamy Veggie Casserole

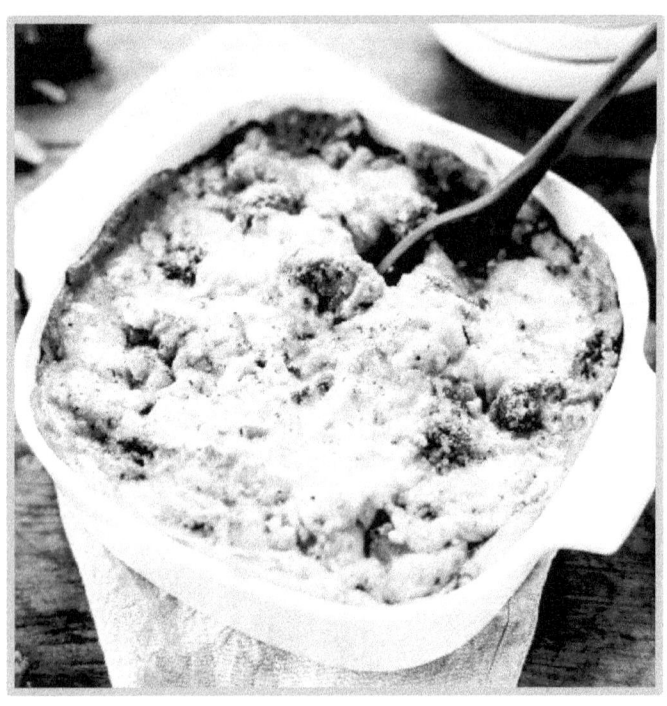

NUTRITION

Calories: 234
Total fat: 18g
Saturated fat: 3g
Sodium: 139mg
Phosphorus: 21mg
Potassium: 210mg
Carbohydrates: 16g
Fiber: 3g
Protein: 3g
Sugar: 5g

PREP TIME
25 min

COOK TIME
35 min

SERVING
4 people

DIRECTIONS

1. Preheat the oven to 375°F.
2. Next is heat 2 tablespoons of olive oil in a large skillet over medium heat. Add the onion and cook for 3 to 4 minutes, stirring, until the onion is tender.
3. Add the flour and stir for 2 minutes.
4. Add the broth to the saucepan, stirring for 3 to 4 minutes, or until the sauce starts to thicken.
5. Add the vegetables to the saucepan. Simmer and cook until vegetables are tender (for six to eight minutes).
6. When the vegetables are done, pour the mixture into a 3-quart casserole dish.
7. Sprinkle the vegetables with the crushed cereal.
8. Bake for 20 to 25 minutes or until the cereal is golden brown and the filling is bubbling. Let cool for 5 minutes and serve.

INGREDIENTS

- ⅓ cup of extra-virgin olive oil, divided
- 1 onion, chopped
- 2 tablespoons of flour
- 3 cups of low-sodium vegetable broth
- 3 cups of frozen California blend vegetables
- 1 cup of crushed crisp rice cereal

113. Vegetable Green Curry

PREP TIME
20 min

COOK TIME
20 min

SERVING
6 people

NUTRITION

Calories: 113
Total fat: 6g
Saturated fat: 1g
Sodium: 174mg
Phosphorus: 117mg
Potassium: 569mg
Carbohydrates: 13g
Fiber: 6g
Protein: 5g
Sugar: 7g

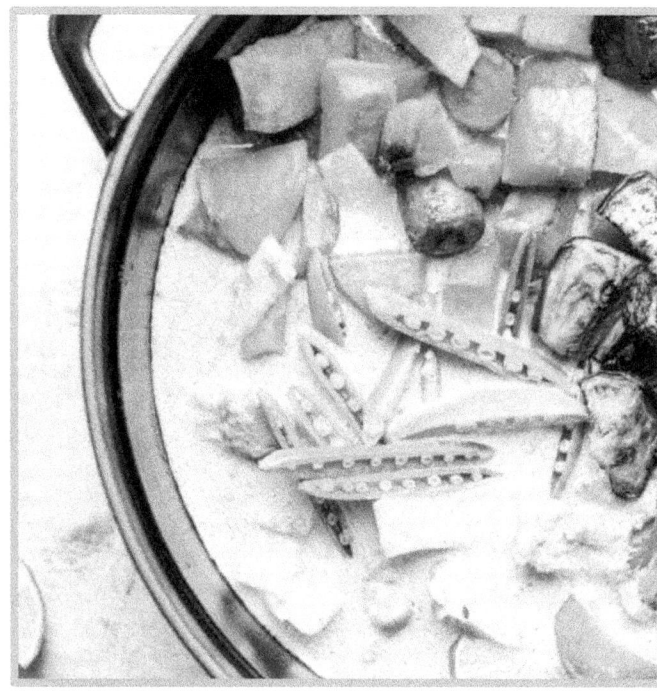

INGREDIENTS

- 2 tablespoons of extra-virgin olive oil
- 1 head of broccoli, cut into florets
- 1 bunch of asparagus, cut into 2-inch lengths
- 3 tablespoons of water
- 2 tablespoons of green curry paste
- 1 medium eggplant
- ⅛ teaspoon of salt
- ⅛ teaspoon of freshly ground black pepper
- ⅔ cup of plain whole-milk yogurt

DIRECTIONS

1. Put olive oil in a large saucepan in medium heat. Add the broccoli and stir-fry for 5 minutes. Add the asparagus and stir-fry for another 3 minutes.
2. Meanwhile, in a small bowl, combine the water with the green curry paste.
3. Add the eggplant, curry-water mixture, salt, and pepper. Stir-fry or until vegetables are all tender.
4. Add the yogurt. Heat through but avoid simmering. Serve.

114. Zucchini Bowl

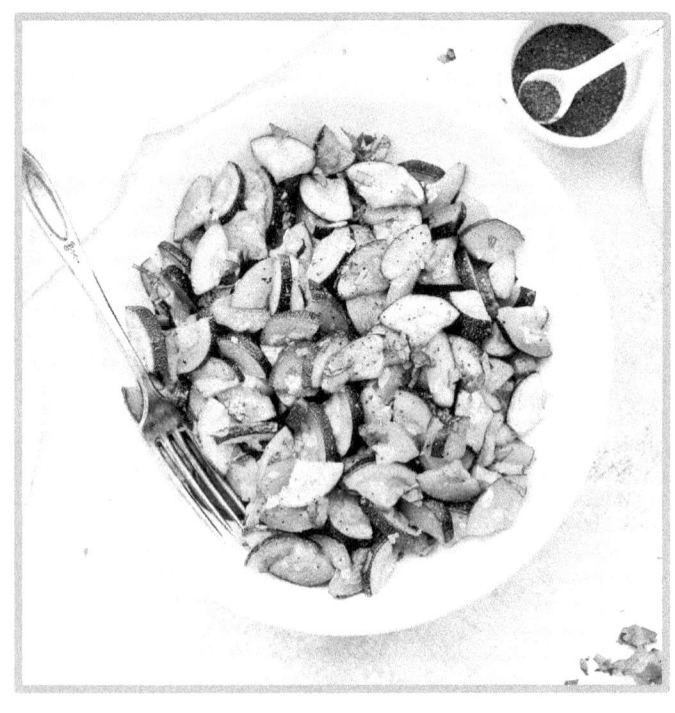

NUTRITION

Calories: 160

Fat: 2g

Carbohydrates: 4g

Protein: 7g

PREP TIME
10 min

COOK TIME
20 min

SERVING
4 people

DIRECTIONS

1. Take a pot and place it over medium heat
2. Add oil and let it heat up
3. Add zucchini, garlic, onion, and stir
4. Cook for 5 minutes
5. Add stock, salt, pepper, and stir
6. Bring to a boil and lower down the heat
7. Simmer for 20 minutes.
8. Remove heat and add coconut milk
9. Use an immersion blender until smooth
10. Ladle into soup bowls and serve
11. Enjoy!

INGREDIENTS

- 1 onion, chopped
- 3 zucchini, cut into medium chunks
- 2 tablespoons coconut milk
- 2 garlic cloves, minced
- 4 cups chicken stock
- 2 tablespoons coconut oil
- Pinch of salt
- Black pepper to taste

115. Nice Coconut Haddock

PREP TIME: 10 min
COOK TIME: 12 min
SERVING: 3 people

NUTRITION

Calories: 299
Fat: 24g
Carbohydrates: 1g
Protein: 20g

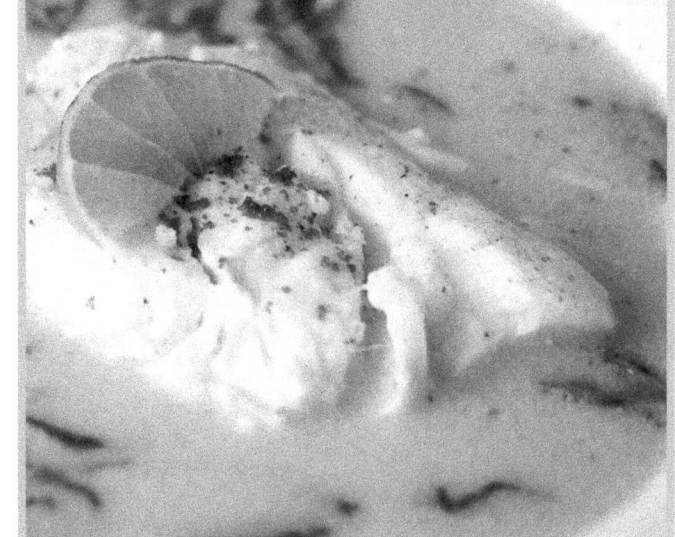

INGREDIENTS

- 4 haddock fillets, 5 ounces each, boneless
- 2 tablespoons of coconut oil, melted
- 1 cup of coconut, shredded and unsweetened
- ¼ cup of hazelnuts, ground
- Salt to taste

DIRECTIONS

1. Preheat your oven to 400°F.
2. Line a baking sheet with parchment paper.
3. Keep it on the side.
4. Pat fish fillets with a paper towel and season with salt.
5. Take a bowl and stir in hazelnuts and shredded coconut.
6. Drag fish fillets through the coconut mix until both sides are coated well.
7. Transfer to a baking sheet.
8. Brush with coconut oil.
9. Bake for about 12 minutes until flaky.
10. Serve and enjoy!

116. Vegetable Rice Casserole

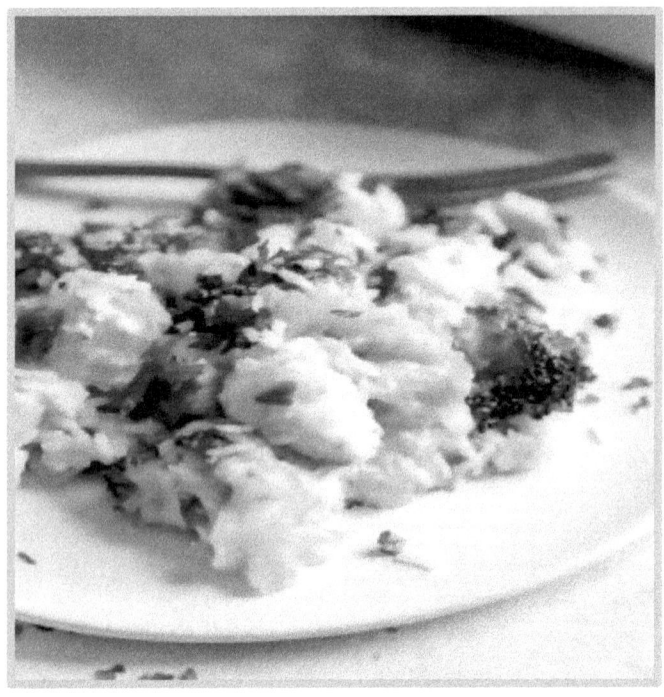

NUTRITION

Calories: 224
Total fat: 3g
Saturated fat: 1g
Cholesterol: 6mg
Sodium: 105mg
Carbohydrates: 41g
Fiber: 2g
Phosphorus: 118mg
Potassium: 176mg
Protein: 6g
Kidney Disease Stage 1

PREP TIME
10 min

COOK TIME
50 min

SERVING
4 people

DIRECTIONS

1. Preheat the oven to 350°F.
2. In a medium skillet over medium-high heat, heat the olive oil.
3. Add the onion and garlic, and sauté until softened, about 3 minutes.
4. Transfer the vegetables to a 9-by-9-inch baking sheet, and stir in the rice and water.
5. Cover the dish and bake until the liquid is absorbed 35 to 40 minutes.
6. Sprinkle the cheese on top and bake an additional 5 minutes to melt.
7. Season the casserole with pepper, and serve.

Substitution tip: Not surprisingly, the cheesy topping on this casserole elevates it to a truly sublime experience. You can also try feta, Cheddar cheese, and goat cheese for different tastes and textures.

INGREDIENTS

- 1 teaspoon of olive oil
- ½ small sweet onion, chopped
- ½ teaspoon of minced garlic
- ½ cup of chopped red bell pepper
- ¼ cup of grated carrot
- 1 cup of white basmati rice
- 2 cups of water
- ¼ cup of grated Parmesan cheese
- Freshly ground black pepper

117. Vegetable Confetti Relish

PREP TIME
25 min

COOK TIME
15 min

SERVING
1 people

NUTRITION

Calories: 230
Fat: 25g
Fiber: 3g
Carbs: 24g
Protein: 43g

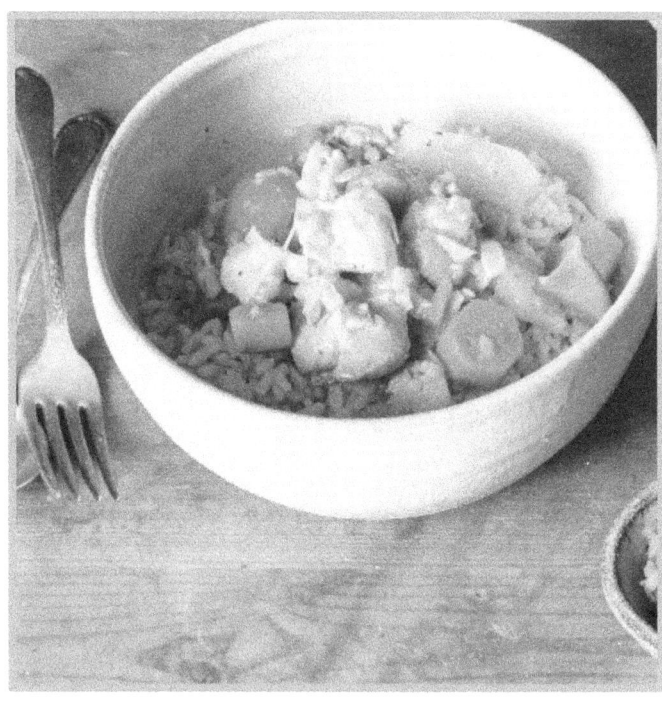

INGREDIENTS

- ½ red bell pepper
- ½ green pepper, boiled and chopped
- 4 scallions, thinly sliced
- ½ tsp. of ground cumin
- 3 tbsp. of vegetable oil
- 1 ½ tbsp. of white wine vinegar
- Black pepper to taste

DIRECTIONS

1. Join all fixings and blend well.
2. Chill in the fridge.
3. You can include a large portion of slashed jalapeno pepper for an increasingly fiery blend

118. Braised Cabbage

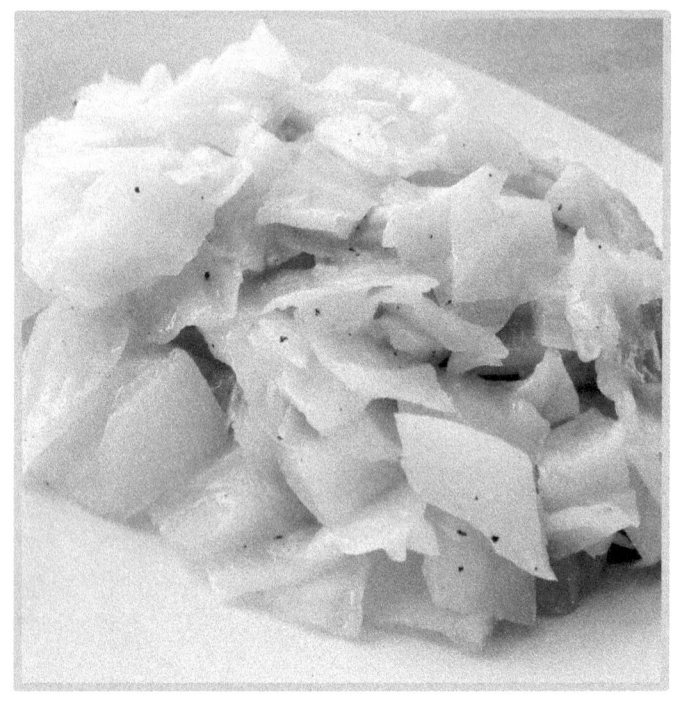

NUTRITION

Calories: 45
Fat: 1.8g
Carbs: 6.6g
Protein: 1.1g
Fiber: 1.9g
Potassium: 136mg
Sodium: 46mg

PREP TIME
10 min

COOK TIME
29 min

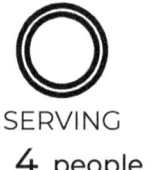

SERVING
4 people

DIRECTIONS

1. In a large skillet, heat oil on medium-high heat.
2. Add garlic and sauté for about 1 minute.
3. Add onion and sauté for about 4–5 minutes.
4. Add cabbage and sauté for about 3–4 minutes.
5. Stir in broth and black pepper and immediately reduce the heat to low.
6. Cook, covered for about 20 minutes.
7. Serve warm.

INGREDIENTS

- 1½ tsp. of olive oil
- 2 minced garlic cloves
- 1 thinly sliced onion
- 3 cups of chopped green cabbage
- 1 cup of low- sodium vegetable broth
- Freshly ground black pepper, to taste

119. Raw Vegetables. Chopped Salad

PREP TIME
15 min

COOK TIME
0 min

SERVING
1 people

NUTRITION

Calories: 111

Total Fat: 2g

Saturated Fat: 1g

Cholesterol: 10mg

Sodium: 58mg

Carbohydrates: 19g

Sugar: 18g

Calcium: 15g

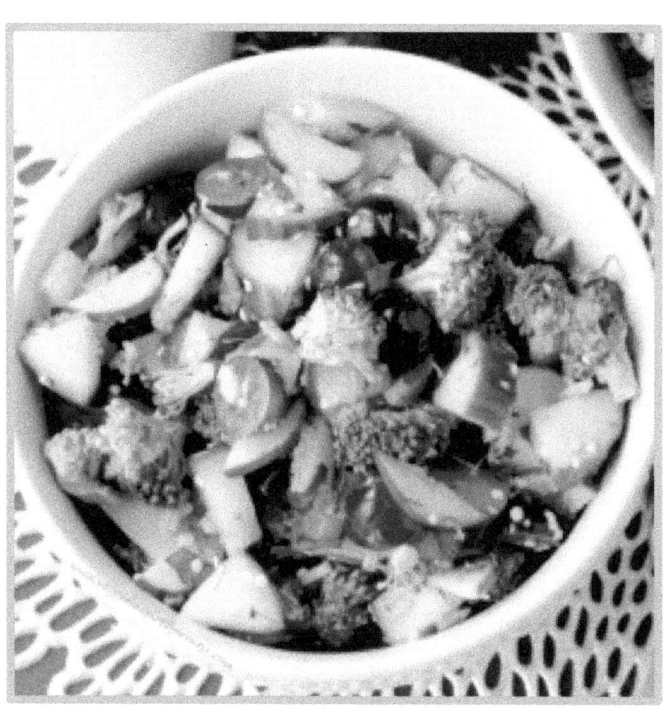

INGREDIENTS

- Chopped raw veggie salad
- 1 orange pepper (minced)
- 1 yellow pepper (small cut)
- 5–8 radishes (halve and cut into thin slices) (about 3/4 cup)
- Small head of broccoli (minced) (about 2 cups)
- 1 seedless cucumber (small cut) (about 2 cups)
- 1 cup of halved red seedless grapes
- 2–3 tablespoons of chopped fresh dill
- 1/4 cup of chopped fresh parsley
- 1/4 cup of raw peeled sunflower seeds
- 1/8 cup of raw hemp hearts (peeled hemp seeds)
- Oil-free dressing
- Garlic clove (chopped)
- 1 tablespoon of red wine vinegar
- 1 tablespoon of apple cider vinegar
- 1 lemon juice
- 1 tbsp. of Dijon-senf
- 1 tbsp. of pure maple syrup
- 1/8 tsp. of pepper (or to taste)

DIRECTIONS

1. Whisk the ingredients—Chopped raw veggie salad, 1 orange pepper, yellow pepper, radishes, small head of broccoli, seedless cucumber, halved red seedless grapes, chopped fresh dill, chopped fresh parsley, raw peeled sunflower seeds, raw hemp hearts, garlic clove, red wine vinegar, apple cider vinegar, lemon, Dijonsenf, pure maple syrup, pepper.

2. Combine all the salad ingredients in a large bowl.

3. Pour the dressing over the chopped vegetables and wrap well.

4. Cover and then refrigerate it for an hour or two and toss the salad once or twice during this time to coat evenly.

5. Enjoy!

120. Broccoli Soup, Green Leaves, And Beans

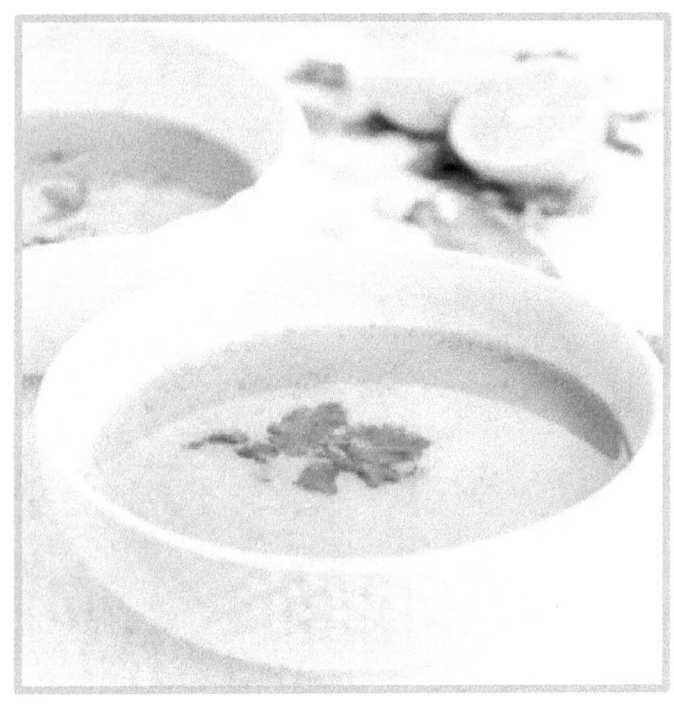

NUTRITION

Calories: 34
Carbohydrate: 6.6g
Fiber: 2.6g
Sugar: 1.7g
Fat: 0.4g

PREP TIME
10 min

COOK TIME
40 min

SERVING
2 people

DIRECTIONS

1. Place a large pot and a lid over medium heat and add the tablespoon of olive oil, onion, garlic. Leave for 5–7 minutes or until the onion is transparent.
2. Add the broccoli and leave for about five minutes or until they change color and start to brown slightly.
3. Add water and spinach. Cover and let it begin to boil over low heat.
4. When the broccoli is soft, add the coriander leaves and stems, the dill (if you are going to use it), and the beans.
5. Blend very carefully with a food processor or in the blender. Add black pepper.
6. Before serving, squeeze the juice of a lemon.
7. You can put lemons on the table so that everyone can put more to their liking.

INGREDIENTS

- 1 tablespoon of olive oil
- 1/2 medium-size onion, cut into large pieces
- 3 cloves of garlic in pieces
- 1 medium-size broccoli head in pieces
- 6 cups of water
- 1 spinach bunches or 3 large fleas of green leaves kale, spinach, etc.
- 1 fist of coriander leaves and stems
- 1 1/2 cups of white beans cooked beans
- Freshly ground black pepper
- 2–3 tablespoons of fresh chopped dill
- Lemon juice to serve

121. Pumpkin Filled With Vegetables and Quinoa

PREP TIME
5 min

COOK TIME
30 min

SERVING
4 people

NUTRITION

Calories: 232

Carbohydrates: 40.4g

Proteins: 8.9g

Lipids: 3.8g

Fiber: 4.4g

Sugar: 0.2g

Cholesterol: 0.0mg

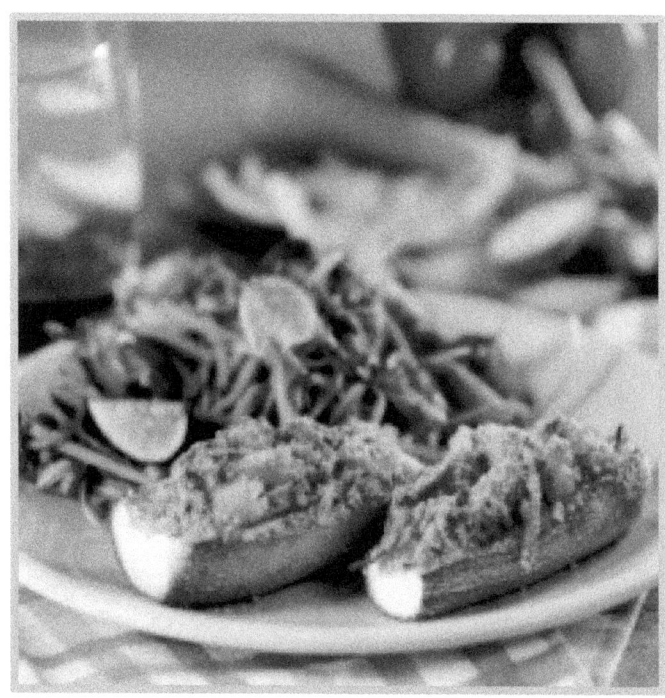

INGREDIENTS

- 2 pieces of Italian pumpkin
- 2 tablespoons of olive oil
- 1 tablespoon of onion
- Cut 2 pieces of carrots into strips
- Cut 1 piece of potato into cubes
- Cut 2 pieces of paprika into strips
- 1 cup of cooked quinoa
- 1 teaspoon of curry
- Enough of ground bread
- pepper

DIRECTIONS

1. Preheat the oven to 180°C.
2. Cut the Italian pumpkin lengthwise and remove the filling place with water in a bowl.
3. Heat over medium heat in a pan, add the oil, quinoa, and onion, add the carrots, potatoes, and paprika and cook for 3 minutes, and pepper curry.
4. Put the pumpkins in a tray and fill with the filling, place on the ground bread and bake for 10 minutes.

122. Vegan Vegetable Mini Tortillas

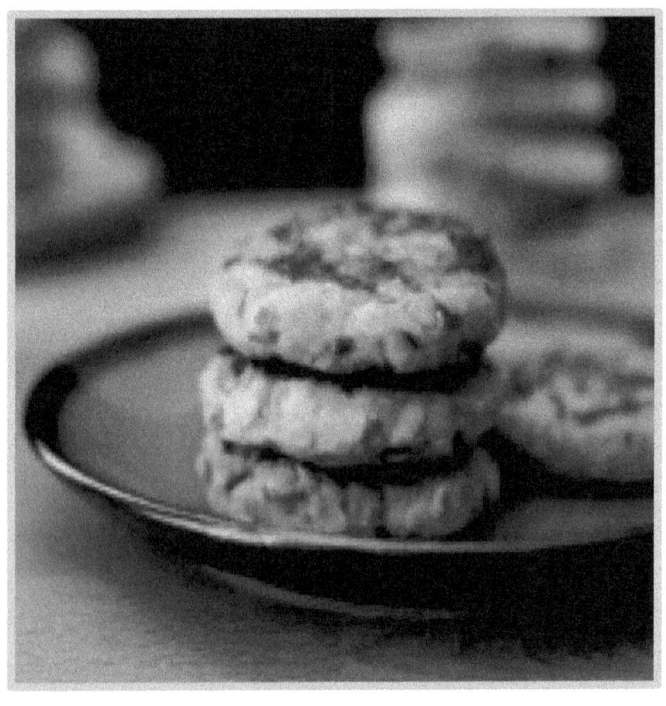

NUTRITION

Calories: 196.09

Carbohydrates: 25.4g

Proteins: 6.92g

PREP TIME
10 min

COOK TIME
40 min

SERVING
5 people

DIRECTIONS

1. Peel potatoes, onions, and carrots. Wash the zucchini and cut all the vegetables into as small as possible (in brunoise).
2. In a pan, fry all the vegetables with a little oil until they are very soft. Comino, pepper, and a few sprigs of chopped parsley and leave over medium heat.
3. We undo the chickpea flour in a little water. It has to be a texture like a beaten egg, so we will be adding the water little by little until it is almost liquid. We add it to the pan of the vegetables and, without stopping to stir, until it is fully integrated. There will be a paste that can be worked with your hands.
4. When the mixture has cooled a little, and we can work by hand, we flour our hands and make balls as twice the size of a meatball. Then we flatten them a bit to give them a hamburger shape, and we put them on the griddle with a drop of oil on both sides.
5. And ready! The vegan vegetable omelets are ready to serve.

INGREDIENTS

- 1 zucchini
- 1 onion
- 2 carrots
- Pinch of pepper
- 1 teaspoon of Parsley
- 3 small potatoes
- 1 tablespoon of olive oil
- Pinch of comino
- 3 tablespoon of chickpea flour

123. Vegetarian Recipe

PREP TIME
10 min

COOK TIME
8 min

SERVING
1 people

NUTRITION

Calories: 111
Total Fat: 2g
Saturated Fat: 1g
Cholesterol: 10mg
Sodium: 58mg
Carbohydrates: 19g
Fiber: 0g
Sugar: 18g
Calcium: 15g

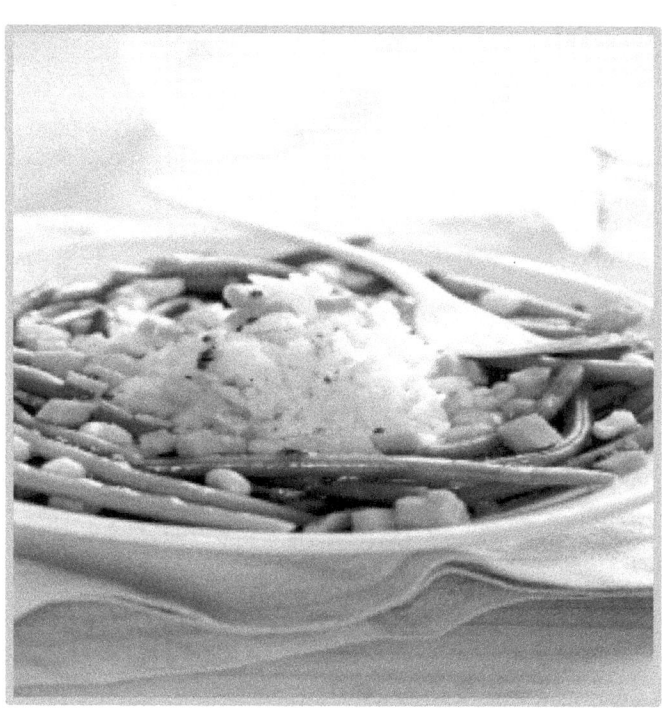

INGREDIENTS

- 1 cup of green beans
- 2 carrots
- Sweet corn
- Cooked rice
- 1 teaspoon of mustard
- A little honey
- Olive oil
- A handful of cooked chickpeas
- 3–4 chopped pistachios

DIRECTIONS

1. You have to mix some green beans and some boiled or steamed carrots, along with sweet corn and cooked rice.

2. To dress it, mix a teaspoon of mustard with a little honey and olive oil. And if you want to turn it into a complete and balanced single dish, you can add a handful of cooked chickpeas and three or four chopped pistachios. Besides being delicious, this vegetarian recipe is one of the best meals to take to work.

124. White Bean Veggie Burgers

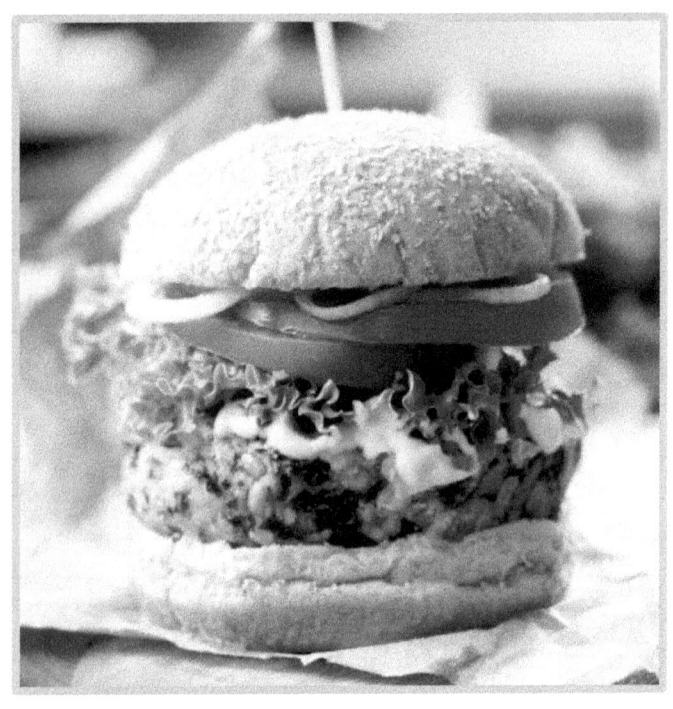

NUTRITION

Calories: 305
Fat: 4g
Carbs: 57g
Protein: 11g
Phosphorus: 181mg
Potassium: 515mg
Sodium: 281mg

PREP TIME
10 min

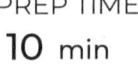
COOK TIME
15 min

SERVING
4 people

DIRECTIONS

1. In a large bowl, mash the beans with a potato masher, leaving a few whole beans as desired. Add the rice, garlic powder, thyme, chipotle pepper, onion, corn, bell pepper, lemon, flour, and egg, and mix well to blend. Season with pepper.
2. Using your hands, form the mixture into four patties. Set your oil on in a skillet on medium heat. Cook the burgers for 5 minutes, until browned on one side, flip, and cook the other side for an additional 5 minutes.

INGREDIENTS

- 1 cup of canned white beans, drained and rinsed
- 1 cup of cooked white rice
- 1 teaspoon of garlic powder
- 2 teaspoons of dried thyme
- ½ teaspoon of ground chipotle pepper
- ½ sweet onion, finely chopped
- ½ cup of fresh or frozen corn
- ½ cup of red bell pepper, finely chopped
- Juice of 1 lemon
- ⅓ cup of all-purpose flour
- 1 large egg
- Freshly ground black pepper
- 2 teaspoons of extra-virgin olive oil

125. Spicy Tofu and Broccoli Stir-Fry

PREP TIME
15 min

COOK TIME
15 min

SERVING
4 people

NUTRITION

Calories: 410

Fat: 18g

Carbs: 51g

Protein: 13g

Phosphorus: 222mg

Potassium: 487mg

Sodium: 51mg

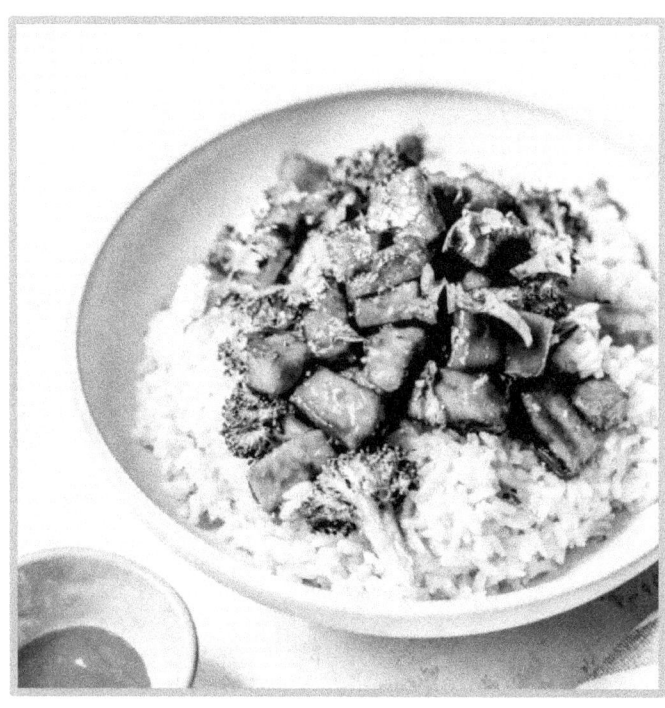

INGREDIENTS

For the sauce:
- 3 garlic cloves
- 2-inch piece of ginger, peeled
- 2 tablespoons of honey
- ¼ cup of rice wine vinegar
- 2 tablespoons of extra-virgin olive oil

For the stir-fry:
- 1 (14-ounce) package of extra-firm tofu
- 1 cup of long-grain white rice
- 2 tablespoons of extra-virgin olive oil
- 2 cups of chopped broccoli
- 1 cup of shredded carrots
- 3 scallions, finely chopped

DIRECTIONS

To make the sauce:
1. Combine the garlic, ginger, honey, vinegar, and olive oil in a food processor, and purée until smooth.

To make the stir-fry:
1. Cut the tofu into small cubes, and press the excess moisture from the tofu using paper towels, repeating several times until dry. In a medium pot, cook the rice according to package directions.
2. Set your oil on in a skillet on medium heat. Add the tofu to the pan in a single layer. Carefully add ¼ of the sauce to the pan and continue to cook, flipping the tofu only once or twice every 4 minutes, until it is well browned. With a slotted spoon, transfer the tofu to a plate lined with paper towels to drain.
3. Add the broccoli to the pan. Cook, covered, often stirring, until fork-tender, about 5 minutes. Add the carrots and continue to cook for an additional 3 minutes, until softened. Add the remaining sauce to the vegetables, return the tofu to the pan, and stir to mix. Garnish with scallions and serve over rice.

126. Barley and Roasted Vegetable Bowl

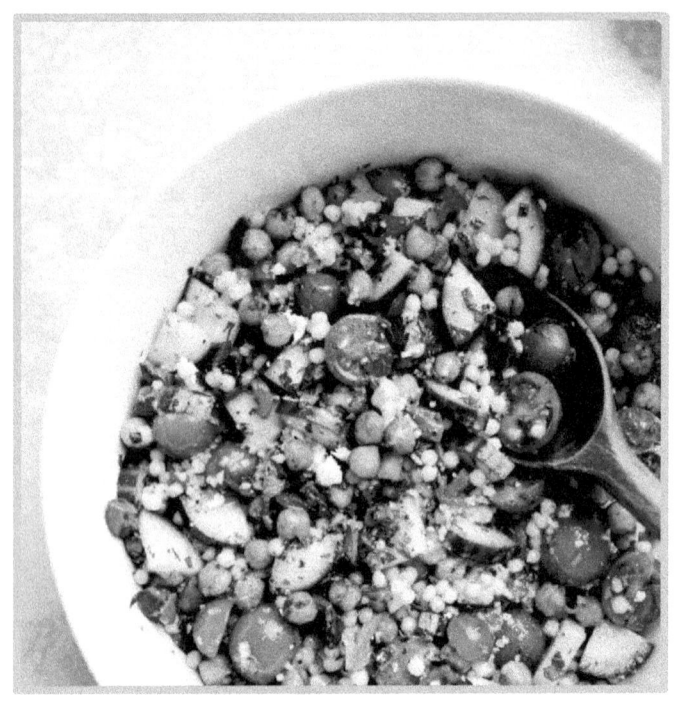

NUTRITION

Calories: 292

Fat: 10g

Carbs: 44g

Protein: 9g

Phosphorus: 201mg

Potassium: 543mg

Sodium: 119mg

PREP TIME
10 min

COOK TIME
30 min

SERVING
4 people

DIRECTIONS

1. Preheat the oven to 425°F. In a medium bowl, toss your onion, bell pepper, zucchini, and eggplant with 1 tablespoon of olive oil and transfer to a baking tray in a single layer. Season with pepper.
2. Roast the vegetables for about 25 minutes, stirring once or twice, until they are browned and tender. Set aside. Meanwhile, in a medium pot, add the barley and 2 cups of water.
3. Bring to a boil, reduce the heat to simmer, cover, and cook for 20 minutes. Turn off the heat and let rest for 10 minutes. Fluff with a fork and drain any remaining water.
4. In a small bowl, whisk the lemon juice, garlic, and remaining tablespoon of olive oil. Toss the vegetables with the barley, and then mix with the lemon-garlic dressing. Right before serving, stir in the basil, feta cheese, and salad greens.

INGREDIENTS

- 2 small Asian eggplants, diced
- 2 small zucchini, diced
- ½ red bell pepper, chopped
- ½ sweet onion, cut into wedges
- 2 tablespoons of extra-virgin olive oil, divided
- Freshly ground black pepper
- 1 cup of barley
- Juice of 1 lemon
- 3 garlic cloves, minced
- ¼ cup of basil leaves, roughly chopped
- ¼ cup of crumbled feta cheese
- 2 cups of arugula or mixed baby salad greens

127. Fragrant Egg Fried Rice

PREP TIME
10 min

COOK TIME
20 min

SERVING
4 people

NUTRITION

Calories: 105.4

Protein: 2.7g

Sodium: 23.2mg

Phosphorus: 4.5m

Potassium: 48.9mg

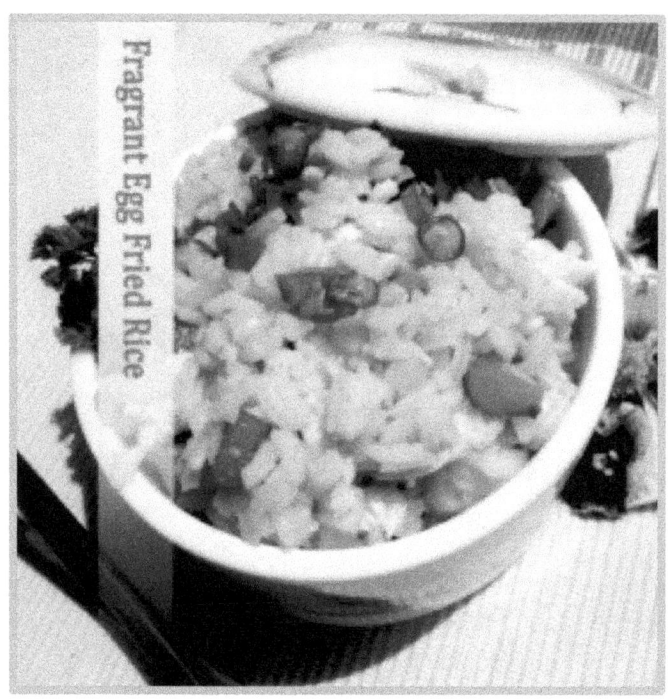

INGREDIENTS

- 1 stalk of lemongrass
- 1 cup of basmati rice
- 1 tbsp. of olive oil
- 1 green onion sliced
- 1-inch piece of ginger peeled, chopped fine
- 1 1/2 tsp. of coriander seeds
- 1 1/2 tsp. of cumin seeds
- 2 cups of low-sodium vegetable stock
- 1/4 cup of chopped cilantro
- 1 diced red pepper
- 1 beaten egg

DIRECTIONS

1. Finely chop the peeled lemongrass.
2. Rinse the rice in cold water and drain through a sieve.
3. Heat the oil in a large stockpot and add the lemongrass, spices, ginger, and onion.
4. Cook for 3 minutes, stirring continuously.
5. Add the rice and cook for 1 more minute, stirring frequently.
6. Add the stock and bring to a boil.
7. Cover pan and simmer 18 minutes or until rice is not crunchy.
8. Remove from heat and fluff with a fork.
9. Add cilantro.

128. Pumpkin Filled With Vegetables and Quinoa

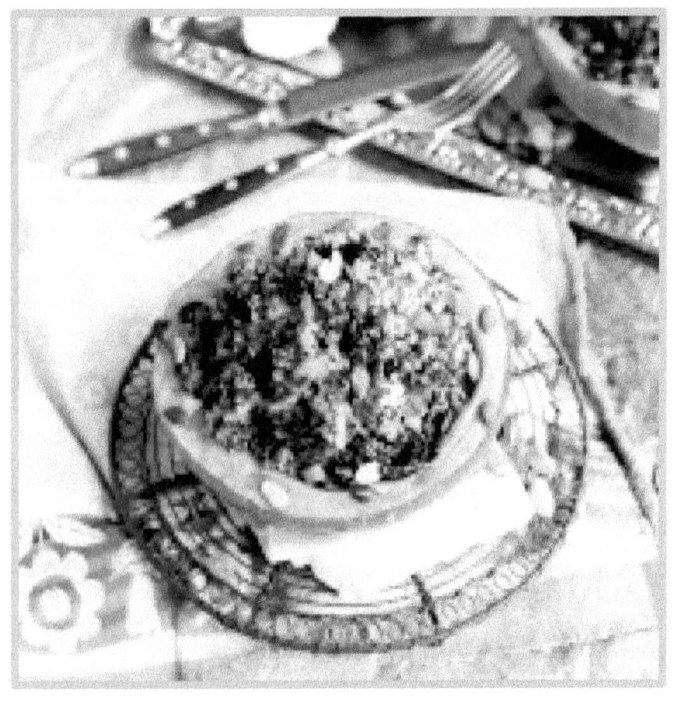

NUTRITION

Calories: 232
Carbohydrates: 40.4g
Proteins: 8.9g
Lipids: 3.8g
Fiber: 4.4g
Sugar: 0.2g

PREP TIME
35 min

COOK TIME
10 min

SERVING
4 people

DIRECTIONS

1. Preheat the oven to 180°C.
2. Cut the Italian pumpkin lengthwise and remove the filling place with water in a bowl.
3. Heat over medium heat in a pan, add the oil, quinoa, and onion, add the carrots, potatoes, and paprika and cook for 3 minutes, season with salt and pepper curry.
4. Put the pumpkins in a tray and fill with the filling, place on the ground bread and bake for 10 minutes.

INGREDIENTS

- 2 pieces of Italian pumpkin
- 2 tablespoons of olive oil
- 1 tablespoon of onion
- Cut 2 pieces of carrots into strips
- Cut 1 piece of potato into cubes
- Cut 2 pieces of paprika into strips
- 1 cup of cooked quinoa
- 1 teaspoon of curry
- Enough of ground bread
- To the taste of salt and pepper

Chapter 12

SEAFOOD

129. Corn and Shrimp Quiche

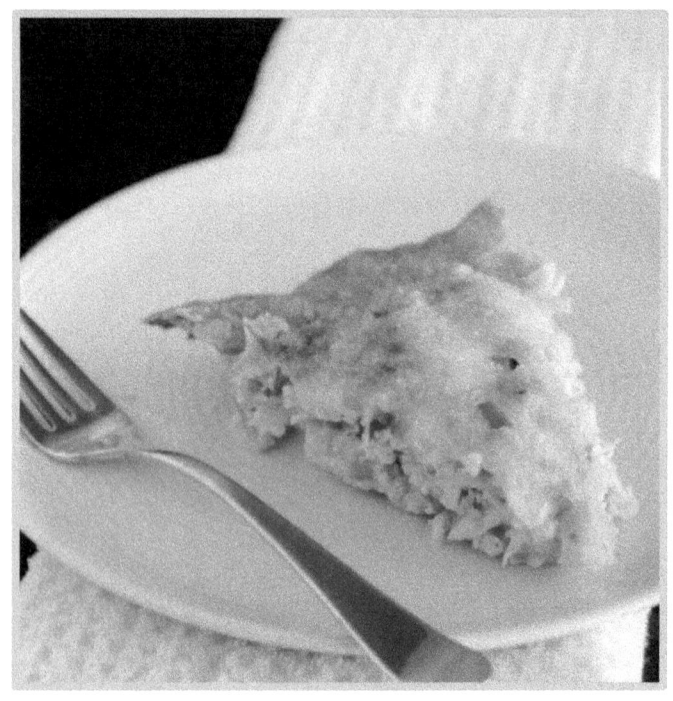

NUTRITION

Calories: 198
Total fat: 10g
Saturated fat: 4g
Sodium: 238mg
Phosphorus: 260mg
Potassium: 261mg
Carbohydrates: 9g
Fiber: 1g
Protein: 20g
Sugar: 2g

PREP TIME
15 min

COOK TIME
50 min

SERVING
6 people

DIRECTIONS

1. Preheat the oven to 350°F. Spray a 9-inch pie pan with nonstick baking spray.
2. In the prepared pan, combine the shrimp and corn. Sprinkle the cheese over the top.
3. In a medium bowl, beat the eggs, almond milk, salt, and pepper. Gently pour into the pan.
4. Bake for 45 to 55 minutes or until the quiche is puffed, set to the touch, and light golden brown on top. Make sure it is cool enough before cutting into wedges to serve.

INGREDIENTS

- 1 cup of small cooked shrimp
- 1½ cups of frozen corn, thawed and drained
- ¾ cup of shredded sharp Colby cheese
- 5 large eggs, beaten
- 1 cup of unsweetened almond milk
- Pinch salt
- ⅛ teaspoon of freshly ground black pepper

130. Ginger Shrimp with Snow Peas

PREP TIME 20 min

COOK TIME 12 min

SERVING 4 people

NUTRITION

Calories: 237
Total fat: 7g
Saturated fat: 1g
Sodium: 469mg
Phosphorus: 350mg
Potassium: 504mg
Carbohydrates: 12g
Fiber: 4g
Protein: 32g
Sugar: 5g

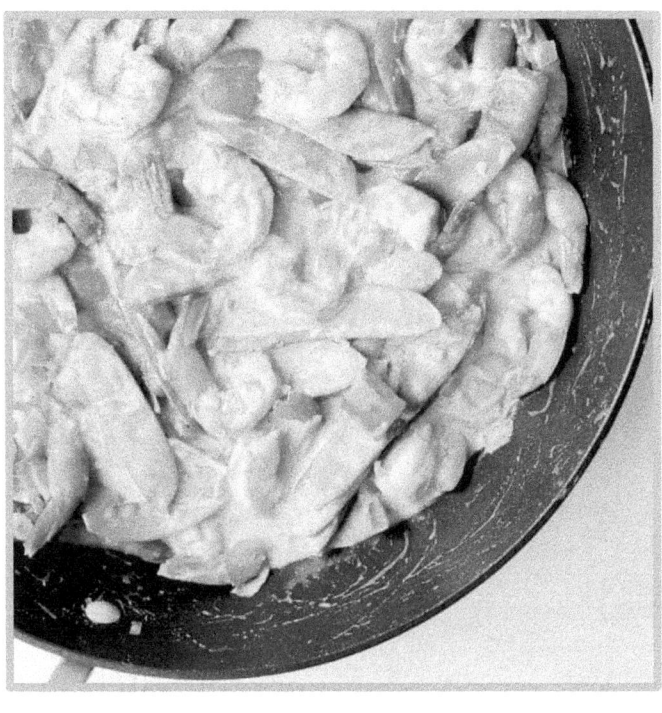

INGREDIENTS

- 2 tablespoons of extra-virgin olive oil
- 1 tablespoon of minced peeled fresh ginger
- 2 cups of snow peas
- 1½ cups of frozen baby peas
- 3 tablespoons of water
- 1 pound of medium shrimp, shelled and deveined
- 2 tablespoons of low-sodium soy sauce
- ⅛ teaspoon of freshly ground black pepper

DIRECTIONS

1. Using a large wok, heat the olive oil over medium heat.
2. Add the ginger and stir-fry for 1 to 2 minutes, until the ginger is fragrant.
3. Add the snow peas and stir-fry for 2 to 3 minutes, until they are tender-crisp.
4. Add the baby peas and the water and stir. Cover the wok and steam for 2 to 3 minutes or until the vegetables are tender.
5. Stir in the shrimp and stir-fry for 3 to 4 minutes, or until the shrimp have curled and turned pink.
6. Add the soy sauce and pepper; stir and serve.

131. Roasted Cod with Plums

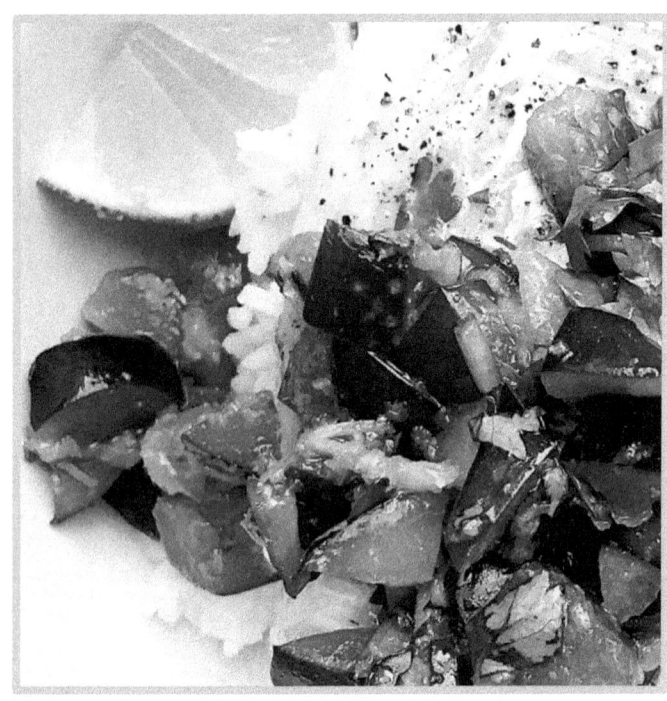

NUTRITION

Calories: 230
Total fat: 9g
Saturated fat: 2g
Sodium: 154mg
Phosphorus: 197mg
Potassium: 437mg
Carbohydrates: 10g
Fiber: 1g
Protein: 27g
Sugar: 8g

PREP TIME
10 min

COOK TIME
20 min

SERVING
4 people

DIRECTIONS

1. Preheat the oven to 375°F. Line a baking sheet with parchment paper.
2. Arrange the plums, cut-side up, along with the fish on the prepared baking sheet. Put the olive oil and lemon juice and sprinkle with the thyme, salt, and pepper.
3. Roast for 15 to 20 minutes or until the fish flakes when tested with a fork and the plums are tender.
4. Serve with the yogurt.

INGREDIENTS

- 6 red plums, halved and pitted
- 1½ pounds cod fillets
- 3 tablespoons extra-virgin olive oil
- 2 tablespoons freshly squeezed lemon juice
- ½ teaspoon dried thyme leaves
- ⅛ teaspoon salt
- ⅛ teaspoon freshly ground black pepper
- ¾ cup plain whole-milk yogurt, for serving

132. Family Hit Curry

NUTRITION

PREP TIME **10** min

COOK TIME **21** min

SERVING **8** people

Calories: 191
Fat: 5.3g
Carbs: 5g
Protein: 29.2g
Fiber: 0g
Potassium: 270mg
Sodium: 199mg

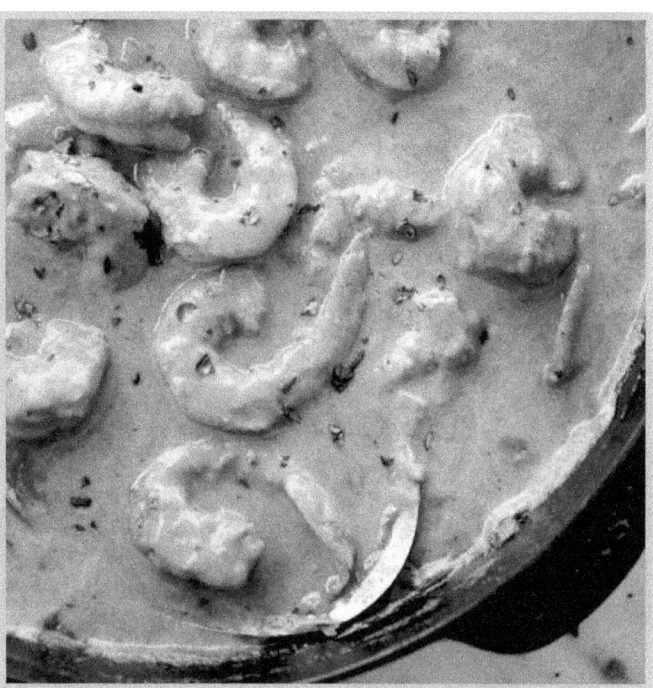

INGREDIENTS

- 1½ tbsp. of canola oil
- 1 finely chopped onion
- 1 tsp. of minced fresh ginger
- 3 minced garlic cloves
- 1 tbsp. of curry paste
- 2 cups of fat-free plain Greek yogurt
- ¼ cup of water
- 1 tsp. of sugar
- 1 pound of cubed cod fillets
- 1 pound of peeled and deveined prawns
- Pinch of salt
- Freshly ground black pepper, to taste
- 2 tbsp. of fresh lemon juice
- ¼ cup of chopped fresh cilantro leaves

DIRECTIONS

1. In a large pan, heat oil on medium heat. Add onion and sauté for about 4–5 minutes.
2. Add ginger, garlic, and curry paste and sauté for about 1 minute.
3. Stir in yogurt, water, and sugar and bring to a boil on high heat.
4. Reduce the heat to medium-low. Simmer for about 5 minutes.
5. Stir in seafood and cook for about 10 minutes or till desired thickness.
6. Stir in salt, black pepper, lemon juice, and cilantro and remove from heat.
7. Serve hot.

133. Homemade Tuna Nicoise

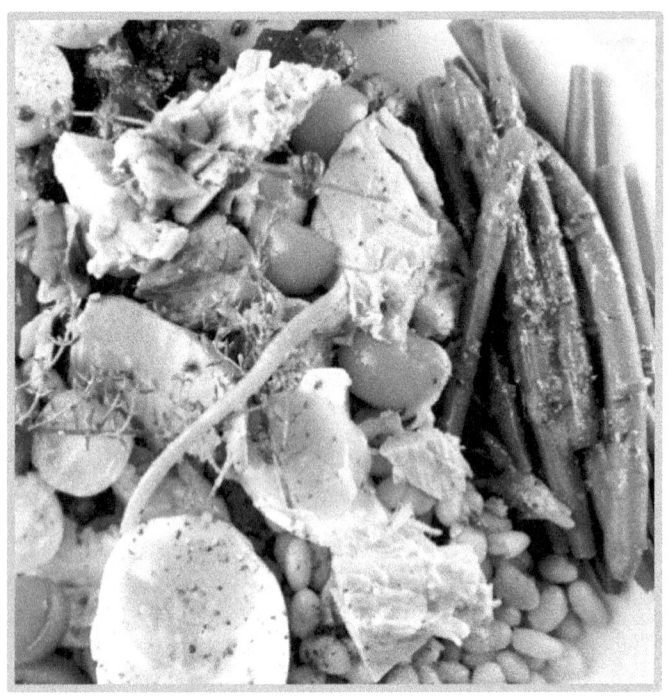

NUTRITION

Calories: 199
Protein: 19g
Carbs: 7g
Fat: 8g
Sodium: 466mg
Potassium: 251mg
Phosphorus: 211mg

PREP TIME
5 min

COOK TIME
10 min

SERVING
2 people

DIRECTIONS

1. Prepare the salad by washing and slicing the lettuce, cucumber, and onion.
2. Add to a salad bowl.
3. Mix 1 tbsp. of oil with the lemon juice, cilantro, and capers for a salad dressing. Set aside.
4. Boil a pan of water on high heat, then lower to simmer and add the egg for 6 minutes. (Steam the green beans over the same pan in a steamer/colander for the 6 minutes.)
5. Remove the egg and rinse under cold water.
6. Peel before slicing in half.
7. Mix the tuna, salad, and dressing in a salad bowl.
8. Toss to coat.
9. Top with the egg and serve with a sprinkle of black pepper.

INGREDIENTS

- 1 egg
- ½ cup of green beans
- ¼ sliced cucumber
- 1 lemon's juice
- 1 tsp. of black pepper
- ¼ sliced red onion
- 1 tbsp. of olive oil
- 1 tbsp. of capers
- 4 oz. of drained canned tuna
- 4 iceberg lettuce leaves
- 1 tsp. of chopped fresh cilantro

134. Cajun Crab

PREP TIME
10 min

COOK TIME
10 min

SERVING
2 people

NUTRITION

Calories: 643

Fat: 51g

Carbohydrates: 3g

Protein: 41g

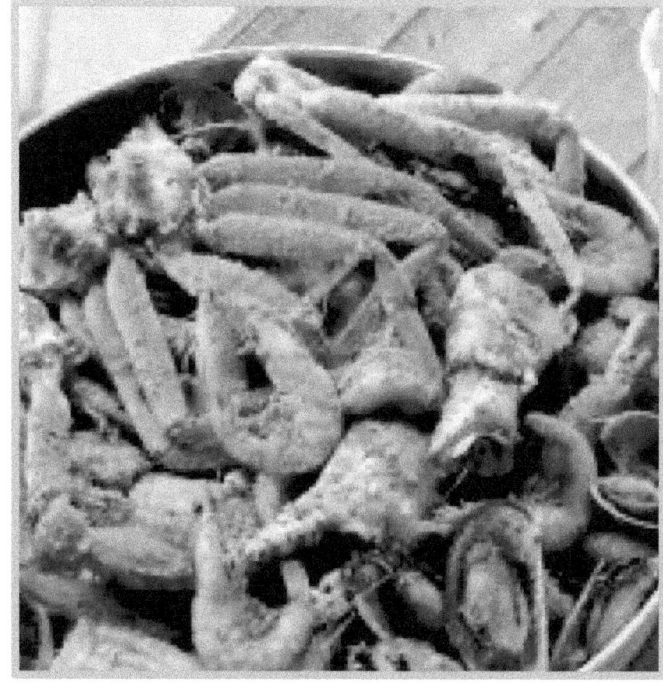

INGREDIENTS

- 1 lemon, fresh and quartered
- 3 tablespoons of Cajun seasoning
- 2 bay leaves
- 4 snow crab legs, precooked and defrosted
- Golden ghee

DIRECTIONS

1. Fill a large pot with salted water about halfway.
2. Bring the water to a boil.
3. Squeeze lemon juice into a pot and toss in remaining lemon quarters.
4. Add bay leaves and Cajun seasoning.
5. Then season for 1 minute.
6. Add crab legs and boil for 8 minutes (make sure to keep them submerged the whole time).
7. Melt ghee in the microwave and use as a dipping sauce, enjoy!

135. Creamy Crab Soup

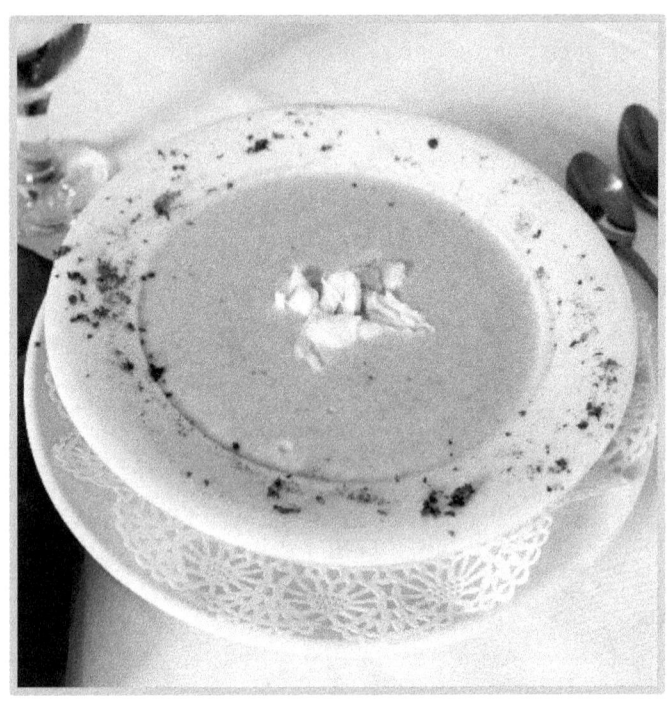

NUTRITION

Calories: 89
Carbohydrate: 10g
Protein: 7g
Sodium: 228mg
Potassium: 237mg
Phosphorus: 83mg
Dietary Fiber: 0.3g
Fat: 3.7g

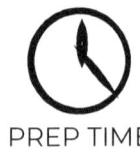

PREP TIME
10 min

COOK TIME
15-20 min

SERVING
7-8 people

DIRECTIONS

1. Melt the butter in a large pan over medium heat.
2. Add the onion to the pot and sauté until transparent, for around 3 minutes.
3. Add the crab meat to the mix and cook for another couple of minutes.
4. Add the chicken broth to the pan mix and bring to a boil.
5. Mix the vegetable or soy cream with the cornstarch and whisk to combine well. Add to the soup and increase the heat to medium-high.
6. Add the dill and pepper and stir frequently until soup comes to a boil.
7. Serve hot.

INGREDIENTS

- 1 tbsp. of low salt butter
- 1 cup of white onion, chopped
- ½ pound of fresh crab meat
- 4 cups of low-salt chicken broth
- 1 cup of soy or vegetable cream
- 2 tbsp. of cornstarch
- ⅛ tsp. of dill
- Kosher pepper

136. Spicy Lime Shrimp

PREP TIME 10 min

COOK TIME 5 min

SERVING 4-5 people

NUTRITION

Calories: 132
Carbohydrate: 3g
Protein: 12g
Sodium: 149mg
Potassium: 202mg
Phosphorus: 128mg
Dietary Fiber: 0.6g
Fat: 8g

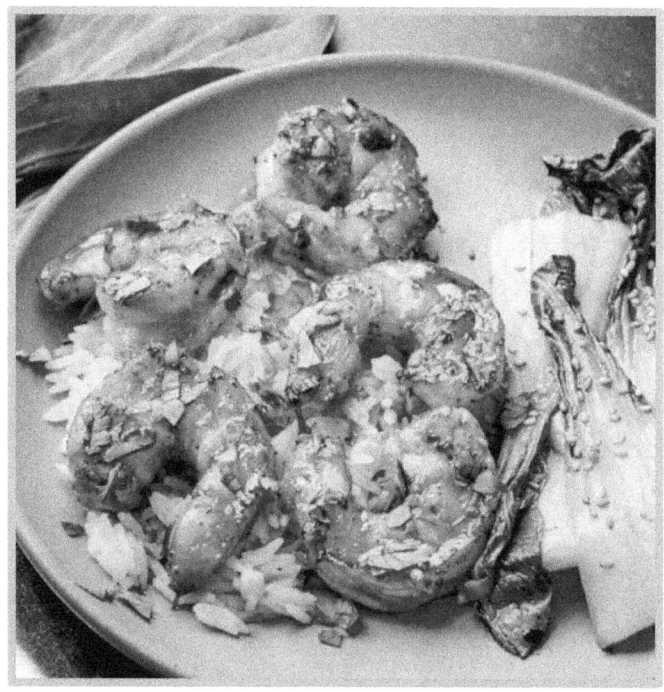

INGREDIENTS

- 32 large shrimp, peeled and deveined
- ¼ cup of lime juice
- 1 garlic clove, minced
- 1 green onion, sliced
- 3 tbsp. of red bell pepper, diced
- 2 tbsp. of fresh cilantro, chopped
- 1 tsp. of jalapeno chili, minced
- ⅛ tsp. of salt
- 1 big cucumber, sliced

DIRECTIONS

1. To make your dressing, combine the lime juice, green onion, jalapeno chili, cilantro, garlic, and oil or salt in a mixing bowl.
2. In a separate mixing bowl, add the shrimps with 3 tbsp of the lime juice marinade. Cover and let in the fridge for 40 minutes.
3. Turn on your oven's broiler. Discard the shrimp from the lime marinade and broil for around 3–4 minutes in total or 2 minutes on each side.
4. Take off the heat and pour the remaining marinade on top.
5. Place over the cucumber slices and serve cold.

137. Seafood Casserole

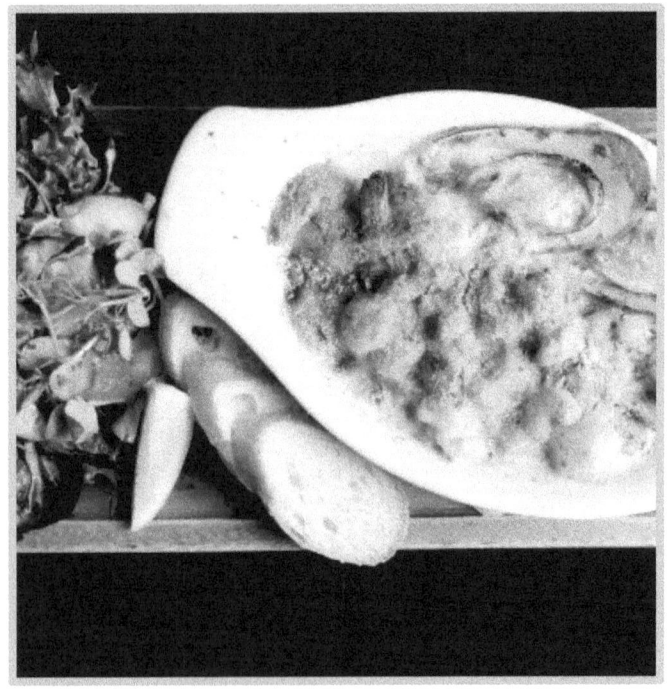

NUTRITION

Calories: 118
Fat: 4g
Carb: 9g
Phosphorus: 102mg
Potassium: 199mg
Sodium: 235mg
Protein: 12g

PREP TIME
20 min

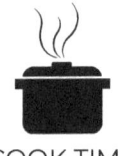

COOK TIME
45 min

SERVING
6 people

DIRECTIONS

1. Preheat the oven to 350°F.
2. Boil the eggplant in a saucepan for 5 minutes. Drain and set aside.
3. Grease a 9-by-13-inch baking sheet with butter and set aside.
4. Heat the olive oil in a large skillet over medium heat.
5. Sauté the garlic, onion, celery, and bell pepper for 4 minutes or until tender.
6. Add the sautéed vegetables to the eggplant, along with the lemon juice, hot sauce, seasoning, rice, and egg.
7. Stir to combine.
8. Fold in the shrimp and crab meat.
9. Spoon the casserole mixture into the casserole dish, patting down the top.
10. Bake for 25 to 30 minutes or until casserole is heated through and rice is tender.
11. Serve warm.

INGREDIENTS

- 2 cups eggplant—peeled and diced into 1-inch pieces
- Butter, for greasing the baking sheet
- 1 tbsp. of olive oil
- ½ sweet onion, chopped
- 1 tsp. of minced garlic
- 1 stalk of celery, chopped
- ½ red bell pepper, boiled and chopped
- 3 tbsps. of freshly squeezed lemon juice
- 1 tsp. of hot sauce
- ¼ tsp. of creole seasoning mix
- ½ cup of uncooked white rice
- 1 large egg
- 4 ounces of cooked shrimp
- 6 ounces of queen crab meat

138. Tilapia Ceviche

PREP TIME
15 min

COOK TIME
5 min

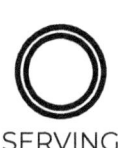

SERVING
1 cup with 6 crackers

NUTRITION

Calories: 220
Protein: 19g
Carbohydrates: 20g
Fat: 7g
Cholesterol: 36mg
Sodium: 168mg
Potassium: 374mg
Phosphorus: 162mg
Fiber: 1.3g

INGREDIENTS

- 1½ pounds of fresh tilapia fillets
- 1 cup of red onion
- ½ cup of red bell pepper
- ¼ cup of cilantro
- 1 cup of pineapple
- 2 tablespoons of canola oil
- ¼ teaspoon of black pepper
- 1¼ cups of fresh lime juice
- 48 saltine crackers with unsalted tops

DIRECTIONS

1. Chop the onion, bell pepper, and cilantro. Also, dice the pineapple, and cube the tilapia into small chunks.
2. Broil tilapia cubes over high heat for about 3 minutes on each side.
3. Cool the tilapia for about 5 minutes, then pour the fresh lime juice on top of it, mixing properly. Ensure all tilapia pieces are coated completely with the lime juice.
4. Combine and mix the bell pepper, onion, pineapple, cilantro, black pepper, and the canola oil with the broiled tilapia mixture.
5. Cover and refrigerate to marinate for about 2 hours.
6. Use six saltine crackers with the unsalted tops for each serving.

139. Fish Tacos

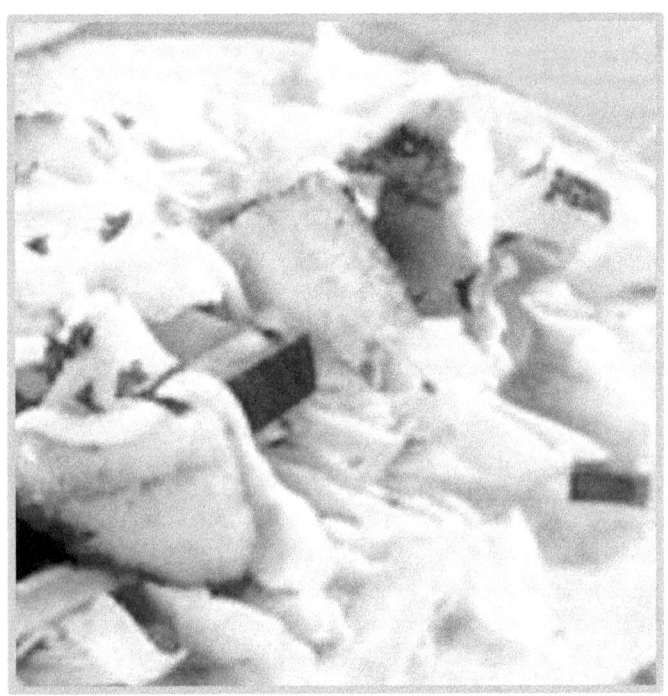

NUTRITION

Calories: 363

Protein: 18g

Carbohydrates: 30g

Fat: 19g

Cholesterol: 40mg

Sodium: 194mg

Potassium: 507mg

Phosphorus: 327mg

Fiber: 4.3g

PREP TIME
10 min

COOK TIME
35 min

SERVING
6 people

DIRECTIONS

1. Shred the cabbage, chop the onion and cilantro, and mince the garlic. Set aside.
2. Use a dish to place in the fish fillets, then squeeze half a lime juice over the fish. Sprinkle the fish fillets with the minced garlic, cumin, black pepper, chili powder, and olive oil. Turn the fish filets to coat with the marinade, then refrigerate for about 15 to 30 minutes.
3. Prepare salsa Blanca by mixing the mayonnaise, milk, sour cream, and the other half of the lime juice. Stir to combine, then place in the refrigerator to chill.
4. Broil in oven, and cover the broiler pan with aluminum foil. Broil the coated fish fillets for about 10 minutes or until the flesh becomes opaque and white and flakes easily. Remove from the oven, slightly cool, and then flake the fish into bigger pieces.
5. Heat the corn tortillas in a pan, one at a time until it becomes soft and warm, then wrap in a dish towel to keep them warm.
6. To assemble the tacos, place a piece of the fish on the tortilla, topping with the salsa blanca, cabbage, cilantro, red onion, and the lime wedges.
7. Serve with hot sauce if you desire.

INGREDIENTS

- 1½ cup of cabbage
- ½ cup of red onion
- ½ bunch of cilantro
- 1 garlic clove
- 2 limes
- 1 pound of cod fillets
- ½ teaspoon of ground cumin
- ½ teaspoon of chili powder
- ¼ teaspoon of black pepper
- 1 tablespoon of olive oil
- ½ cup of mayonnaise
- ¼ cup of sour cream
- 2 tablespoons of milk
- 12 (6-inch) corn tortillas

140. Jambalaya

PREP TIME
10 min

COOK TIME
75 min

SERVING
12 people

NUTRITION

Calories: 294

Protein: 20g

Carbohydrates: 31g

Fat: 10g

Cholesterol: 137mg

Sodium: 186mg

Potassium: 300mg

Phosphorus: 197mg

Fiber: 0.8g

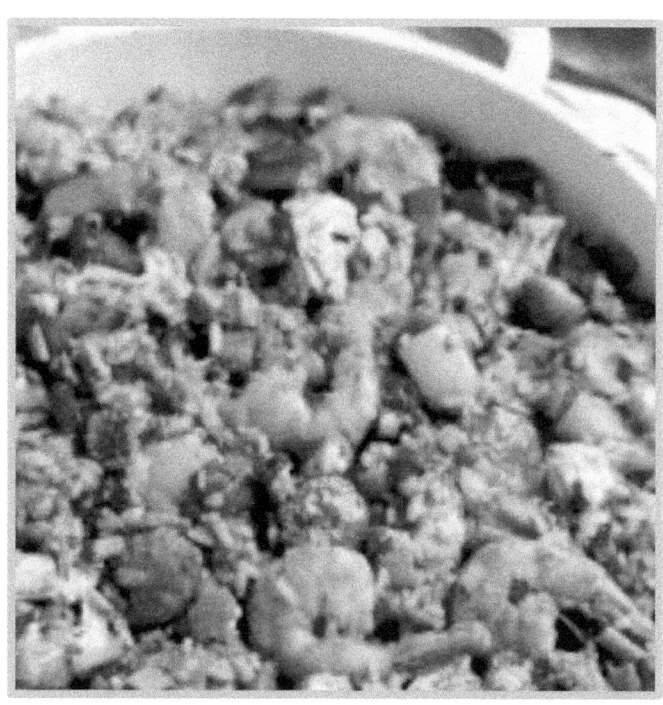

INGREDIENTS

- 2 cups of onion
- 1 cup of bell pepper
- 2 garlic cloves
- 2 cups of uncooked converted brown rice
- ½ teaspoon of black pepper
- 8 ounces of canned low-sodium tomato sauce
- 2 cups of low-sodium beef broth
- 2 pounds of raw shrimp
- ½ cup of unsalted margarine

DIRECTIONS

1. Preheat oven to 350°F.
2. Chop the onion, bell pepper, garlic, then peel the shrimp.
3. Combine and mix all the ingredients in a large bowl except the margarine.
4. Pour into a 9 x 13-inch baking sheet and evenly spread out.
5. Slice the margarine, placing over the top of the ingredients.
6. Cover with foil or lid, and bake for about 1 hr 15 minutes.
7. Serve hot.

141. Asparagus Shrimp Linguini

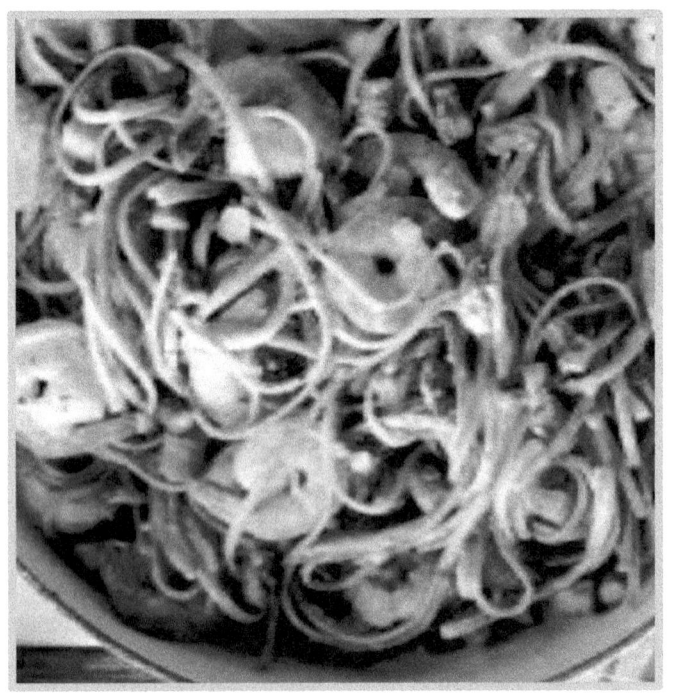

NUTRITION

Calories: 544

Protein: 21g

Carbohydrates: 43g

Fat: 32g

Cholesterol: 188mg

Sodium: 170mg

Potassium: 402mg

Phosphorus: 225mg

Fiber: 2.4g

PREP TIME
10 min

COOK TIME
35 min

SERVING
1 ½ cup

DIRECTIONS

1. Preheat oven to 350°F.
2. Cook the linguini in boiling water until it becomes tender, then drain.
3. Place the asparagus on a baking sheet, then spread two tablespoons of oil over the asparagus. Bake for about 7 to 8 minutes or until it is tender.
4. Remove baked asparagus from the oven and place it on a plate. Cut the asparagus into pieces of medium-sized once cooled.
5. Mince the garlic and chop the parsley.
6. Melt ½ cup of butter in a large skillet with the minced garlic.
7. Stir in the cream cheese, mixing as it melts.
8. Stir in the parsley and basil, then simmer for about 5 minutes. Mix either in boiling water or dry white wine, stirring until the sauce becomes smooth.
9. Add the cooked shrimp and asparagus, then stir and heat until it is evenly warm.
10. Toss the cooked pasta with the sauce and serve.

INGREDIENTS

- 8 ounces of uncooked linguini
- 1 tablespoon of olive oil
- 1¾ cups of asparagus
- ½ cup of unsalted butter
- 2 garlic cloves
- 3 ounces of cream cheese
- 2 tablespoons of fresh parsley
- ¾ teaspoon of dried basil
- ⅔ cup of dry white wine
- ½ pound of peeled and cooked shrimp

142. Tuna Noodle Casserole

PREP TIME
10 min

COOK TIME
35 min

SERVING
2 people

NUTRITION

Calories: 415

Protein: 22g

Carbohydrates: 39g

Fat: 19g

Cholesterol: 88mg

Sodium: 266mg

Potassium: 400mg

Phosphorus: 306mg

Fiber: 3.2g

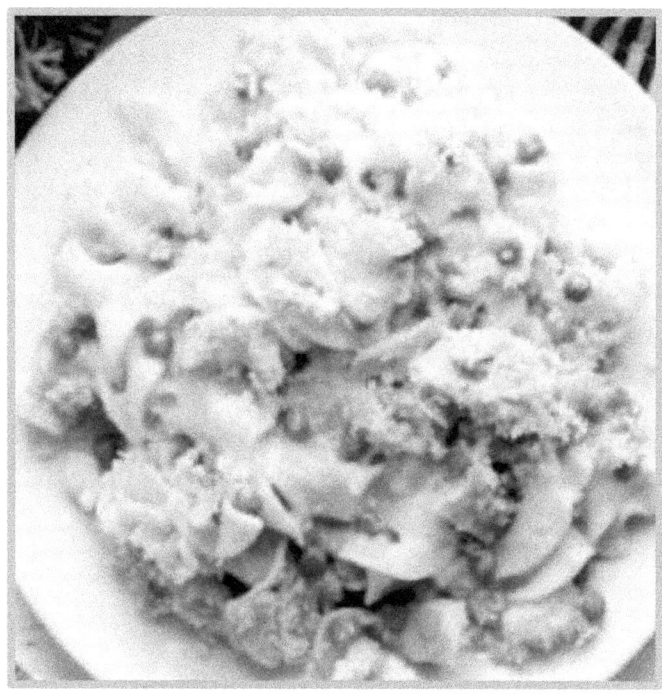

INGREDIENTS

- 2 ounces of wide uncooked egg noodles
- 5 ounces of canned tuna in water
- ½ cup of sour cream
- ¼ cup of cottage cheese
- ½ cup of fresh sliced mushrooms
- ½ cup of frozen green peas
- 1 tablespoon of unsalted butter
- ¼ cup of unseasoned bread crumbs

DIRECTIONS

1. Preheat oven to 350°F.
2. Boil egg noodles based on the package instructions and drain. Also, drain and flake the tuna.
3. Combine and mix the sour cream, cottage cheese, mushrooms, tuna, and peas in a medium bowl.
4. Stir the drained noodle into the tuna mixture, and place it in a small casserole dish that has been sprayed with a non-stick cooking spray.
5. Melt butter, stir into the bread crumbs, then sprinkle over the mixture of noodles in step 4.
6. Bake for about 20 to 25 minutes or until the bread crumbs start to brown.
7. Divide into two and serve.

143. Oven-Fried Southern Style Catfish

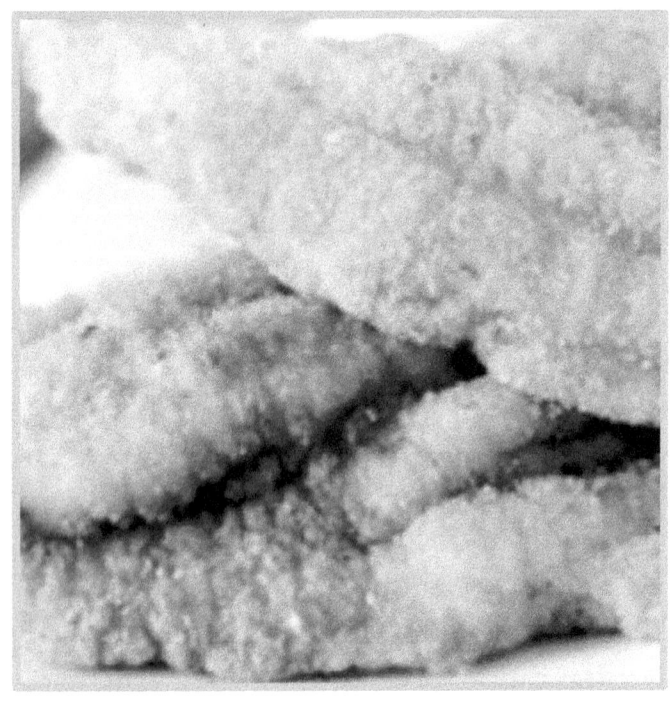

NUTRITION

Calories: 250

Protein: 22g

Carbohydrates: 19g

Fat: 10g

Cholesterol: 53mg

Sodium: 124mg

Potassium: 401mg

Phosphorus: 262mg

Fiber: 1.2g

PREP TIME
10 min

COOK TIME
35 min

SERVING
4 people

DIRECTIONS

1. Heat oven to 450°F.
2. Use cooking spray to spray a non-stick baking sheet.
3. Using a bowl, beat the egg white until very soft peaks are formed. Don't over-beat.
4. Use a sheet of wax paper and place the flour over it.
5. Use a different sheet of wax paper to combine and mix the cornmeal, panko, and the Cajun seasoning.
6. Cut the catfish fillet into four pieces, then dip the fish in the flour, shaking off the excess.
7. Dip coated fish in the egg white, rolling into the cornmeal mixture.
8. Place the fish on the baking pan. Repeat with the remaining fish fillets.
9. Use cooking spray to spray over the fish fillets. Bake for about 10 to 12 minutes or until the sides of the fillets become browned and crisp.

INGREDIENTS

- 1 egg white
- ½ cup of all-purpose flour
- ¼ cup of cornmeal
- ¼ cup of panko bread crumbs
- 1 teaspoon of salt-free Cajun seasoning
- 1 pound of catfish fillets

144. Cilantro-Lime Cod

PREP TIME
10 min

COOK TIME
35 min

SERVING
4 people

NUTRITION

Calories: 292
Protein: 20g
Carbohydrates: 1g
Fat: 23g
Cholesterol: 57mg
Sodium: 228mg
Potassium: 237mg
Phosphorus: 128mg
Calcium: 14mg

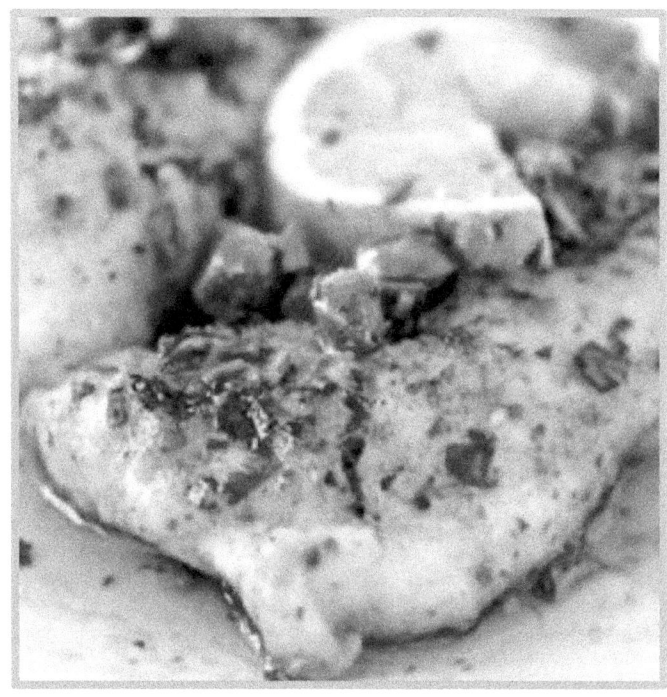

INGREDIENTS

- ½ cup of mayonnaise
- ½ cup of fresh chopped cilantro
- 2 tablespoon of lime juice
- 1 pound of cod fillets

DIRECTIONS

1. Combine and mix the mayonnaise, cilantro, and lime juice in a medium bowl, remove ¼ cup to another bowl and put aside. To be served as fish sauce.
2. Spread the remaining mayonnaise mixture over the cod fillets.
3. Use cooking spray to spray a large skillet, then heat over medium-high heat.
4. Place in the cod fillets, and cook for about 8 minutes or until the fish becomes firm and moist, turning just once.
5. Serve with the ¼ cilantro-lime sauce.

145. Shrimp Quesadilla

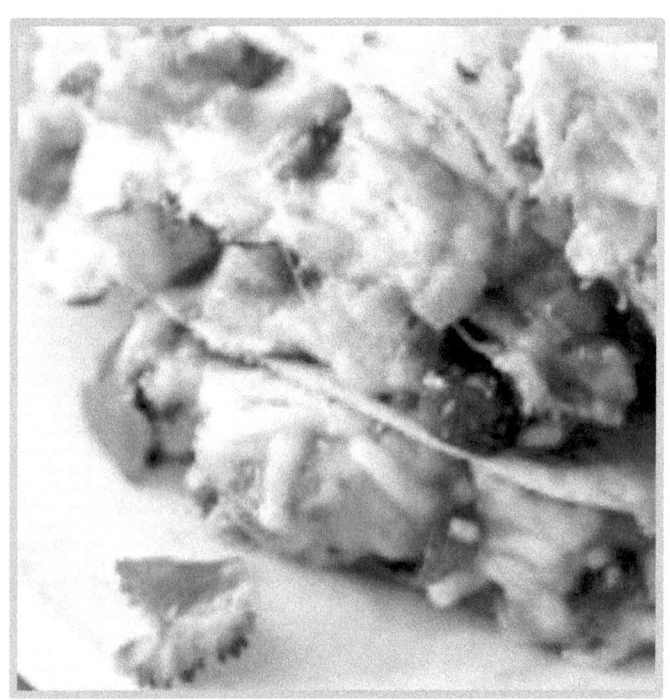

NUTRITION

Calories: 318
Protein: 20g
Carbohydrates: 26g
Fat: 15g
Cholesterol: 118mg
Sodium: 398mg
Potassium: 276mg
Phosphorus: 243mg
Fiber: 1.2g

PREP TIME
15 min

COOK TIME
10 min

SERVING
2 people

DIRECTIONS

1. Peel the shrimp, rinse, and then cut into pieces of bite-size. Dice the cilantro.
2. Use a zip-lock bag to combine and mix the cilantro, lemon juice, cumin, and cayenne pepper to make the marinade. Add the pieces of shrimp and put aside to marinate for about 5 minutes.
3. Heat a skillet over medium heat and add the shrimp with the marinade. Stir-fry for about 1 to 2 minutes or until the shrimp is orange in color. Remove the skillet from heat and spoon out the shrimp, leaving marinade.
4. Add the sour cream to the skillet with the leftover marinade. Stir to mix.
5. Use a large skillet or microwave to heat the tortillas, then spread two teaspoons of salsa over each tortilla. Top with ½ of the shrimp mixture, sprinkling with one tablespoon of cheddar cheese.
6. Spoon out one tablespoon of the sour cream mixture from step 4 on top of the shrimp, fold the tortilla into half, turning over in skillet to heat, then remove from the pan. Repeat the same process with the second tortilla and with the remaining shrimp, cheese, and marinade.
7. Cut each of the tortillas into four pieces, and serve.

INGREDIENTS

- 5 ounces of raw shrimp
- 2 tablespoons of cilantro
- 1 tablespoon of lemon juice
- ¼ teaspoon of ground cumin
- ⅛ teaspoon of cayenne pepper
- 2 flour burrito-sized tortillas
- 2 tablespoons of sour cream
- 4 teaspoons of salsa
- 2 tablespoons of shredded jalapeno cheddar cheese

146. Maryland Crab Cakes

PREP TIME
5 min

COOK TIME
15 min

SERVING
6 people

NUTRITION

Calories: 158
Protein: 17g
Carbohydrates: 2g
Fat: 9g
Cholesterol: 112mg
Sodium: 337mg
Potassium: 268mg
Phosphorus: 177mg
Fiber: 0.3g

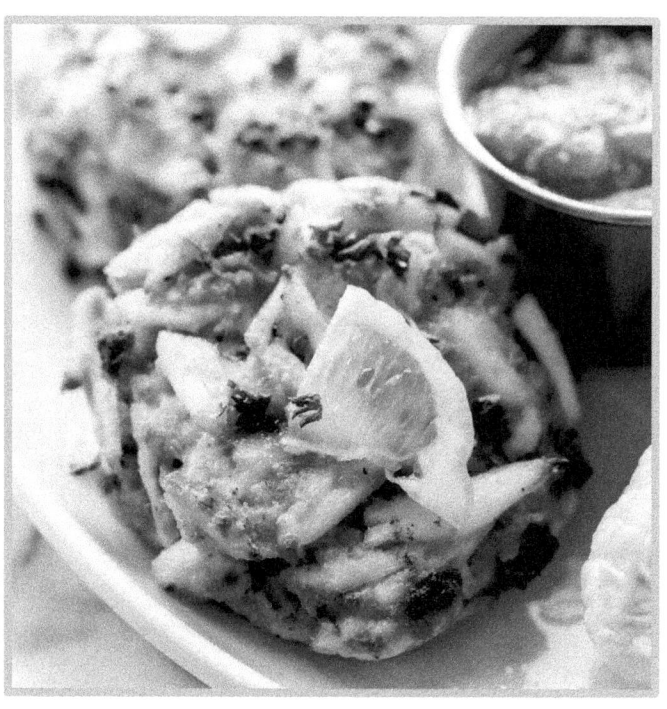

INGREDIENTS

- 1 pound of lump crab meat
- 1 slice of white bread
- 1 tablespoon of mayonnaise
- 1 teaspoon of yellow mustard
- 1 teaspoon of 30%-less-sodium Old Bay seasoning
- 1 tablespoon of fresh parsley
- ⅛ teaspoon of cayenne pepper
- 1 large egg
- 2 tablespoons of olive oil

DIRECTIONS

1. Pick through the crab meat in a medium bowl, removing any shell pieces.
2. Cut the slice of bread into cubes.
3. Add in all the ingredients to the except the olive oil. Mix slightly until all the ingredients are combined. Don't over mix.
4. Portion out six crab cakes using ⅓ cup, with each portion being ¾ inch thick. Store in the refrigerator for one hour.
5. Heat oil or cooking spray in a heavy skillet and fry both sides of the crab for 5 minutes each or until it becomes brown.

147. Citrus Grilled Glazed Salmon

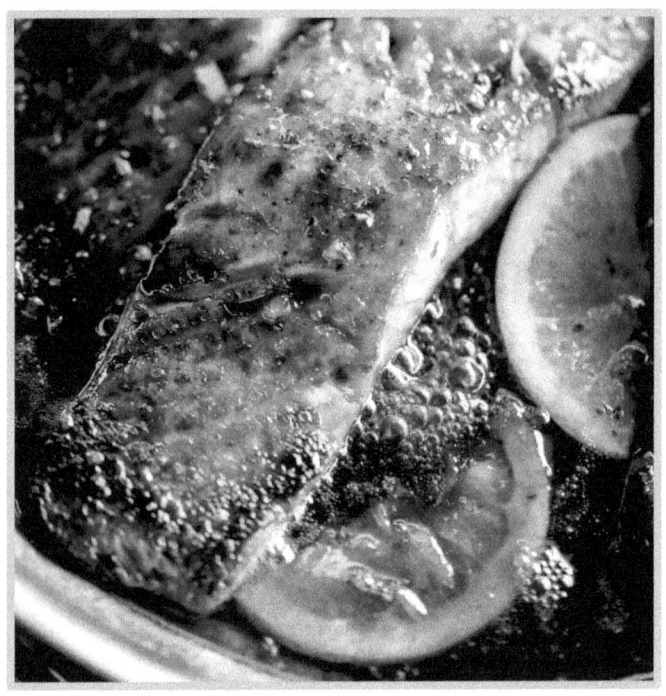

NUTRITION

Calories: 294
Protein: 23g
Carbohydrates: 1g
Fat: 22g
Cholesterol: 68mg
Sodium: 190mg
Potassium: 439mg
Phosphorus: 280mg
Fiber: 0.2g

PREP TIME
10 min

COOK TIME
20 min

SERVING
6 people

DIRECTIONS

1. Crush the garlic.
2. Combine all ingredients in a small saucepan, excluding the salmon, heat to a boil, then reduce the heat to low—Cook for about 5 minutes.
3. Preheat grill, then place the salmon with its skin side down on a sheet of foil that is a little bigger than the fish. Fold up the edges so that the sauce remains with the salmon on the grill. Place on top of the grill, the foil, and fish, then top the salmon with the sauce mixture from step 2.
4. Cover grill and cook for about 12 minutes or until the salmon has cooked (don't flip the salmon).
5. Cut the salmon into six servings.

INGREDIENTS

- 2 garlic cloves
- 1½ tablespoons of lemon juice
- 2 tablespoons of olive oil
- 1 tablespoon of unsalted butter
- 1 tablespoon of Dijon mustard
- 2 dashes of cayenne pepper
- 1 teaspoon of dried basil leaves
- 1 teaspoon of dried dill
- 1 tablespoon of capers
- 24 ounces of salmon filet

148. Omega-3 Rich Salmon

PREP TIME
10 min

COOK TIME
25 min

SERVING
2 people

NUTRITION

Calories: 265

Fat: 19.2g

Carbs: 0.5g

Protein: 22.3g

Fiber: 0g

Potassium: 23mg

Sodium: 146mg

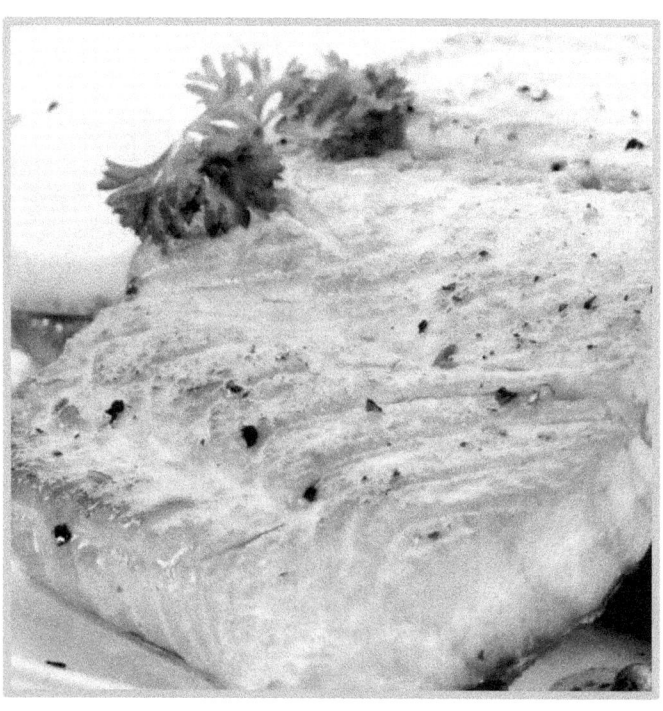

INGREDIENTS

- 2 (4-ounce) skinless, boneless salmon fillets
- 2 tbsp. of fresh lemon juice
- 1 tbsp. of olive oil
- ¼ tsp. of crushed dried oregano
- Pinch of salt
- Freshly ground black pepper, to taste

DIRECTIONS

1. Preheat the oven to 425°F. Line a baking sheet with parchment paper.
2. Place the salmon fillets onto the prepared baking sheet.
3. Drizzle with lemon juice and oil evenly and sprinkle with oregano, salt, and black pepper.
4. Bake for about 20–25 minutes.
5. Serve hot.

149. Wholesome Salmon Meal

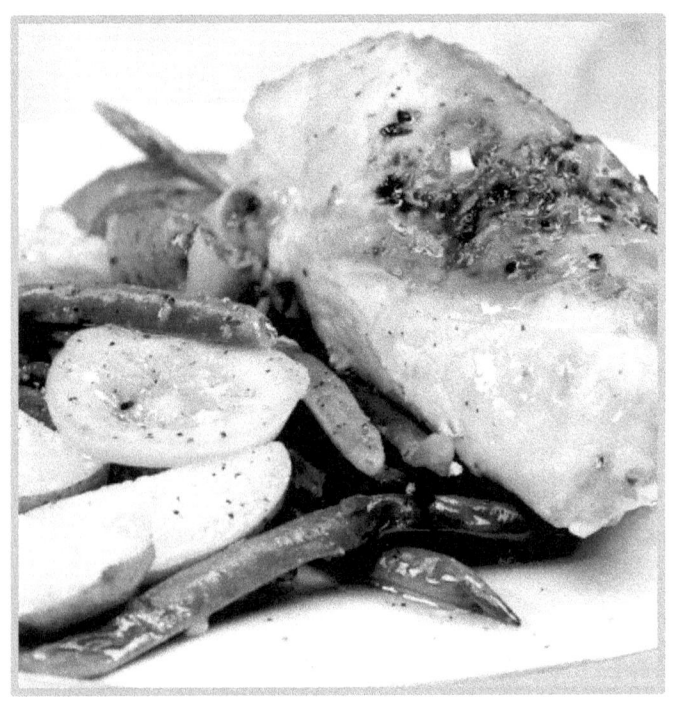

NUTRITION

Calories: 233
Fat: 14.5g
Carbs: 2.5g
Protein: 22.9g
Fiber: 0.8g
Potassium: 173mg
Sodium: 71mg

PREP TIME 10 min

COOK TIME 25 min

SERVING 6 people

DIRECTIONS

1. Preheat the oven to 425°F. Grease an 11x7-inch baking sheet.
2. Place the salmon fillets in the prepared baking sheet in a single layer and sprinkle with black pepper generously.
3. In a bowl, mix the remaining ingredients.
4. Place the mixture over salmon fillets evenly.
5. Bake for about 22 minutes.
6. Remove from the oven and keep aside to cool slightly.
7. Cut the salmon into small chunks and mix with the veggie mixture.
8. Serve warm.

INGREDIENTS

- 4 (6-ounce) (1-inch thick) skinless salmon fillets
- Freshly ground black pepper, to taste
- 2 cups of finely chopped zucchini, chopped finely
- 1 cup of halved cherry tomatoes
- 1 tbsp. of olive oil
- 1 tbsp. of fresh lemon juice

150. Succulent Tilapia

PREP TIME
10 min

COOK TIME
15 min

SERVING
4 people

NUTRITION

Calories: 149

Fat: 6.7g

Carbs: 1.1g

Protein: 21.4g

Fiber: 0g

Potassium: 17mg

Sodium: 107mg

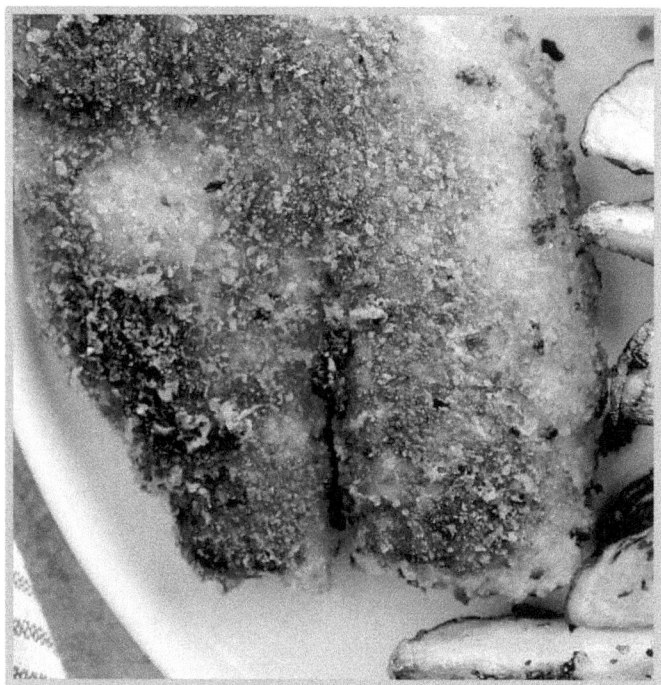

INGREDIENTS

- 2 tbsp. of unsalted margarine
- 4 minced garlic cloves
- 1 tsp. of chopped fresh parsley
- Freshly ground black pepper, to taste
- Pinch of Mrs. Dash salt-free herb seasoning
- 4 (4-ounce) tilapia fillets

DIRECTIONS

1. Preheat the oven to 350°F. Line a shallow baking sheet with a piece of foil.
2. In a large nonstick skillet, add margarine, garlic, parsley, black pepper, and seasoning on low heat.
3. Cook till melted completely, stirring continuously.
4. Remove from heat.
5. At the bottom of a prepared baking sheet, spread a little of the garlic sauce evenly.
6. Arrange the tilapia fillets over the garlic sauce.
7. Coat the top of each tilapia fillet with the garlic sauce evenly.
8. Bake for about 12–15 minutes.

151. Festive Tilapia

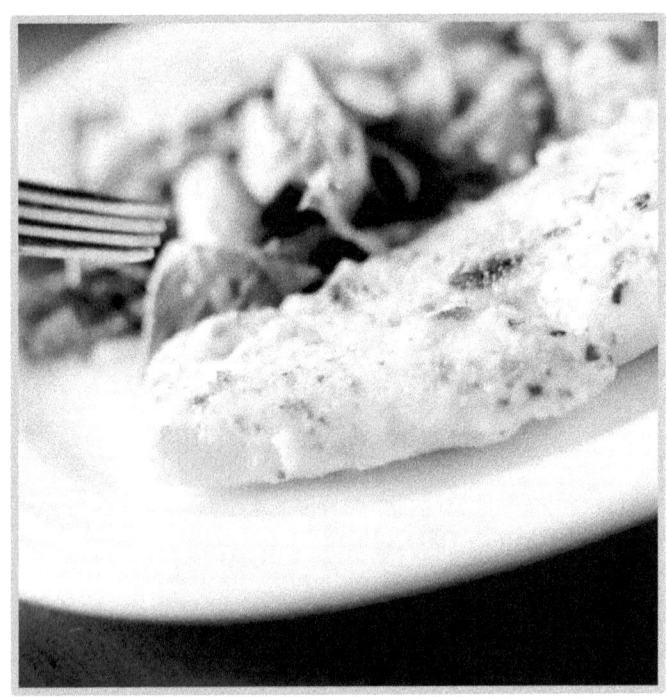

NUTRITION

Calories: 176
Fat: 9.1g
Carbs: 1.2g
Protein: 22.9g
Fiber: 0g
Potassium: 7mg
Sodium: 156mg

PREP TIME
10 min

COOK TIME
3 min

SERVING
8 people

DIRECTIONS

1. Preheat the broiler. Grease the broiler pan.
2. In a large bowl, mix all ingredients except tilapia fillets. Keep aside.
3. Place the fillets onto prepared broiler pan in a single layer.
4. Broil the fillets for about 2–3 minutes.
5. Remove from the oven and top the fillets with cheese mixture evenly.
6. Broil for about 2 minutes more.

INGREDIENTS

- 1/3 cup of shredded low-fat Parmesan cheese
- 2 tbsp. of low-sodium mayonnaise
- ¼ cup of softened unsalted butter
- 2 tbsp. of fresh lemon juice
- 2 pound of tilapia fillets
- ¼ tsp. of crushed dried thyme
- Freshly ground black pepper, to taste

Chapter 13

POLTRY AND MEAT

152. Curried Chicken Stir-Fry

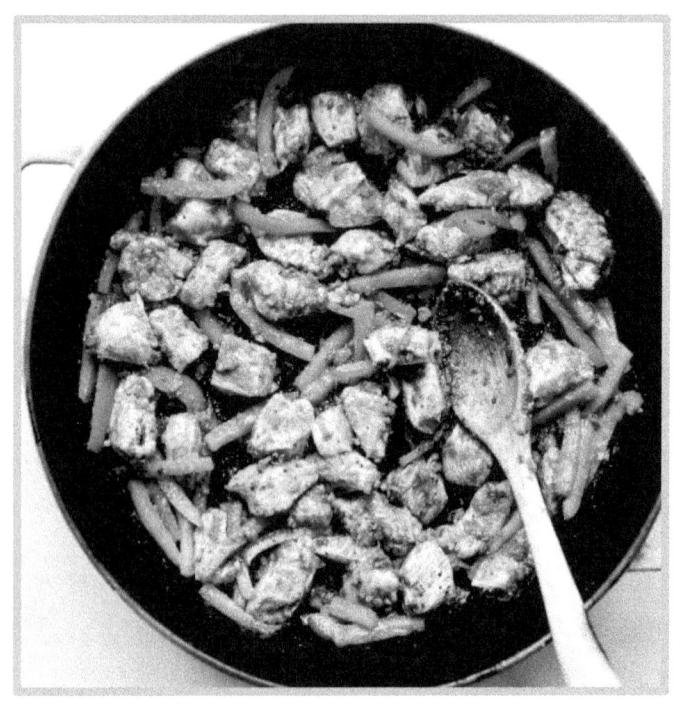

NUTRITION

Calories: 215
Total fat: 7g
Saturated fat: 1g
Sodium: 98mg
Phosphorus: 146mg
Potassium: 374mg
Carbohydrates: 19g
Fiber: 2g
Protein: 19g
Sugar: 16g

PREP TIME
20 min

COOK TIME
15 min

SERVING
6 people

DIRECTIONS

1. In a medium bowl, toss the chicken, curry powder, salt, and pepper and set aside.
2. In a small saucepan, heat the reserved pineapple juice over low heat. Let it reduce, occasionally stirring, while you make the rest of the stir-fry.
3. Heat the large skillet with olive oil in medium heat. Add the chicken. Stir-fry for 3 for 4 minutes or until the chicken is light brown; it doesn't have to completely cook. Transfer the chicken to a plate.
4. Put the onion to the skillet and cook for 3 minutes, stirring, until the onion is crisp-tender. Check to make sure the pineapple liquid isn't burning and continue to stir it. Add bell peppers then stir-fry it for another 3 minutes, until crisp-tender.
5. Put the chicken back to the skillet, add the pineapple tidbits and cook, stirring, for 3 to 4 minutes or until the chicken is cooked through.
6. Add the thickened pineapple juice to the skillet and stir. Serve.

INGREDIENTS

- 12 ounces of chicken breasts, 1-inch cubes, boneless skinless
- 2 teaspoons of curry powder
- ⅛ teaspoon of salt
- ⅛ teaspoon of freshly ground black pepper
- 1 (20-ounce) can of pineapple tidbits, strained, reserving juice
- 2 tablespoons of extra-virgin olive oil
- 1 yellow onion, chopped
- 2 red bell peppers, chopped

153. Thai-Style Chicken Salad

PREP TIME
10 min

COOK TIME
20 min

SERVING
6 people

NUTRITION

Calories: 415
Total fat: 31g
Saturated fat: 5g
Sodium: 119mg
Phosphorus: 239mg
Potassium: 408mg
Carbohydrates: 9g
Fiber: 3g
Protein: 28g
Sugar: 3g

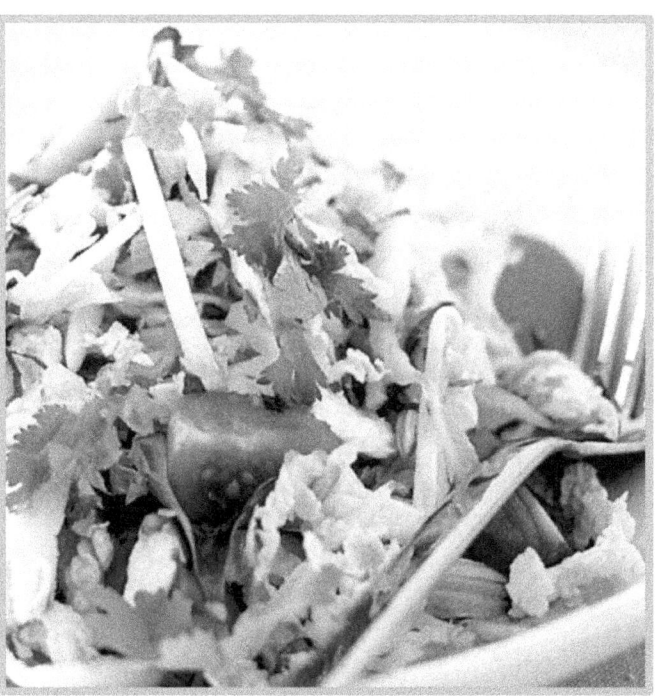

INGREDIENTS

- 3 cups (1 pound) cooked chicken, shredded
- 1 (10-ounce) package shredded cabbage with carrots
- 2 limes
- ⅓ cup extra-virgin olive oil
- ¼ cup peanut butter
- ¼ teaspoon freshly ground black pepper
- ¼ cup chopped peanuts

DIRECTIONS

1. Combine the chicken and cabbage and toss to mix in a large bowl.
2. In a small bowl, zest one of the limes. Juice both of the limes into the bowl. Add the olive oil, peanut butter, and pepper and mix with a whisk.
3. Drizzle the dressing over the salad and toss. Top with the peanuts and serve.

Ingredient Tip: If you like spicy food, add 1 or 2 minced jalapeño peppers to this salad. You could also add minced chipotle peppers in adobo sauce; just a teaspoon of each will add lots of heat.

154. Flavorful Pork Chop

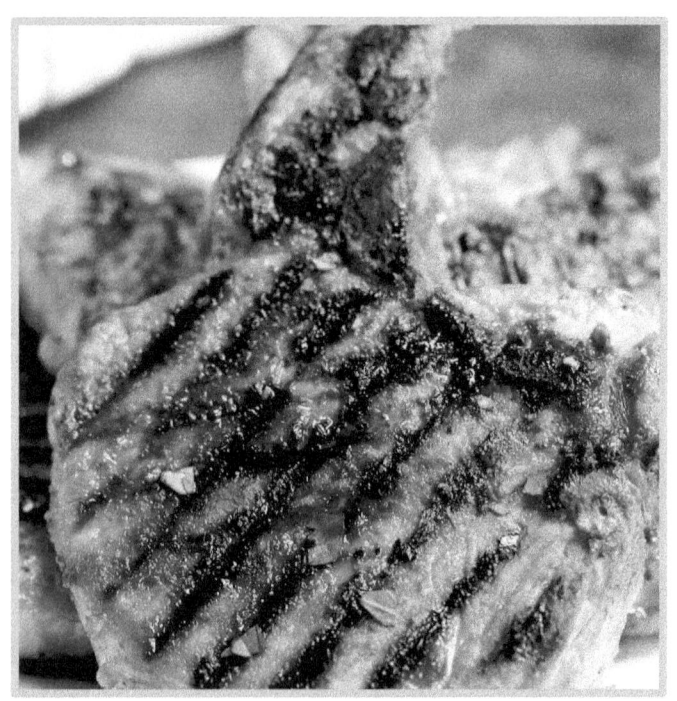

NUTRITION

Calories: 267
Fat: 13.5g
Carbs: 0.9g
Protein: 35.9g
Fiber: 0g
Potassium: 20mg
Sodium: 41mg

PREP TIME
6 min

COOK TIME
14 min

SERVING
4 people

DIRECTIONS

1. In a large bowl, mix all ingredients except chops.
2. Add chops and coat with mixture generously.
3. Cover and keep aside to marinate for about 30–45 minutes.
4. Preheat the grill to medium-high heat. Grease the grill grate.
5. Grill for about 6 minutes per side.

INGREDIENTS

- ¼ cup of minced fresh basil
- 2 minced garlic cloves
- 2 tbsp. of olive oil
- 2 tbsp. of fresh lemon juice
- Pinch of salt
- Freshly ground black pepper, to taste
- 4 bone-in pork loin chops

155. Creamy Chicken

PREP TIME
10 min

COOK TIME
15 min

SERVING
2 people

NUTRITION

Calories: 206
Fat: 10.5g
Carbs: 1.2g
Protein: 26.1g
Fiber: 0g
Potassium: 43mg
Sodium: 144mg

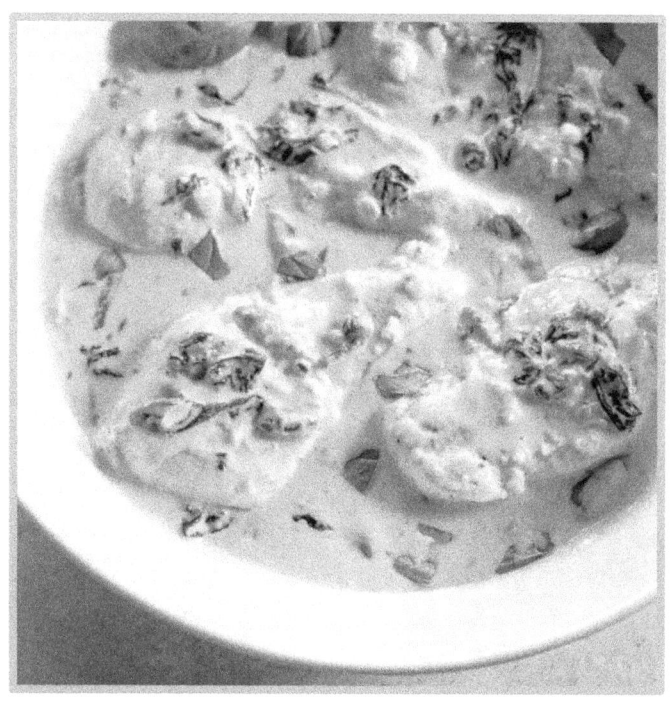

INGREDIENTS

- 3 tbsp. of unsalted butter
- 2 pound of cut into 1-inch thick strips skinless, boneless chicken breasts
- 4 minced garlic cloves
- ½ tsp. of ground ginger
- ½ tsp. of ground coriander
- ½ tsp. of ground cumin
- ¼ tsp. of crushed red pepper flakes
- ½ cup of chicken broth
- 1/3 cup of low-fat sour cream
- 1 tbsp. of chopped fresh parsley

DIRECTIONS

1. In a large skillet, melt butter on medium-high heat.
2. Add chicken and cook for about 5–6 minutes.
3. Add garlic and spices and cook for 1 minute.
4. Add broth and bring to a boil. Reduce the heat to medium-low.
5. Simmer for about 5 minutes, stirring occasionally.
6. Stir in cream and simmer, occasionally stirring for about 3 minutes.
7. Serve hot with the garnishing of parsley.

156. Fabulous Chicken

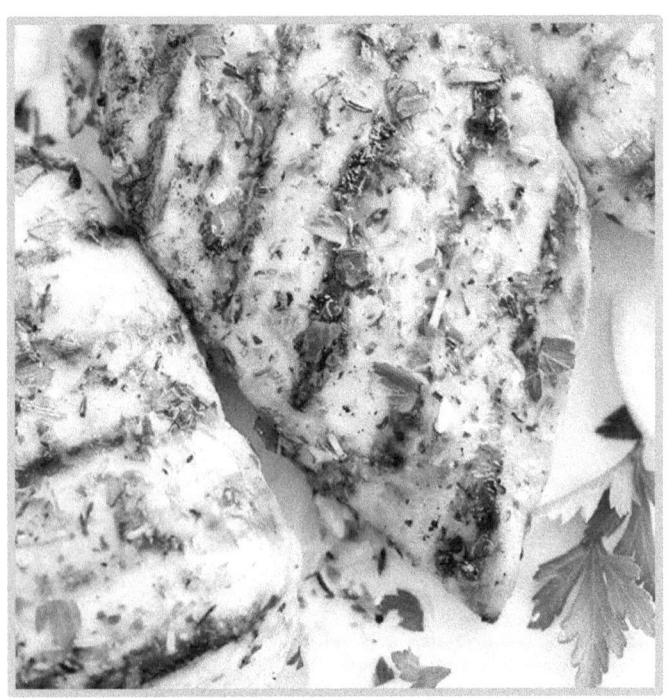

NUTRITION

Calories: 279
Fat: 11.2g
Carbs: 18.8g
Protein: 26.4g
Fiber: 3.8g
Potassium: 145mg
Sodium: 60mg

PREP TIME
10 min

COOK TIME
15 min

SERVING
8 people

DIRECTIONS

1. In a bowl, mix broth, vinegar, and cornstarch.
2. In a large skillet, heat oil on medium-high heat.
3. Add garlic and basil and sauté for about 1 minute.
4. Add chicken and sprinkle with salt and black pepper.
5. Cook for about 12–15 minutes. Transfer the chicken into a bowl.
6. In the same skillet, add pears and cook for about 4–5 minutes.
7. Add broth mixture and bring to a boil, cook for about 1 minute.
8. Reduce the heat to low.
9. Stir in chicken and cook for about 3–4 minutes.

INGREDIENTS

- 1 cup of low-sodium chicken broth
- 3 tbsp. of balsamic vinegar
- 2 tsp. of cornstarch
- 2 tbsp. of olive oil
- 4 minced garlic cloves
- 2 tbsp. of minced fresh basil
- 4 (4-ounce) skinless, boneless chicken breasts
- Pinch of salt
- Freshly ground black pepper, to taste
- 2 cored and sliced pears

157. Divine Ground Chicken

PREP TIME
10 min

COOK TIME
21 min

SERVING
5 people

NUTRITION

Calories: 164
Fat: 6.2g
Carbs: 2.9g
Protein: 23.5g
Fiber: 0.7g
Potassium: 161mg
Sodium: 99mg

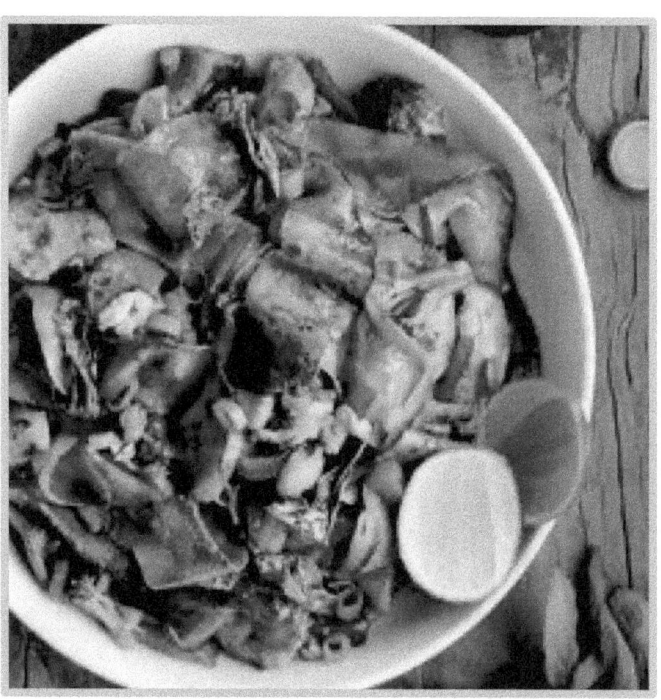

INGREDIENTS

- 1¼ pound of lean ground chicken
- 1 small sliced onion
- 2 tsp. of minced garlic
- 1 tsp. of ground cumin
- 1 tsp. of ground coriander
- 1/8 tsp. of ground turmeric
- 1/8 tsp. of cayenne pepper
- Pinch of salt
- Freshly ground black pepper
- 1 chopped medium tomato
- 1 cup of water
- ¼ cup of chopped fresh cilantro, chopped

DIRECTIONS

1. Heat a nonstick skillet on medium-high heat.
2. Add chicken, onion and garlic and cook for about 5–6 minutes or till browned.
3. Remove any excess fat from the skillet.
4. Add spices and tomato cook for about 2 minutes.
5. Stir in water and bring to a gentle boil.
6. Reduce the heat to medium-low and simmer, covered for about 10–15 minutes.
7. Stir in cilantro and serve immediately.

158. Comforting Chicken Chili

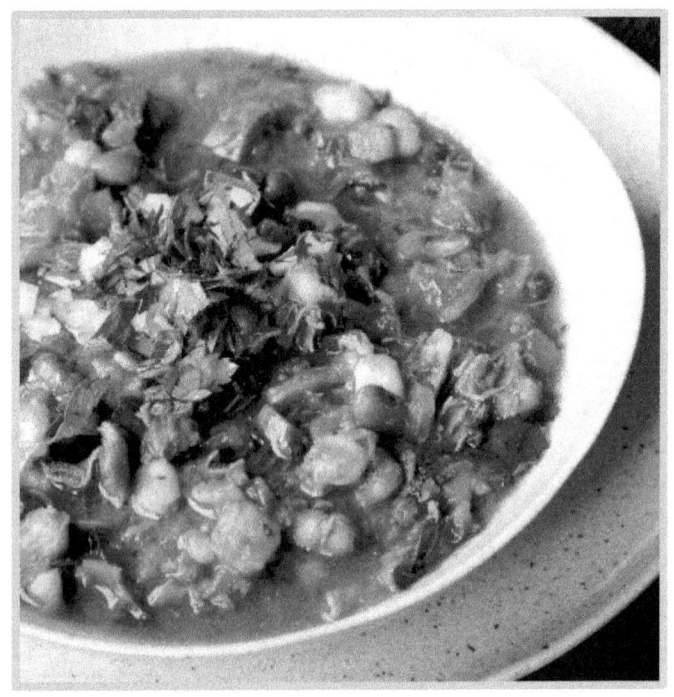

NUTRITION

Calories: 155
Fat: 6.7g
Carbs: 7.4g
Protein: 17.1g
Fiber: 1.6g
Potassium: 275mg
Sodium: 123mg

PREP TIME
10 min

COOK TIME
120 min

SERVING
12 people

DIRECTIONS

1. In a large pan, heat oil on medium heat.
2. Add onion and bell pepper and sauté for about 5–7 minutes.
3. Add garlic, jalapeño pepper, herbs, spices, and black pepper and sauté for about 1 minute.
4. Add chicken and cook for about 4–5 minutes.
5. Stir in tomato paste and cook for about 2 minutes.
6. Add broth and water and bring to a boil.
7. Reduce the heat to low and simmer, covered for about 1-1½ hours or till the desired doneness.
8. Serve hot.

INGREDIENTS

- 2 tbsp. of olive oil
- 1 chopped large onion
- 1 seeded and chopped medium green bell pepper
- 1 seeded and chopped medium red bell pepper
- 4 minced garlic cloves
- 1 chopped jalapeño pepper
- 1 tsp. of crushed dried basil
- 1 tsp. of crushed dried thyme
- 1 tbsp. of red chili powder
- 1 tbsp. of ground cumin
- 2 pound of lean ground chicken
- 8-ounce of low-sodium tomato paste
- 2 cups of low-sodium chicken broth
- 2 cups of water

159. Simple Lamb Chops

PREP TIME
35 min

COOK TIME
5 min

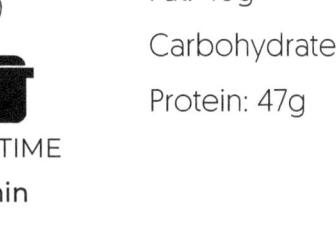

SERVING
3 people

NUTRITION

Calories: 566

Fat: 40g

Carbohydrates: 2g

Protein: 47g

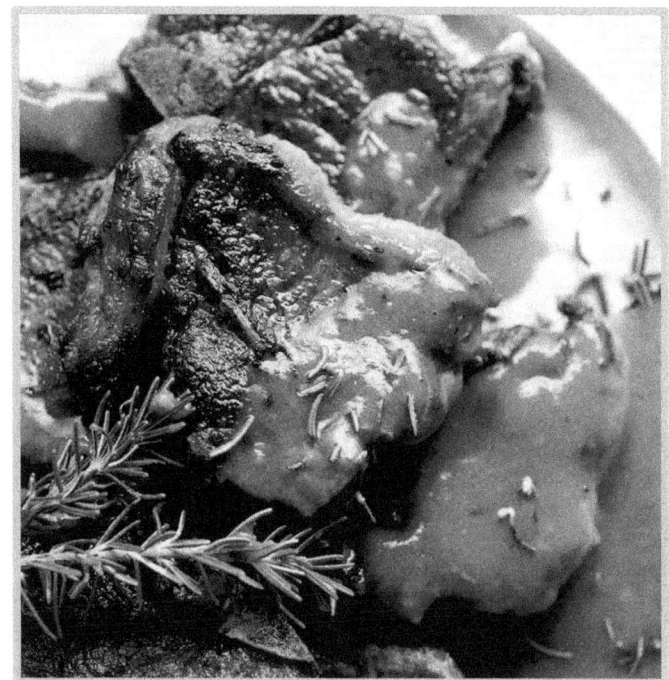

INGREDIENTS

- ¼ cup of olive oil
- ¼ cup of mint, fresh and chopped
- 8 lamb rib chops
- 1 tablespoon of garlic, minced
- 1 tablespoon of rosemary, fresh and chopped

DIRECTIONS

1. Add rosemary, garlic, mint, olive oil into a bowl and mix well.
2. Keep a tablespoon of the mixture on the side for later use.
3. Toss lamb chops into the marinade, letting them marinate for 30 minutes.
4. Take a cast-iron skillet and place it over medium-high heat.
5. Add lamb and cook for 2 minutes per side for medium-rare.
6. Let the lamb rest for a few minutes and drizzle the remaining marinade.
7. Serve and enjoy!

160. Beer Pork Ribs

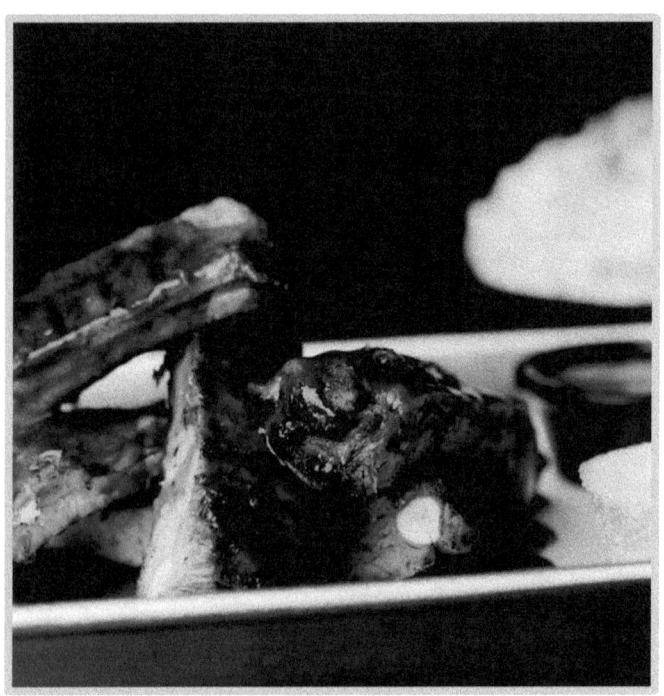

NUTRITION

Calories: 301

Carbohydrate: 36g

Protein: 21g

Sodium: 729mg

Potassium: 200mg

Phosphorus: 209mg

Dietary Fiber: 0g

Fat: 18g

PREP TIME
35 min

COOK TIME
8 hours

SERVING
6 people

DIRECTIONS

1. Wrap the pork ribs with vegetable oil and place one unit on the bottom of your slow cooker with half of the minced garlic and the onion powder. Place the other rack on top with the rest of the garlic and onion powder.
2. Pour over the root beer and cover the lid.
3. Let simmer for 8 hours on low heat.
4. Take off and finish optionally in a grilling pan for a nice sear.

INGREDIENTS

- 2 pounds of pork ribs, cut in two units/racks
- 18 oz. of root beer
- 2 cloves of garlic, minced
- 2 tbsps. of onion powder
- 2 tbsps. of vegetable oil (optional)

161. Mexican Steak Tacos

PREP TIME
10 min

COOK TIME
15 min

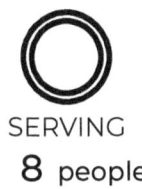

SERVING
8 people

NUTRITION

Calories: 230

Carbohydrate: 19.5g

Protein: 15g

Sodium: 486.75g

Potassium: 240mg

Phosphorus: 268mg

Dietary Fiber: 0.1g

Fat: 11g

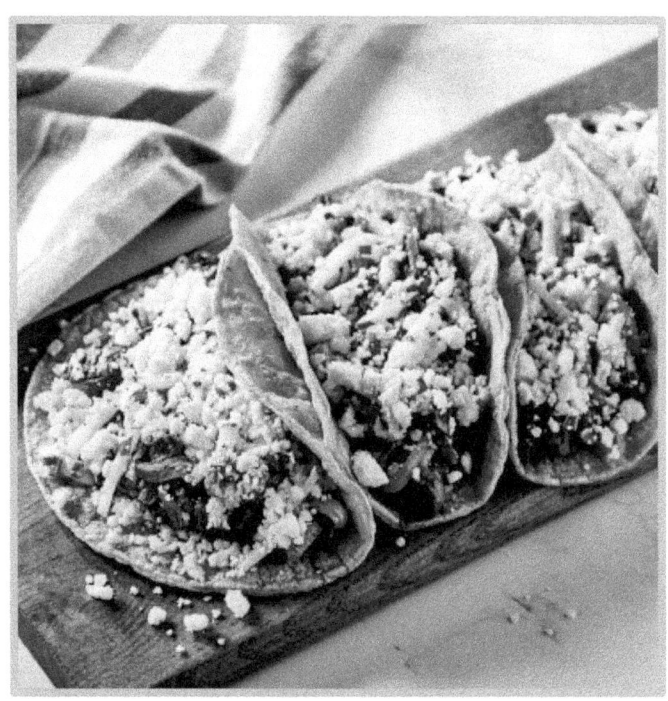

INGREDIENTS

- 1 pound of flank or skirt steak
- ¼ cup of fresh cilantro, chopped
- ¼ cup white onion, chopped
- 3 limes, juiced
- 3 cloves of garlic, minced
- 2 tsp. of garlic powder
- 2 tbsps. of olive oil
- ½ cup of Mexican or mozzarella cheese, grated
- 1 tsp. of Mexican seasoning
- 8 medium-sized (6") corn flour tortillas

DIRECTIONS

1. Combine the juice from two limes, Mexican seasoning, and garlic powder in a dish or bowl, and marinate the steak with it for at least half an hour in the fridge.
2. In a separate bowl, combine the chopped cilantro, garlic, onion, and juice from one lime to make your salsa. Cover and keep in the fridge.
3. Heat the olive oil in a medium pan. Slice steak into thin strips and cook for approx. 3 minutes on each side.
4. Preheat your oven to 350°F/180°C.
5. Distribute the steak strips evenly in each tortilla. Top with a tablespoon of the grated cheese on top.
6. Wrap each taco in aluminum foil and bake in the oven for approx. 7–8 minutes or until cheese is melted.
7. Serve warm with your cilantro salsa.

162. Mexican Chorizo Sausage

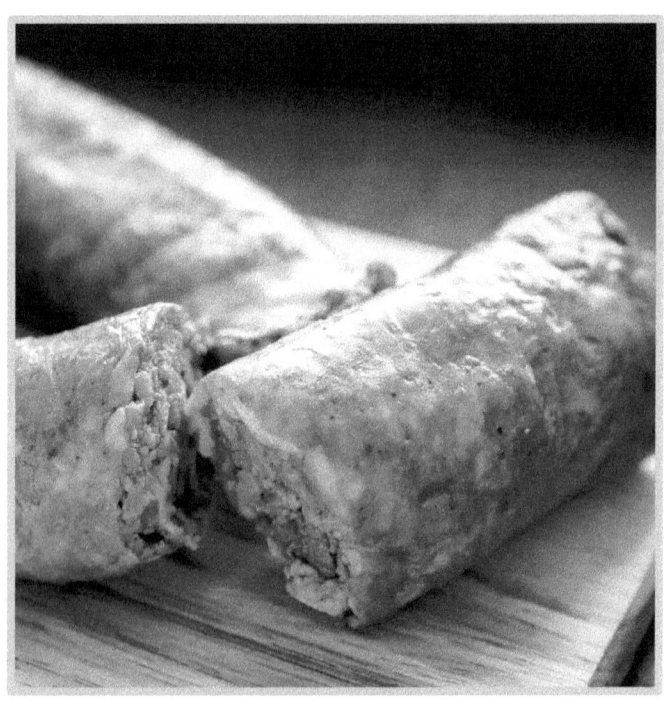

NUTRITION

Calories: 134
Carbohydrate: 0g
Protein: 10g
Sodium: 40mg
Potassium: 138mg
Phosphorus: 128mg
Dietary Fiber: 0g
Fat: 7g

PREP TIME 15 min

COOK TIME 15 min

SERVING 16 people

DIRECTIONS

1. In a large mixing bowl, combine the ground pork with the seasonings, brandy, and vinegar and mix with your hands well.
2. Place the mixture into a large Ziploc bag and leave in the fridge overnight, for all the flavors to blend with each other and for lightly curing the sausage.
3. Form into 15-16 patties of equal size.
4. Heat the oil in a large pan and fry the patties for approx. 5–7 minutes on each side, or until the meat inside is no longer pink and there is a light brown crust on top.
5. Serve hot.

INGREDIENTS

- 2 pounds of boneless pork but, coarsely ground
- 3 tbsps. of red wine vinegar
- 2 tbsps. of smoked paprika
- ½ tsp. of cinnamon
- ½ tsp. of ground cloves
- ¼ tsp. of coriander seeds
- ¼ tsp. ground ginger
- 1 tsp. of ground cumin
- 3 tbsps. of brandy

163. Caribbean Turkey Curry

PREP TIME
10 min

COOK TIME
90 min

SERVING
6 people

NUTRITION

Calories: 275

Protein: 26g

Carbohydrates: 9g

Fat: 13g

Cholesterol: 82mg

Sodium: 122mg

Potassium: 277mg

Phosphorus: 193mg

Calcium: 24mg

Fiber: 0.2g

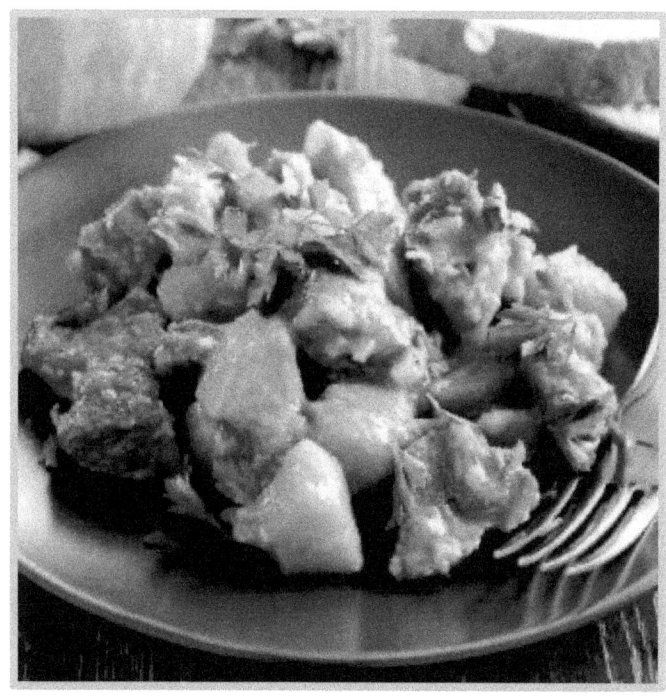

INGREDIENTS

- 3 1/2 lbs. of turkey breast, with skin
- 1/4 cup of butter, melted
- 1/4 cup of honey
- 1 tbsp. of mustard
- 2 tsp. of curry powder
- 1 tsp. of garlic powder

DIRECTIONS

1. Place the turkey breast in a shallow roasting pan.
2. Insert a meat thermometer to monitor the temperature.
3. Bake the turkey for 1.5 hours at 350°F until its internal temperature reaches 170°F.
4. Meanwhile, thoroughly mix honey, butter, curry powder, garlic powder, and mustard in a bowl.
5. Glaze the cooked turkey with this mixture liberally.
6. Let it sit for 15 minutes for absorption.
7. Slice and serve.

164. Lemon and Fruit Pork Kebabs

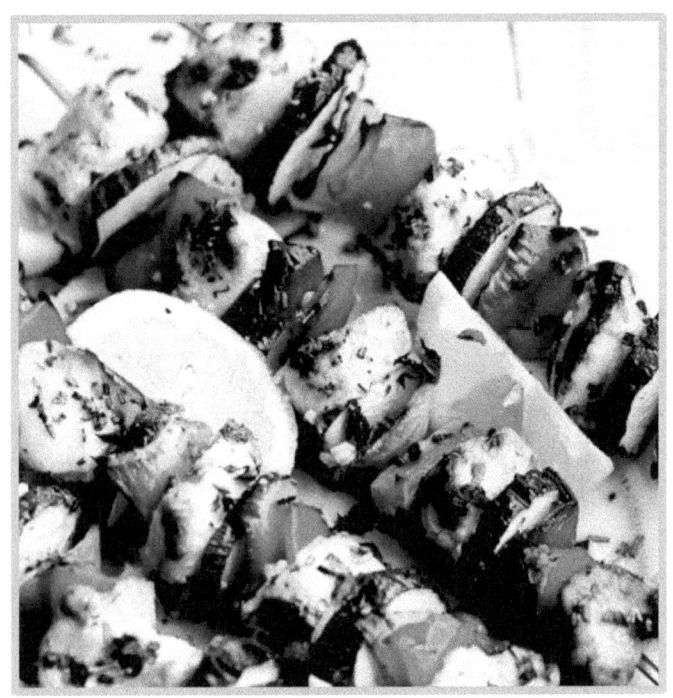

NUTRITION

Calories: 273
Total fat: 13g
Saturated fat: 3g
Sodium: 118mg
Potassium: 471mg
Phosphorus: 158mg
Carbohydrates: 22g
Fiber: 2g
Protein: 18g
Sugar: 17g

PREP TIME 20 min

COOK TIME 10 min

SERVING 4 people

DIRECTIONS

1. Prepare and preheat the grill to medium coals and set a grill 6 inches from the coals.
2. Thread the pork cubes, pineapple, peach cubes, and scallion pieces onto 4 (10-inch) metal skewers. Drizzle the kebabs with olive oil and set aside.
3. In a small saucepan, stir together the reserved pineapple juice, lemon juice, mustard, cornstarch, and brown sugar and bring to a simmer over medium heat. Simmer for 2 to 3 minutes or until the sauce boils and thickens. Remove from heat.
4. Place the kebabs on the grill. Grill for 8 to 10 minutes, turning frequently and brushing with the sauce until the pork registers at least 145°F internal temperature. Use all of the sauce.
5. Remove the kebabs from the heat and let stand for 5 minutes before serving.
6. Pork can be cooked to medium-well and still be considered food safe. Cook it to at least 145°F, measured with a meat thermometer, and let the pork stand for 5 minutes. This wait time will raise the temperature to 150°F and maintain its juiciness.

INGREDIENTS

- 8 ounces of boneless pork loin chops, cubed
- 1 cup of canned pineapple chunks, drained, reserving ¼ cup juice
- 2 peaches, peeled and cubed
- 4 scallions, white and green parts, cut into 2-inch pieces
- 2 tablespoons of olive oil
- 1 lemon juice
- 2 tablespoons of mustard
- 1 tablespoon of cornstarch
- 2 teaspoons of packed brown sugar

165. Chicken Stew

PREP TIME
20 min

COOK TIME
50 min

SERVING
6 people

NUTRITION

Calories: 141

Fat: 8g

Carb: 5g

Phosphorus: 53mg

Potassium: 192mg

Sodium: 214mg

Protein: 9g

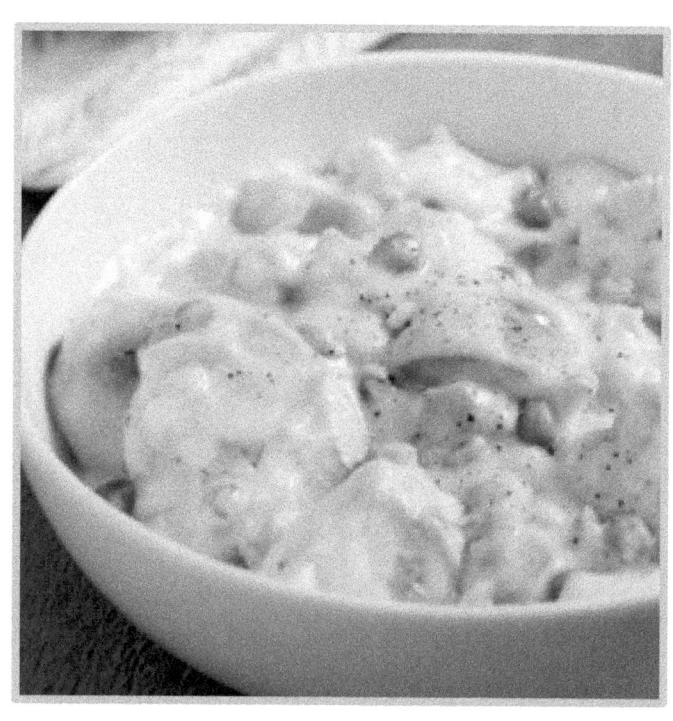

INGREDIENTS

- 1 tbsp. of olive oil
- 1 pound of chicken thighs - boneless, skinless (1-inch cubes)
- ½ sweet onion, chopped
- 1 tbsp. of minced garlic
- 2 cups of chicken stock
- 1 cup, plus 2 tbsp. of water
- 1 sliced carrot
- 2 stalks of celery, sliced
- 1 turnip, sliced thin
- 1 tbsp. of chopped fresh thyme
- 1 tsp. of chopped fresh rosemary
- 2 tsp. of cornstarch
- Ground black pepper to taste

DIRECTIONS

1. Place a large saucepan on medium heat and add the olive oil.
2. Sauté the chicken for 6 minutes or until it is lightly browned, stirring often.
3. Add the onion and garlic, and sauté for 3 minutes.
4. Add 1 cup of water, chicken stock, carrot, celery, and turnip and bring the stew to a boil.
5. Reduce the heat to low and simmer for 30 minutes or until the chicken is cooked through and tender.
6. Add the thyme and rosemary and simmer for 3 minutes more.
7. In a small bowl, stir together the 2 tbsp. of water and the cornstarch
8. Add the mixture to the stew.
9. Stir to incorporate the cornstarch mixture for 3 to 4 minutes or until the stew thick
10. Remove from the heat and season with

166. Asian Style Pan-Fried Chicken

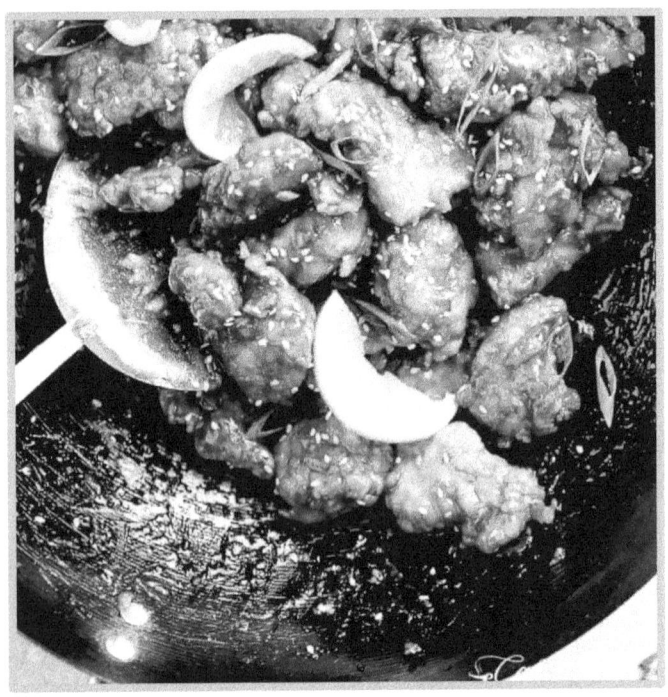

NUTRITION

Calories: 198

Protein: 17g

Sodium: 119mg

Potassium: 218mg

Phosphorus: 148mg

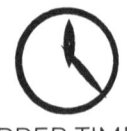

PREP TIME
10 min

COOK TIME
20 min

SERVING
4 people

DIRECTIONS

1. Mix the soy sauce, ginger, rice wine, and chicken.
2. Toss everything together and allow it to marinate for 15 minutes.
3. Toss the chicken one more time and then drain off the liquid. One at a time, dip the chicken pieces into the cornstarch so that they are coated.
4. Heat 1.5 teaspoons of oil on medium-high in a medium skillet.
5. Add in half of the chicken to the skillet and cook until it has turned golden brown on one side, around 3 to 5 minutes. Turn the chicken over and continue to cook until the chicken has cooked through and browned. Place on a plate lined with a paper towel to cool and to absorb excess oil.
6. Add in the remaining oil and cook the rest of the chicken thighs.
7. Serve the chicken with a garnish of lemon. Enjoy!

INGREDIENTS

- 1 lemon, cut into wedges
- 3 tsp. of canola oil, divided
- 1/2 cup of cornstarch
- 1 tsp. of low sodium soy sauce
- 1-inch piece of minced ginger
- 1 tsp. of dry rice wine
- 12 oz. of chicken thighs, boneless and skinless

167. Curried Chicken with Cauliflower

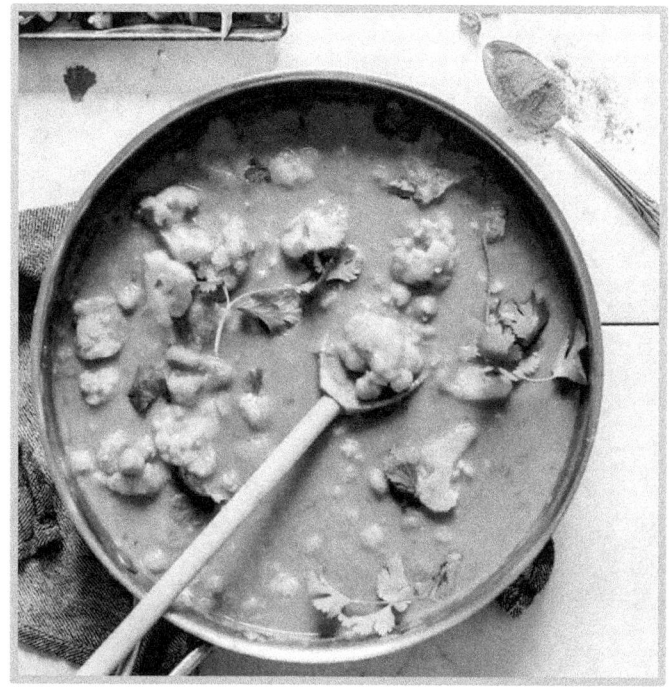

PREP TIME 20 min

COOK TIME 150 min

SERVING 6 people

NUTRITION

Calories: 175

Protein: 16g

Sodium: 77mg

Potassium: 486mg

Phosphorus: 152mg

INGREDIENTS

- Lime juice of 2 limes
- 1/2 tsp. of dried oregano
- Cauliflower head, cut into florets
- 4 tsp. of EVOO, divided
- 6 chicken thighs, bone-in
- 1/2 tsp. of pepper, divided
- 1/4 tsp. of paprika
- 1/2 tsp. of ground cumin
- 3 tbsp. of curry powder

DIRECTIONS

1. Mix a quarter of a tsp. of pepper, paprika, cumin, and curry in a small bowl.
2. Add the chicken thighs to a medium bowl and drizzle with 2 tsp. of olive oil and sprinkle in the curry mixture.
3. Toss them together so that the chicken is well coated.
4. Cover this up and refrigerate it for at least 2 hours.
5. Now set your oven to 400°F.
6. Toss the cauliflower, remaining oil, and the oregano together in a medium bowl. Arrange the cauliflower and chicken across a baking sheet in one layer.
7. Allow this to bake for 40 minutes. Stir the cauliflower and flip the chicken once during the cooking time. The chicken should be browned, and the juices should run clear. The temperature of the chicken should reach 165°F.
8. Serve with some lime juice. Enjoy!

168. Red and Green Grapes Chicken Salad with Curry

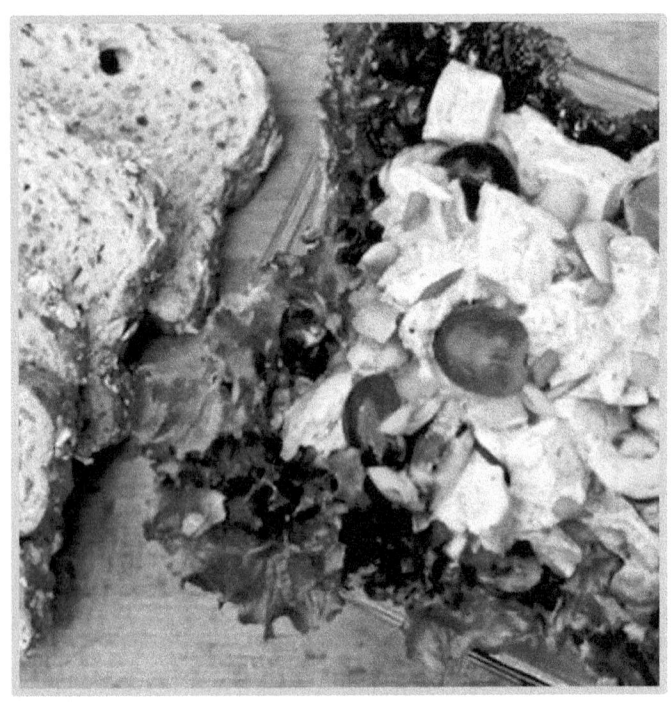

NUTRITION

Calories: 235
Protein: 13g
Sodium: 160mg
Potassium: 200mg
Phosphorus: 115mg

PREP TIME
5 min

COOK TIME
0 min

SERVING
2 people

DIRECTIONS

1. Cut the chicken into small dices and chop celery, onion, and apple. Drain and cut chestnuts.
2. Put together the chicken pieces, celery, onion, apple, grapes, water chestnuts, pepper, curry powder, and mayonnaise.
3. Serve it in a big salad bowl. Enjoy!

INGREDIENTS

- 1 apple
- 1/4 bowl of seedless, red grapes
- 1/4 bowl of seedless, green grapes
- 4 cooked skinless and boneless chicken breasts
- 1 piece of celery
- 1/2 bowl of onion
- 1/2 bowl of canned water chestnuts
- 1/2 tsp. of curry powder
- 3/4 cup of mayonnaise
- 1/8 tsp. of black pepper

169. Grilled Chicken Pizza

PREP TIME
20 min

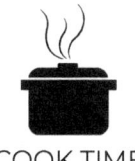

COOK TIME
15 min

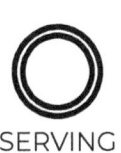

SERVING
2 people

NUTRITION

Calories: 320

Protein: 22g

Sodium: 520mg

Potassium: 250mg

Phosphorus: 220mg

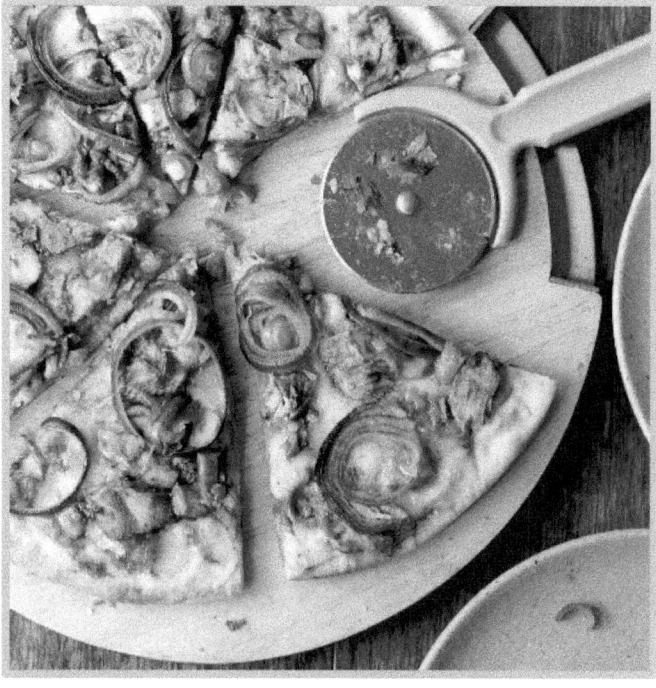

INGREDIENTS

- 2 pita bread
- 3 tbsp. of low sodium BBQ sauce
- 1/4 bowl of red onion
- 4 oz. of cooked chicken
- 2 tbsp. of crumbled feta cheese
- 1/8 tsp. of garlic powder

DIRECTIONS

1. Preheat oven at 350°F (that is 175°C).
2. Place 2 pitas on the pan after you have put non-stick cooking spray on it.
3. Spread BBQ sauce (2 tablespoons) on the pita.
4. Cut the onion and put it on pita. Cube chicken and put it on the pitas.
5. Put also both feta and the garlic powder over the pita.
6. Bake for 12 minutes. Serve and enjoy!

170. Chicken Breast and Bok Choy

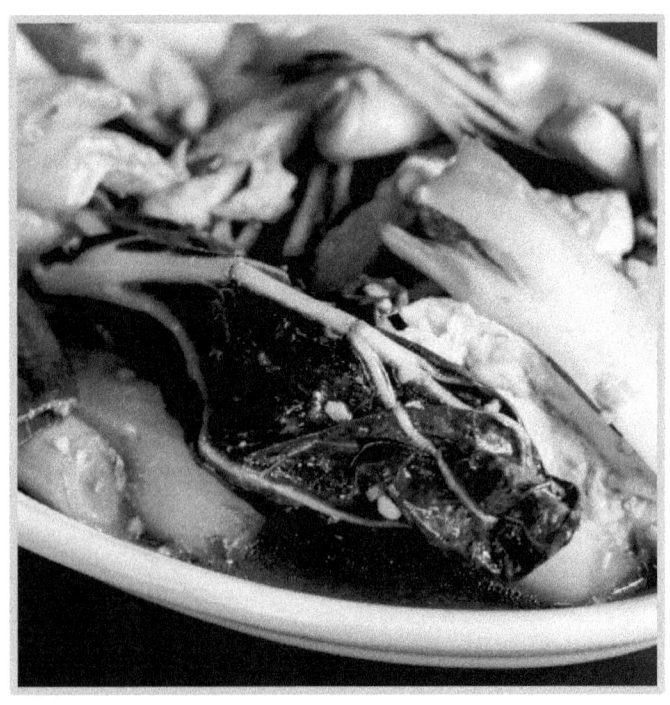

NUTRITION

Calories: 164

Protein: 24g

Sodium: 356mg

Potassium: 189mg

Phosphorus: 26mg

PREP TIME
10 min

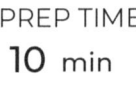

COOK TIME
30 min

SERVING
4 people

DIRECTIONS

1. Start by setting your oven to 425°F.
2. Mix the thyme, olive oil, and mustard in a small bowl.
3. Take four 18 inch long pieces of parchment paper and fold them in half. Cut them like you would make a heart. Open each of the pieces and lay them flat.
4. In each parchment piece, place .5 cup of bok choy, a few slices of leek, and a small handful of carrots.
5. Lay the chicken breast on top and season with some pepper.
6. Brush the chicken breasts with the marinade and top each one with a slice of lemon.
7. Fold the packets up, and roll down the edges to seal the packages.
8. Allow them to cook for 20 minutes. Let them rest of 5 minutes, and make sure you open them carefully when serving. Enjoy!

INGREDIENTS

- 4 slices of lemon
- Pepper, to taste
- 4 chicken breasts, boneless and skinless
- 1 tbsp. of Dijon mustard
- 1 small leek, thinly sliced
- 2 julienned carrots
- 2 cups of thinly sliced bok choy
- 1 tbsp. of chopped thyme
- 1 tbsp. of EVOO

171. Baked Herbed Chicken

PREP TIME 10 min

COOK TIME 60 min

SERVING 6 people

NUTRITION

Calories: 226
Protein: 16g
Sodium: 120mg
Potassium: 158mg
Phosphorus: 114mg

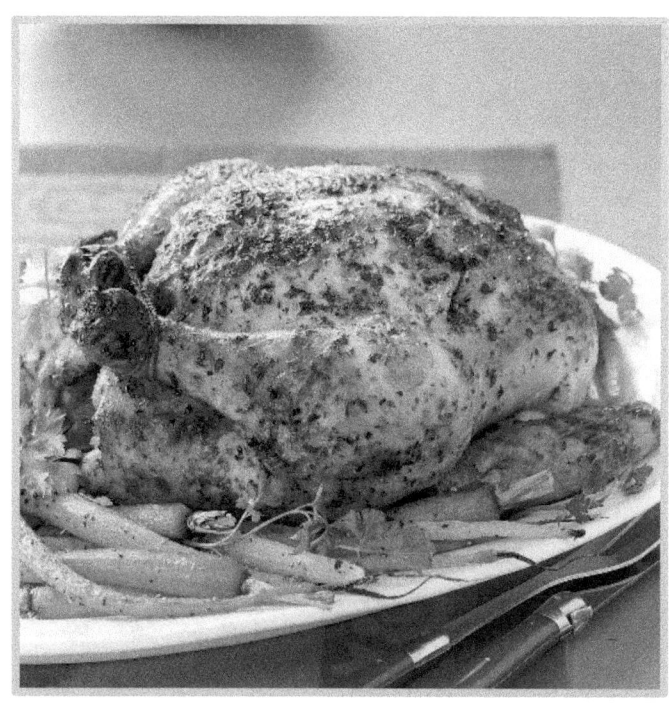

INGREDIENTS

- 1/4 tsp. of pepper
- 6 chicken thighs, bone-in
- 1 tbsp. of chopped oregano
- 1 tsp. of lemon zest
- 1 tbsp. of chopped parsley
- 4 garlic cloves, minced
- 4 tbsp. of butter at room temperature

DIRECTIONS

1. Start by setting your oven to 425°F.
2. Add the lemon zest, parsley, oregano, garlic, and butter to a small bowl and mix well, making sure that everything is distributed evenly throughout the butter.
3. Lay the chicken on a baking pan and gently pull the skin back, but leaving it attached.
4. Brush the thigh meat with some of the butter mixture and lay the skin back over the meat. Sprinkle on some pepper.
5. Bake the chicken for 40 minutes. The skin should be crispy, and the juices should be clear. Also, the chicken should reach 165°F.
6. Allow the chicken to rest for 5 minutes before serving. Enjoy!

172. Chicken and Cabbage Stir-Fry

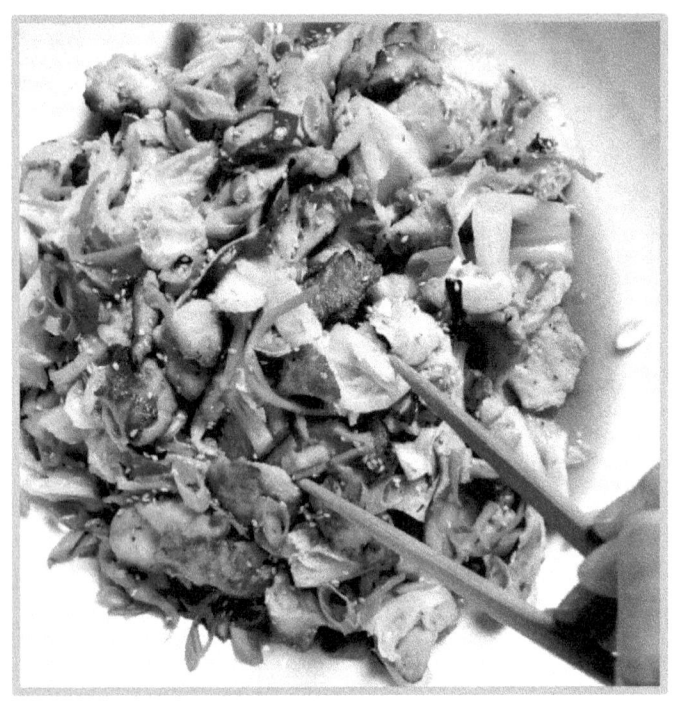

NUTRITION

Calories: 96

Protein: 15g

Sodium: 156mg

Potassium: 140mg

Phosphorus: 15mg

PREP TIME
5 min

COOK TIME
8 min

SERVING
4 people

DIRECTIONS

1. Add the oil to a large skillet and heat. Add in the chicken and cook well, often stirring until it is cooked through and browned.
2. Add the cabbage into the skillet and cook for another 2 to 3 minutes. The cabbage should become tender, but it should still be green and crisp.
3. In a separate bowl, combine the water, garlic, ginger, and cornstarch. Pour this into the skillet and cook everything until the sauce has thickened up about 1 minute.
4. Season with some pepper. Serve and enjoy!

INGREDIENTS

- Pepper, to taste
- 1/4 cup of water
- 1/2 tsp. of garlic powder
- 1 tbsp. of cornstarch
- 3 cups of thinly sliced cabbage
- 1 tsp. of ground ginger
- 10 oz. of thinly sliced boneless, skinless chicken breast
- 1 tsp. of canola oil

173. Herb Crusted Pork Tenderloin

PREP TIME
10 min

COOK TIME
105 min

SERVING
6 people

NUTRITION

Calories: 219.4

Protein: 28.9g

Sodium: 61.7mg

Phosphorus: 28.2mg

Potassium: 434.0mg

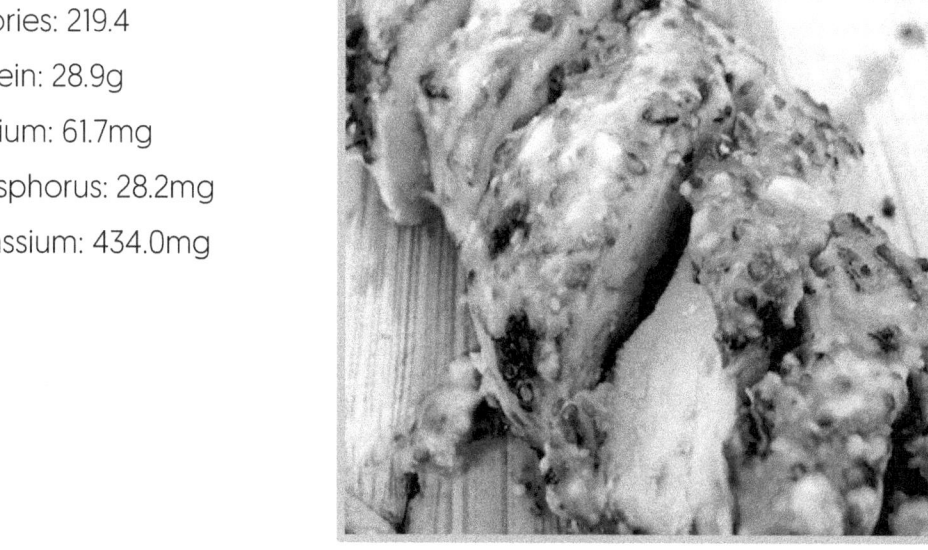

INGREDIENTS

- 4 lb. of boneless pork loin untrimmed
- 2 tbsp. of olive oil
- 4 garlic cloves, minced
- 1 tsp. of dried thyme
- 1 tsp. of dried basil
- 1 tsp. of dried rosemary

DIRECTIONS

1. Preheat oven to 450°F.
2. Place the pork loin on a rack in a roasting pan.
3. Combine the remaining ingredients in a small bowl.
4. Rub the pork loin with the paste.
5. Roast the pork for 30 minutes.
6. Reduce heat to 375°F and roast for an additional hour or until internal temperature reaches 160°F.
7. Allow to sit for 20 minutes before carving.

174. Pork and Plum Tenderloin

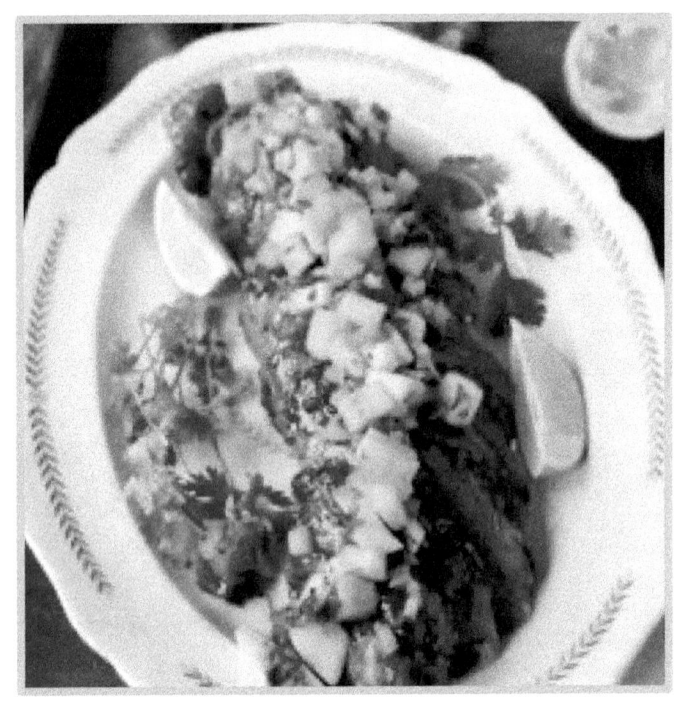

NUTRITION

Calories: 242.8

Protein: 26.6g

Sodium: 57.5mg

Phosphorus: 26.9mg

Potassium: 536.7mg

PREP TIME 20 min

COOK TIME 40 min

SERVING 4 people

DIRECTIONS

1. Preheat oven to 400°F.
2. Brush tenderloin with oil.
3. Rub garlic into the meat and place the meat on a rack in a shallow roasting pan.
4. Roast for 30 minutes or until internal temperature is 160°F.
5. For the salsa, put pulse plums, grapes, sugar, jalapeno, lemon juice, and ginger in a food processor.
6. Process until roughly chopped.
7. Transfer to a small saucepan and cook over medium heat for 2 minutes.
8. To serve, slice meat and serve with warm salsa.

INGREDIENTS

- 12 oz. of pork tenderloin
- 2 tsp. of olive oil
- 1 cup of grapes
- 2 garlic cloves, minced
- 3 fresh plums, pitted and chopped
- 3 tbsp. of lemon juice
- 2 tbsp. of sugar
- 1 seeded jalapeno pepper
- 1 tsp. of grated fresh ginger
- 1/2 cup of blueberries

175. Exceptional Steak

PREP TIME
15 min

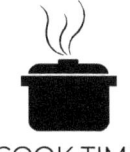
COOK TIME
31 min

SERVING
16 people

NUTRITION

Calories: 166

Fat: 7.2g

Carbs: 0.2g

Protein: 23.7g

Fiber: 0g

Potassium: 295mg

Sodium: 70mg

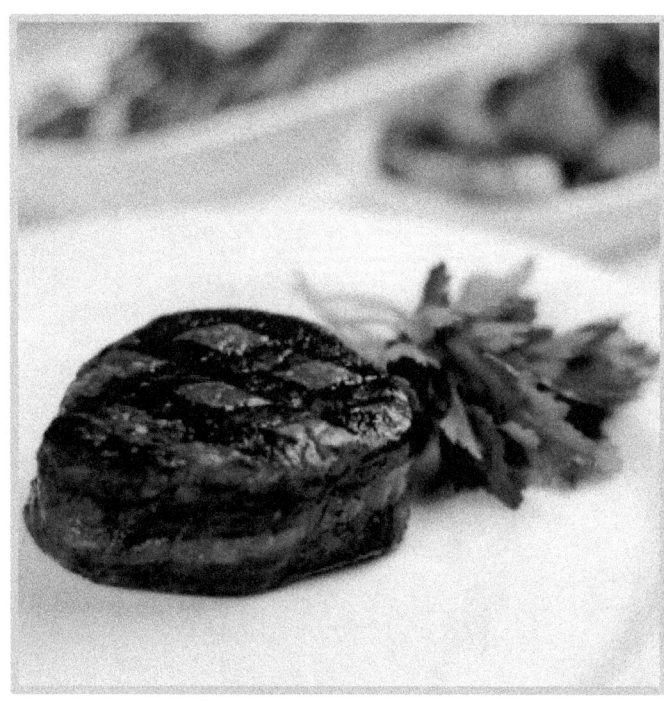

INGREDIENTS

- ¼ tsp. of ground cumin
- 1 tsp. of red chili powder
- Pinch of salt
- Freshly ground black pepper, to taste
- 1¼-pound of trimmed flank steak

DIRECTIONS

1. Preheat the grill to medium heat. Grease the grill grate.
2. In a large bowl, mix all ingredients except steak.
3. Add steak and coat with spice mixture generously.
4. Place the steak on grill over medium coals.
5. Grill for about 17–21 minutes, flipping once in the middle way.
6. Remove the steak from grill and keep aside for about 5–10 minutes before slicing.
7. With a sharp knife, cut the steak into desired size slices.

176. Chicken and Leek Salad

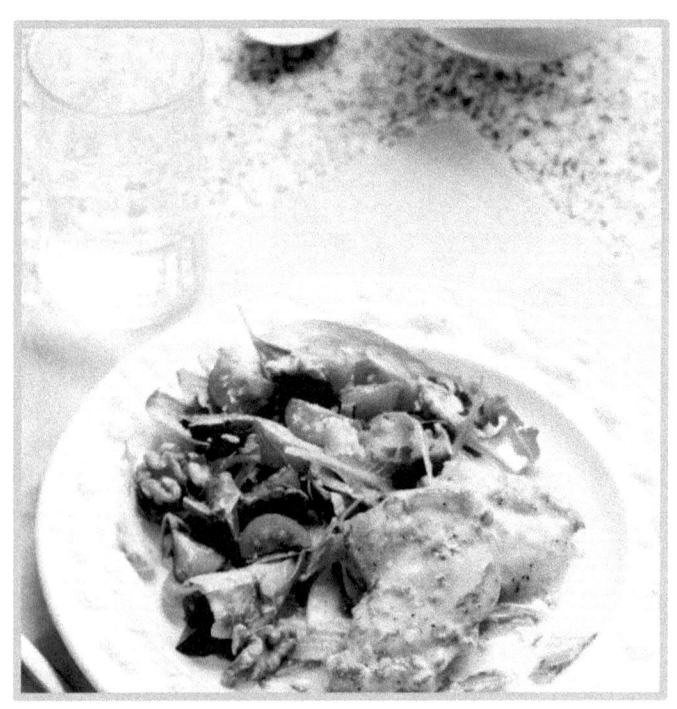

NUTRITION

Calories: 290

Total Fat: 14g

Cholesterol: 88mg

Sodium: 82mg

Potassium: 223mg

Protein: 27g

PREP TIME
15 min

COOK TIME
30 min

SERVING
16 people

DIRECTIONS

1. Rinse chicken breast fillets, pat dry, and season with salt and pepper. Heat 1 tbsp. of oil in a pan; roast the chicken meat for 4–5 minutes, turning it over. Then place in an ovenproof dish and cook in a Preheated oven at 110°C (circulating air 90°C, gas: stage 1–2) in about 8–10 minutes.
2. Meanwhile, fresh leek, wash and cut diagonally into rings, heat 1 tbsp. of oil in the pan. Brown leeks in medium heat for about 5 minutes, season with salt and pepper, remove from heat and let cool for 5 minutes. While doing so, wash apples, quarter them, core them, cut them into thin slices and drizzle with lemon juice.
3. Whisk the vegetable stock, vinegar, salt, pepper, mustard, maple syrup, and remaining oil and stir in the yogurt.
4. Take the roasted chicken from the oven and let it cool for 5 minutes. Mix the leek with the apple slices, spread on plates, and drizzle with the dressing. Slice chicken breasts in slices and place on plates. Sprinkle chicken and leek salad with paprika and sesame seeds and serve.

INGREDIENTS

- 450g chicken breast fillet
- Salt
- Pepper
- 2 tbsps. of olive oil
- 3 bars leek
- 2 small apples (300g)
- ½ lemons (juice)
- 50ml of vegetable stock
- 2 tbsps. of red wine vinegar
- 1 tsp. of mustard
- 1 tsp. of maple syrup
- 50g yogurt (3.5% fat)
- 1 tsp. of paprika
- 1 tbsp. of light sesame seeds (15g)

Chapter 14

DESSERT

177. Buttery Pound Cake

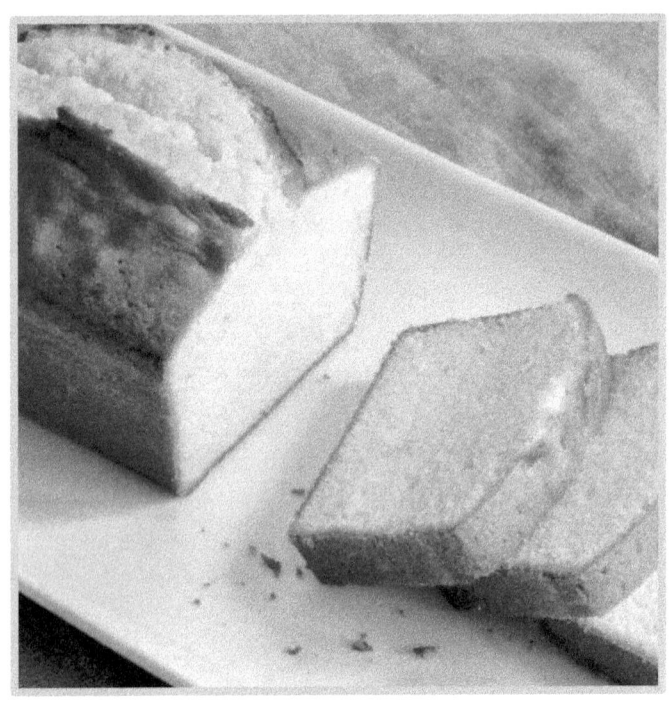

NUTRITION

Calories: 389
Fat: 20g
Carbohydrates: 50g
Phosphorus: 67mg
Potassium: 57mg
Sodium: 28mg
Protein: 5g

PREP TIME
20 min

COOK TIME
75 min

SERVING
20 people

DIRECTIONS

1. Preheat the oven to 325°F.
2. Grease your Bundt pan (10-inch) with butter and dust with flour; set aside.
3. Use a large bowl; make sure to beat the butter and sugar with a hand mixer for about 4 minutes or until very fluffy and pale.
4. Add the eggs, one at a time, beating well after each addition and scraping down the sides of the bowl.
5. Beat in the vanilla.
6. Add the flour and rice milk, alternating in 3 additions, with the flour first and last.
7. Spoon the batter into the Bundt pan.
8. Bake to 1 hour and 15 minutes or until the top of the cake is golden brown and the cake springs back when lightly pressed.
9. Cool the cake in the Bundt pan on a wire rack for 10 minutes.
10. Remove the cake from the pan to a wire rack and cool completely before serving.

INGREDIENTS

- Unsalted butter, for greasing the baking pan
- All-purpose flour, for dusting the baking pan
- 2 cups of unsalted butter, at room temperature
- 3 cups of granulated sugar
- 6 eggs, at room temperature
- 1 tablespoon of pure vanilla extract
- 4 cups of all-purpose flour
- ¾ cup of unsweetened rice milk

178. Pudding Glass with Banana and Whipped Cream

PREP TIME 10 min

COOK TIME 8 min

SERVING 2 people

NUTRITION

Calories: 255

Protein: 3g

Sodium: 275mg

Potassium: 50mg

Phosphorus: 40mg

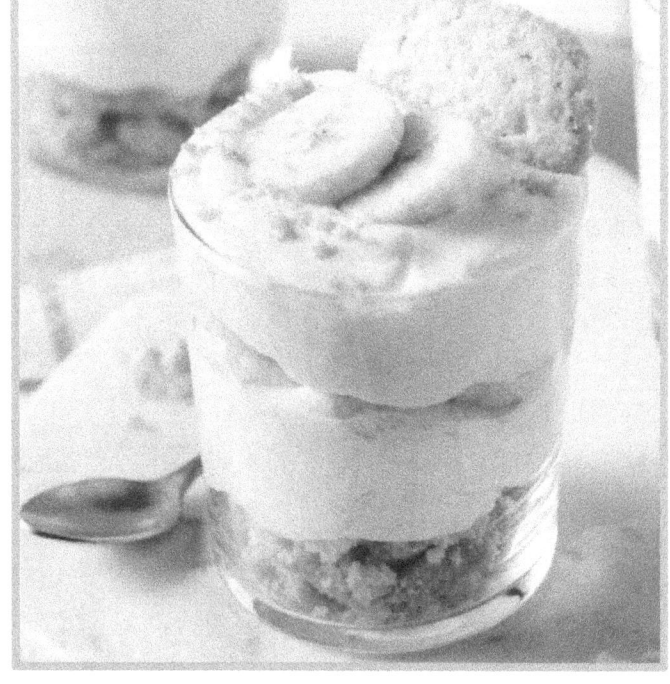

INGREDIENTS

- 2 portions of banana cream pudding mix
- 2 1/2 cups of rice milk
- 8 oz. of dairy whipped cream
- 12 oz. of vanilla wafers

DIRECTIONS

1. Put vanilla wafers in a pan, and in another bowl, mix banana cream pudding and rice milk.
2. Boil the ingredients, blending them slowly.
3. Pour the mixture over the wafers and make 2 or 3 layers.
4. Put the pan in the fridge for one hour and afterward spread the whipped topping over the dessert.
5. Put it back in the fridge for 2 hours and serve it cool in transparent glasses. Serve and enjoy!

179. Chocolate Beet Cake

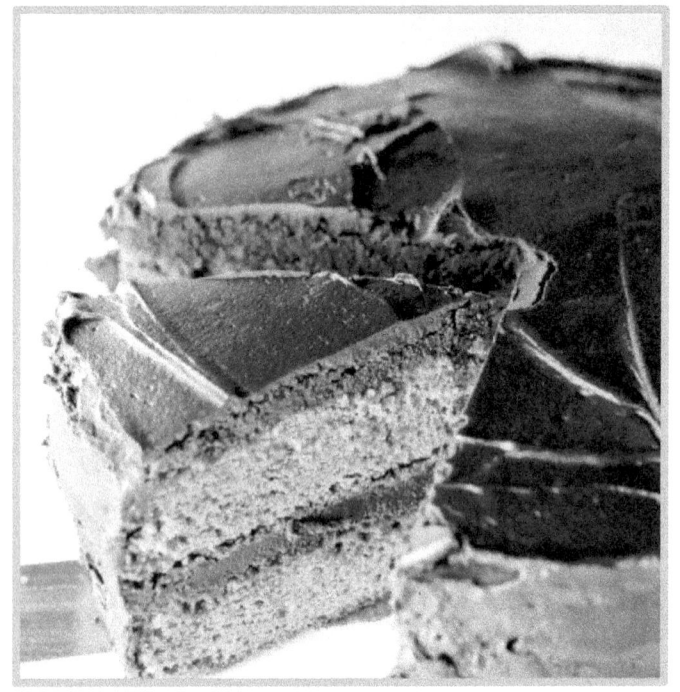

NUTRITION

Calories: 270

Protein: 6g

Sodium: 109mg

Potassium: 299mg

Phosphorus: 111mg

PREP TIME
10 min

COOK TIME
50 min

SERVING
12 people

DIRECTIONS

1. Set your oven to 325°F. Grease two 8 inch cake pans.
2. Mix the baking powder, flour, and sugar. Set aside.
3. Chop up the chocolate as finely as you can and melt using a double boiler. A microwave can also be used, but don't let it burn.
4. Allow it to cool and then mix in the oil and eggs.
5. Mix all of the wet ingredients into the flour mixture and combine everything until well mixed.
6. Fold the beets in and pour the batter in the cake pans.
7. Let them bake for 40 to 50 minutes. To know it's done, the toothpick should come out clean when inserted into the cake.
8. Remove from the oven and allow them to cool.
9. Once cool, invert over a plate to remove.
10. This is great when served with whipped cream and fresh berries. Enjoy!

INGREDIENTS

- 3 cups of grated beets
- 1/4 cup of canola oil
- 4 eggs
- 4 oz. of unsweetened chocolate
- 2 tsp. of Phosphorus-free baking powder
- 2 cups of all-purpose flour
- 1 cup of sugar

180. Strawberry Pie

PREP TIME
25 min

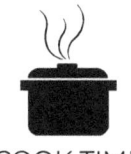

COOK TIME
3 hours

SERVING
8 people

NUTRITION

Calories: 265

Protein: 3g

Sodium: 143mg

Potassium: 183mg

Phosphorus: 44mg

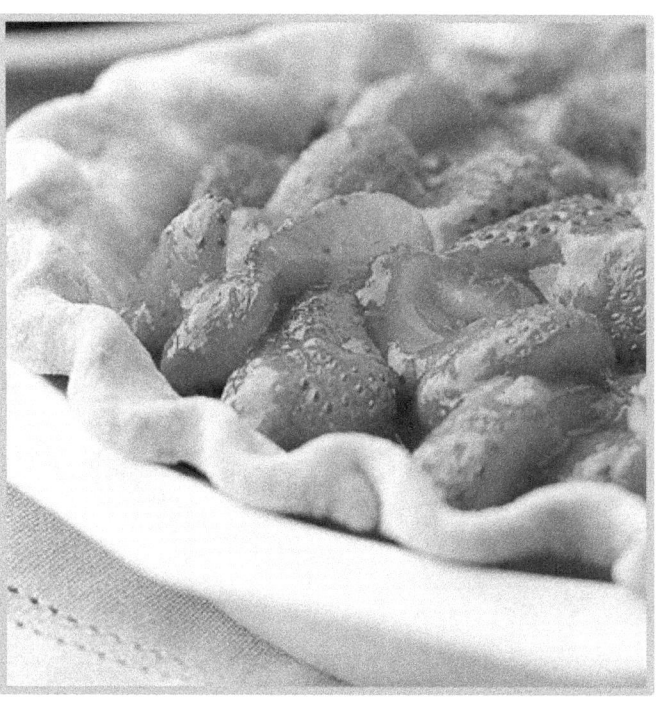

INGREDIENTS

For the Crust:
- 1 1/2 cups of Graham cracker crumbs
- 5 tbsp. of unsalted butter, at room temperature
- 2 tbsp. of sugar

For the Pie:
- 1 1/2 tsp. of gelatin powder
- 3 tbsp. of cornstarch
- 3/4 cup of sugar
- 5 cups of sliced strawberries, divided
- 1 cup of water

DIRECTIONS

For the crust:
1. Heat your oven to 375°F. Grease a pie pan.
2. Combine the butter, crumbs, and sugar and then press them into your pie pan.
3. Bake the crust for 10 to 15 minutes, until lightly browned.
4. Take out of the oven and let it cool completely.

For the pie:
1. Crush up a cup of strawberries.
2. Using a small pot, combine the sugar, water, gelatin, and cornstarch.
3. Bring the mixture in the pot up to a boil, lower the heat, and simmer until it has thickened.
4. Add in the crushed strawberries in the pot and let it simmer for another 5 minutes until the sauce has thickened up again.
5. Set it off the heat and pour it into a bowl.
6. Cool until it comes to room temperature.
7. Toss the remaining berries with the sauce so that it is well distributed and pour into the pie crust and spread it into an even layer.
8. Refrigerate the pie until cold. This will take about Serve and enjoy!

181. Grape Skillet Galette

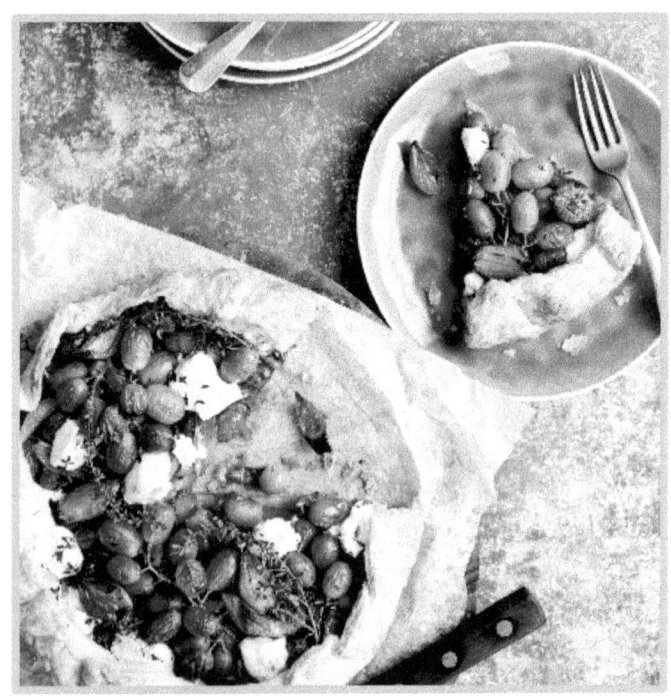

NUTRITION

Calories: 172

Protein: 2g

Sodium: 65mg

Potassium: 69mg

Phosphorus: 21mg

PREP TIME
20 min

COOK TIME
120 min

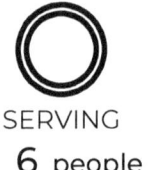

SERVING
6 people

DIRECTIONS

For the crust:
1. Add the sugar and the flour to a food processor and mix for a few seconds.
2. Place in the butter and pulse until it looks like a coarse meal.
3. Add in the rice milk and combine until the dough forms.
4. Place the dough on a clean surface and shape it into a disc.
5. Wrap it with a plastic wrap and place it in the fridge for 2 hours.

For the galette:
1. Set your oven to 425°F.
2. Mix the cornstarch and sugar and toss the grapes in.
3. Unwrap the dough and roll out on a floured surface.
4. Press it into a 14-inch circle and place it in a cast-iron skillet.
5. Add the grape filling in the center and spread out to fill, leaving a 2-inch crust. Fold the edge over.
6. Brush the crust with egg white and cook for 20 to 25 minutes. The crust should be golden.
7. Allow to rest for 20 minutes before you serve. Enjoy!

INGREDIENTS

For the Crust:
- 1/2 cup of unsweetened rice milk
- 4 tbsp. of cold butter
- 1 tbsp. of sugar
- 1 cup of all-purpose flour

For the Galette:
- 1 tbsp. of cornstarch
- 1/3 cup of sugar
- 1 egg white
- 2 cups of halved seedless grapes

182. Pumpkin Cheesecake

PREP TIME
20 min

COOK TIME
50 min

SERVING
2 people

NUTRITION

Calories: 364

Protein: 5g

Sodium: 245mg

Potassium: 125mg

Phosphorus: 65mg

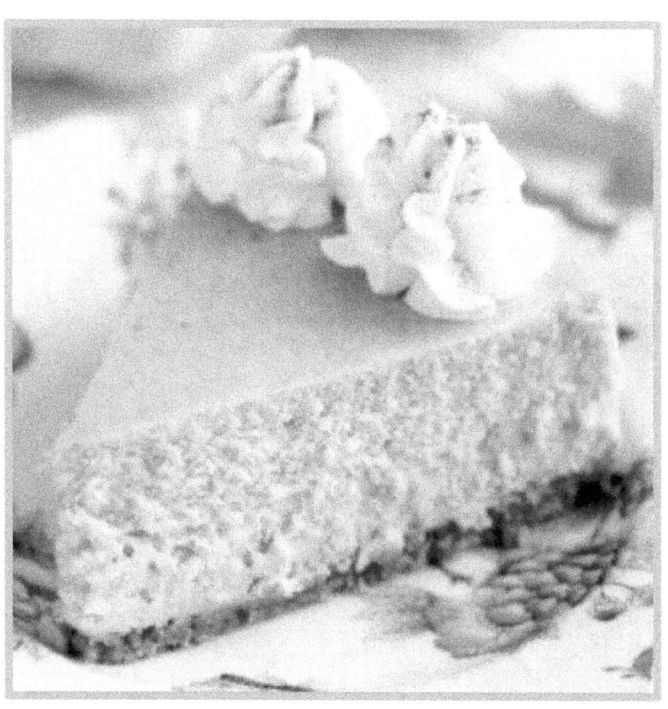

INGREDIENTS

- 1 egg white
- 1 wafer crumb, 9-inch pie crust
- 1/2 small bowl of granular sugar
- 1 tsp. of vanilla extract
- 1 tsp. of pumpkin pie flavoring
- 1/2 bowl of pumpkin cream
- 1/2 small bowl of liquid egg substitute
- 8 tbsp. of frozen topping, for desserts
- 16 oz. of cream cheese

DIRECTIONS

1. Brush pie crust with egg white and cook for 5 minutes in a Preheated oven from 375°F from 375°F now down to 350°F.
2. In a large cup, put together sugar, vanilla, and cream cheese, beating with a mixer until smooth.
3. Beat the egg substitute and add pumpkin cream with pie flavoring: blend everything until softened.
4. Put the pumpkin mixture in a pie shell and bake for 50 minutes to set the center.
5. Then let the pie cool down and then put it in the fridge. When you wish to, serve it in 8 slices, putting some topping on it. Serve and enjoy!

183. Small Chocolate Cakes

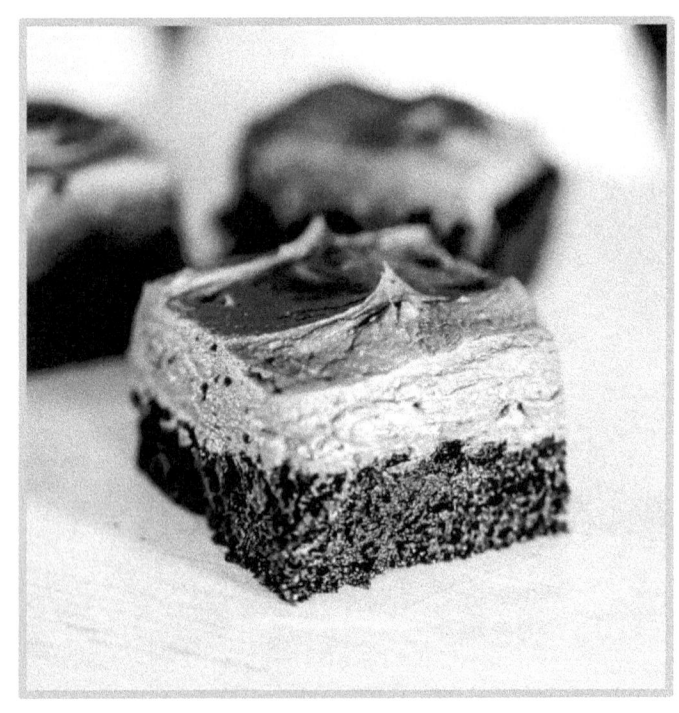

NUTRITION

Calories: 95

Protein: 1g

Sodium: 162mg

Potassium: 15mg

Phosphorus: 80mg

PREP TIME
5 min

COOK TIME
15 min

SERVING
2 people

DIRECTIONS

1. Use a transparent kitchen cooking bag and put inside both lemon cake mix, angel food mix, and chocolate chips.
2. Mix everything together and add water to prepare a small cupcake.
3. Put the mix in a mold to prepare a cupcake containing the ingredients and put in microwave for a one-minute high temperature.
4. Slip the cupcake out of the mold and put it on a dish, let it cool, and put some more chocolate crumbs on it. Serve and enjoy!

INGREDIENTS

- 1 box of angel food cake mix
- 1 box of lemon cake mix
- Water
- Non-stick cooking spray or batter
- Dark chocolate small squared chops and chocolate powder

184. Strawberry Whipped Cream Cake

PREP TIME
10 min

COOK TIME
20 min

SERVING
2 people

NUTRITION

Calories: 355

Protein: 4g

Sodium: 275mg

Potassium: 145mg

Phosphorus: 145mg

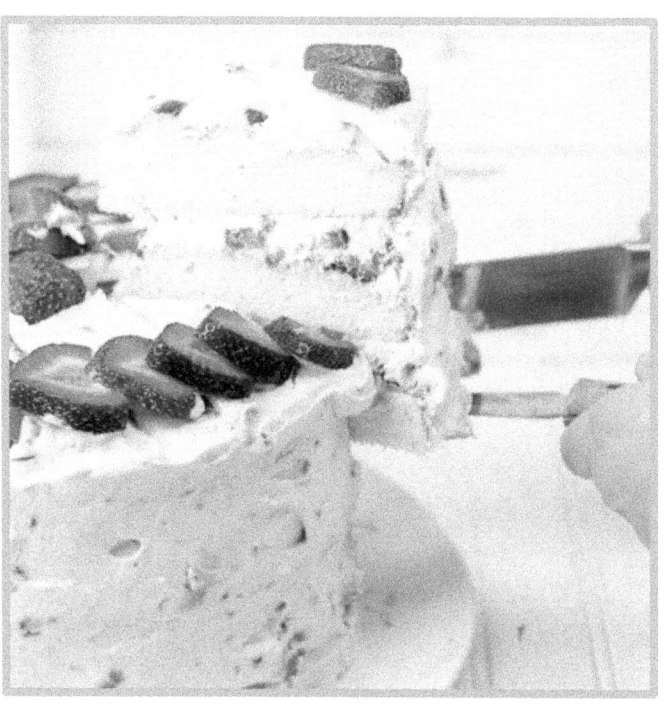

INGREDIENTS

- 1 pint of whipping cream
- 2 tbsp. of gelatin
- 1/2 glass of cold water
- 1 glass of boiling water
- 3 tbsp. of lemon juice
- 1 orange glass juice
- 1 tsp. of sugar
- 3/4 cup of sliced strawberries
- 1 large angel food cake or light sponge cake

DIRECTIONS

1. Put the gelatin in cold water, then add hot water and blend. Add orange and lemon juice, also add some sugar and go on blending.
2. Refrigerate and leave it there until you see it is starting to gel.
3. Whip half portion of cream and add it to the mixture along with strawberries, put wax paper in the bowl, and cut the cake in small pieces.
4. In between the pieces, add the whipped cream and put everything in the fridge for one night.
5. When you take out the cake, add some whipped cream on top and decorate with some more fruit. Serve and enjoy!

185. Sweet Cracker Pie Crust

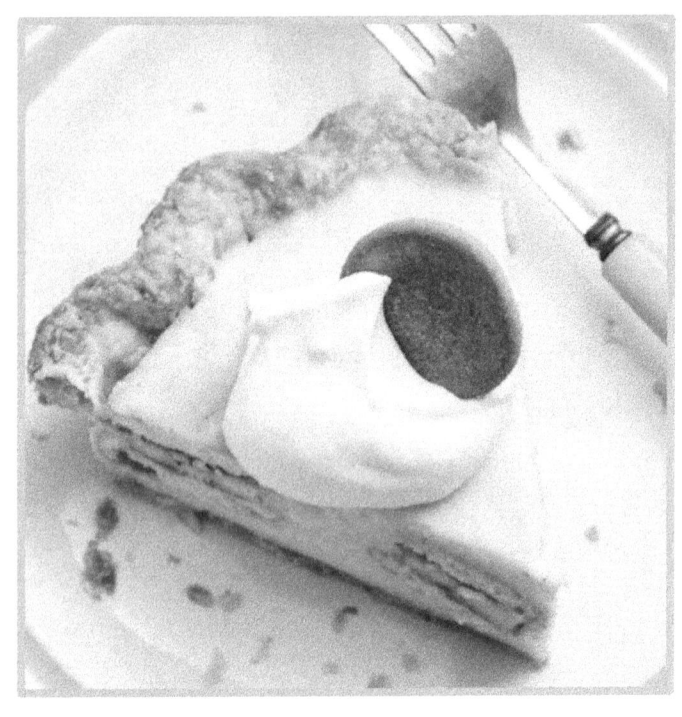

NUTRITION

Calories: 205

Protein: 2g

Sodium: 208mg

Potassium: 67mg

Phosphorus: 22mg

PREP TIME
5 min

COOK TIME
10 min

SERVING
2 people

DIRECTIONS

1. Mix sweet cracker crumbs, butter, and sugar.
2. Put in the over Preheat at 375°F.
3. Bake for 7 minutes, putting it in a greased pie.
4. Let the pie cool before adding any kind of filling. Serve and enjoy!

INGREDIENTS

- 1 bowl of gelatin cracker crumbs
- 1/4 small cup of sugar
- Unsalted butter

186. Old-Fashioned Apple Kuchen

PREP TIME
25 min

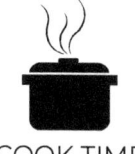
COOK TIME
60 min

SERVING
16 people

NUTRITION

Calories: 368

Fat: 16g

Carbohydrates: 53g

Phosphorus: 46mg

Potassium: 68mg

Sodium: 15mg

Protein: 3g

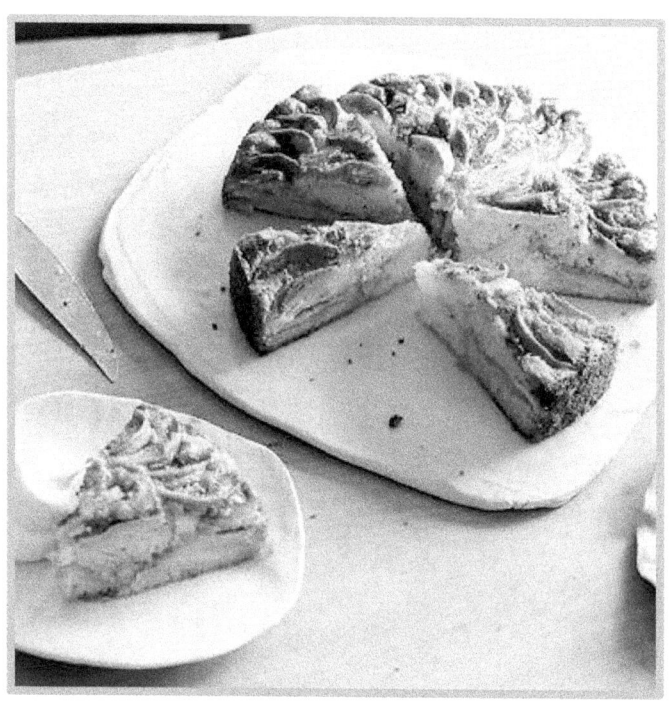

INGREDIENTS

- Unsalted butter, for greasing the baking sheet
- 1 cup of unsalted butter, at room temperature
- 2 cups of granulated sugar
- 2 eggs, beaten
- 2 teaspoons of pure vanilla extract
- 2 cups of all-purpose flour
- 1 teaspoon of Ener-G baking soda substitute
- 2 teaspoons of ground cinnamon
- ½ teaspoon of ground nutmeg
- Pinch ground allspice
- 2 large apples (about 3 cups) peeled, cored, and diced

DIRECTIONS

1. Preheat the oven to 350°F.
2. Grease a 9-by-13-inch glass baking sheet; set aside.
3. Cream together the butter and sugar with a hand mixer until light and fluffy, for about 3 minutes.
4. Add the eggs and vanilla and beat until combined, scraping down the sides of the bowl, about 1 minute.
5. Stir the flour, baking soda substitute, cinnamon, nutmeg, and allspice all together using a large bowl.
6. Add all the dry ingredients in your wet ingredients, then stir to combine everything.
7. Stir in the apple and spoon the batter into the baking sheet.
8. Bake for about 1 hour or until the cake is golden.
9. Cool the cake on a wire rack.
10. Serve warm or chilled.

187. Carob Angel Food Cake

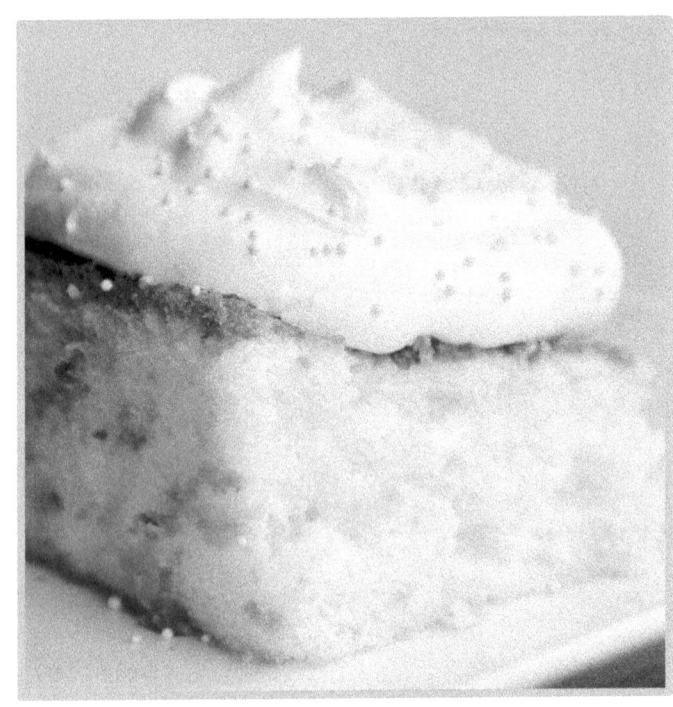

NUTRITION

Calories: 113
Fat: 0g
Carbohydrates: 25g
Phosphorus: 11mg
Potassium: 108mg
Sodium: 42mg
Protein: 3g

PREP TIME
30 min

COOK TIME
30 min

SERVING
16 people

DIRECTIONS

1. Preheat the oven to 375°F.
2. Sift the all-purpose flour, carob flour, and ¾ cup of the sugar together in a medium bowl then set aside.
3. Beat your egg whites then cream of tartar with a hand mixer for about 5 minutes or until soft peaks form.
4. Add the remaining ¾ cup sugar by the tablespoon to the egg whites until all the sugar is used up and stiff peaks form.
5. Fold in the flour mixture and vanilla.
6. Prepare the angel food cake pan and spoon the batter into it.
7. Run a knife through the batter to remove any air pockets.
8. Bake the cake for about 30 minutes or until the top springs back when pressed lightly.
9. Invert the pan onto a wire rack to cool.
10. Remove the cake from the pan.

INGREDIENTS

- ¾ cup of all-purpose flour
- ¼ cup of carob flour
- 1½ cups of sugar, divided
- 12 large egg whites, at room temperature
- 1½ teaspoons of cream of tartar
- 2 teaspoons of vanilla

188. Elegant Lavender Cookies

PREP TIME
10 min

COOK TIME
15 min

SERVING
24 cookies

NUTRITION

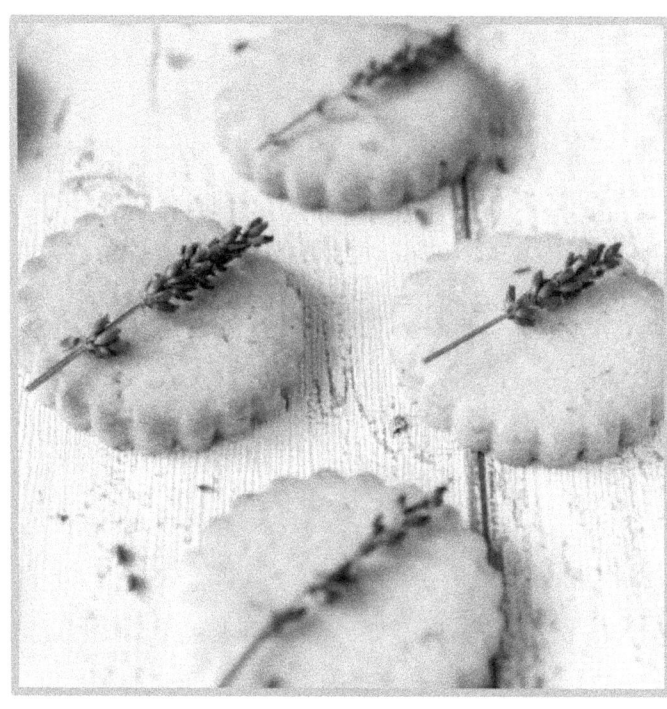

INGREDIENTS

- 5 dried organic lavender flowers, the entire top of the flower
- ½ cup of granulated sugar
- 1 cup of unsalted butter, at room temperature
- 2 cups of all-purpose flour
- 1 cup of rice flour

DIRECTIONS

1. Strip the tiny lavender flowers off the main stem carefully and place the flowers and granulated sugar into a food processor or blender. Pulse until the mixture is finely chopped.
2. Beat your egg whites, then cream of tartar with cream together the butter and lavender sugar until it is very fluffy in a medium bowl.
3. Mix the flours into the creamed mixture until the mixture resembles fine crumbs.
4. Gather the dough together into a ball and then roll it into a long log.
5. Wrap the cookie dough in plastic and refrigerate it for about 1 hour or until firm.
6. Preheat the oven to 375°F.
7. Slice the chilled dough into ¼-inch rounds and refrigerate it for 1 hour or until firm.
8. Bake for 15 to 18 minutes or until your cookies are very pale, golden brown.
9. Let the cookies cool.
10. Store the cookies at room temperature in a sealed container for up to 1 week.

189. Gingerbread Loaf

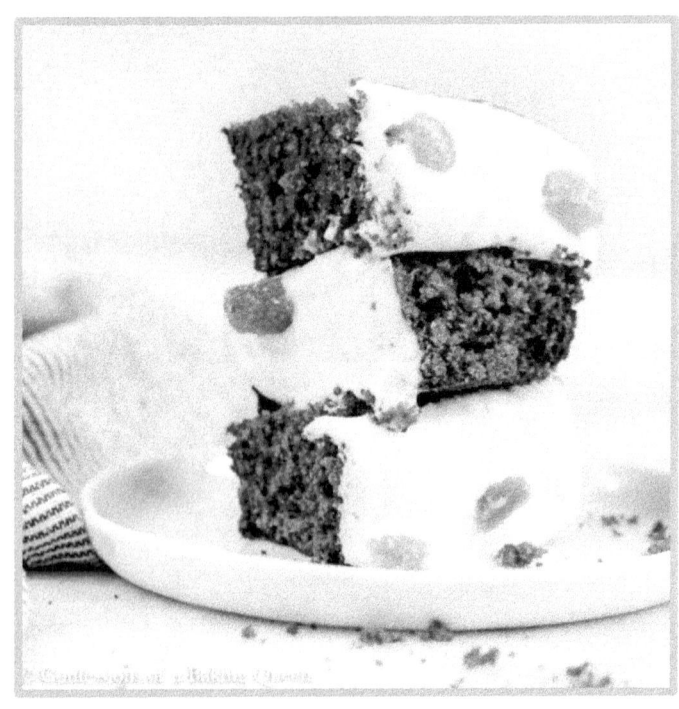

NUTRITION

Calories: 232
Fat: 5g
Carbohydrates: 42g
Phosphorus: 54mg
Potassium: 104mg
Sodium: 18mg
Protein: 4g

PREP TIME 20 min

COOK TIME 60 min

SERVING 16 people

DIRECTIONS

1. Preheat the oven to 350°F.
2. Prepare a 9-by-13-inch baking sheet and grease it with butter; set aside.
3. In a large bowl, sift together the flour, baking soda substitute, cinnamon, and allspice.
4. Stir the sugar into the flour mixture.
5. In a medium bowl, whisk together the milk, egg, olive oil, molasses, and ginger until well blended.
6. In the flour mixture, put a hole in the middle and pour in the wet ingredients.
7. Mix until combined, but do not overmix.
8. Use baking sheet to pour the batter into and bake for about 1 hour or until a wooden pick inserted in the middle comes out clean.
9. Dust it with powdered sugar
10. Serve warm.

INGREDIENTS

- Unsalted butter, for greasing the baking sheet
- 3 cups of all-purpose flour
- ½ teaspoon of Ener-G baking soda substitute
- 2 teaspoons of ground cinnamon
- 1 teaspoon of ground allspice
- ¾ cup of granulated sugar
- 1¼ cups of plain rice milk
- 1 large egg
- ¼ cup of olive oil
- 2 tablespoons of molasses
- 2 teaspoons of grated fresh ginger
- Powdered sugar, for dusting

190. Rhubarb Crumble

NUTRITION

- Calories: 450
- Fat: 23g
- Carbohydrates: 60g
- Phosphorus: 51mg
- Potassium: 181mg
- Sodium: 10mg
- Protein: 4g

PREP TIME 15 min
COOK TIME 30 min
SERVING 6 people

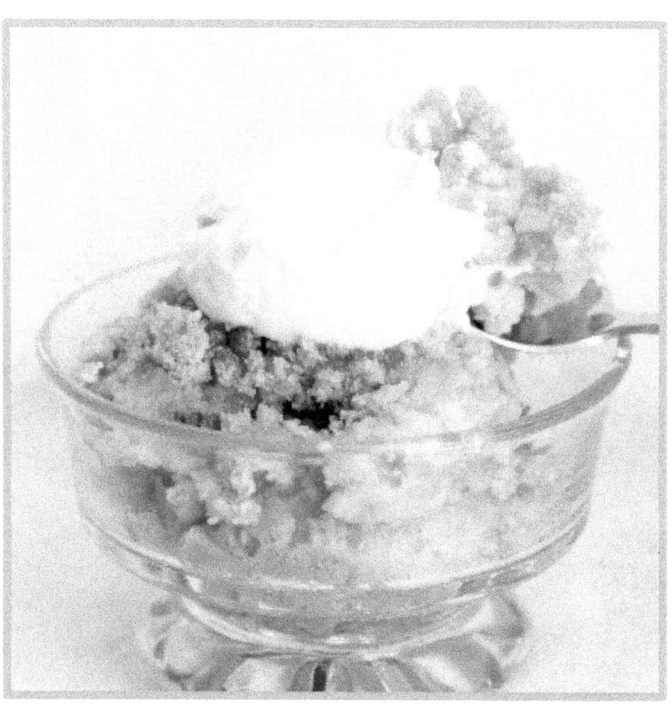

INGREDIENTS

- Unsalted butter, for greasing the baking sheet
- 1 cup of all-purpose flour
- ½ cup of brown sugar
- ½ teaspoon of ground cinnamon
- ½ cup of unsalted butter, at room temperature
- 1 cup of chopped rhubarb
- 2 apples, peeled, cored, and sliced thin
- 2 tablespoons of granulated sugar
- 2 tablespoons of water

DIRECTIONS

1. Preheat the oven to 325°F.
2. Grease the 8-by-8-inch lightly in a baking sheet with butter then set aside.
3. Combine the flour, sugar, and cinnamon until well combined in a small bowl.
4. Add the butter and rub the mixture between your fingers until it resembles coarse crumbs.
5. In a medium saucepan, mix the rhubarb, apple, sugar, and water over medium heat and cook for about 20 minutes or until the rhubarb is soft.
6. Put the fruit mixture in the baking sheet and evenly top with the crumble.
7. Bake the crumble for 20 to 30 minutes or until golden brown.
8. Serve hot.

191. Honey Bread Pudding

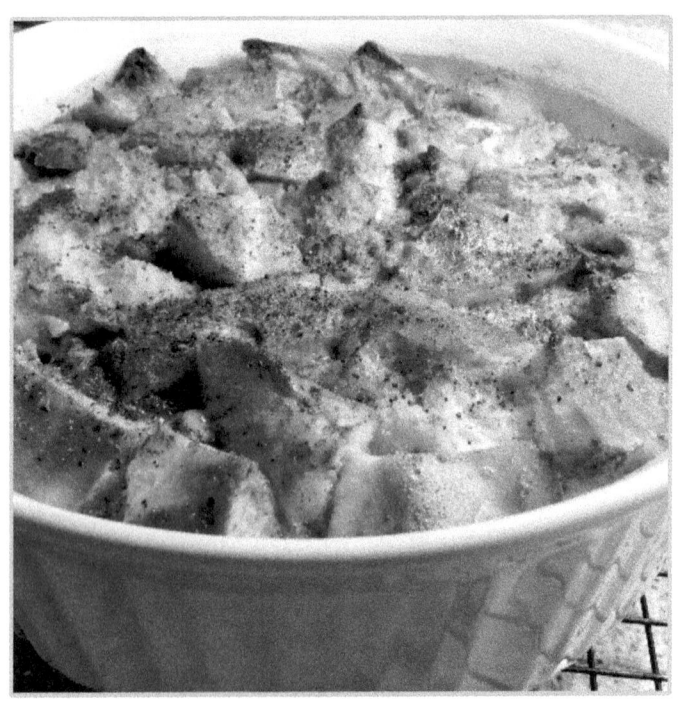

NUTRITION

Calories: 167
Fat: 3g
Carbohydrates: 30g
Phosphorus: 95mg
Potassium: 93mg
Sodium: 189mg
Protein: 6g

PREP TIME
15 min

COOK TIME
40 min

SERVING
6 people

DIRECTIONS

1. Grease the 8-by-8-inch lightly in a baking sheet with butter then set aside.
2. Whisk together the rice milk, eggs, egg whites, honey, and vanilla in a medium bowl.
3. Add the bread cubes and stir until the bread is coated.
4. Transfer the mixture to the baking sheet and cover with plastic wrap.
5. Store the dish in the refrigerator at least 3 hours.
6. Preheat the oven to 325°F.
7. Take the plastic wrap from the baking sheet and bake the pudding for 35 to 40 minutes or until golden brown and a knife inserted in the center comes out clean.
8. Serve warm.

INGREDIENTS

- Unsalted butter, for greasing the baking sheet
- 1½ cups of plain rice milk
- 2 eggs
- 2 large egg whites
- ¼ cup of honey
- 1 teaspoon of pure vanilla extract
- 6 cups of cubed white bread

192. Vanilla-Infused Couscous Pudding

PREP TIME
20 min

COOK TIME
20 min

SERVING
6 people

NUTRITION

Calories: 334

Fat: 1g

Carbohydrates: 77g

Phosphorus: 119mg

Potassium: 118mg

Sodium: 41mg

Protein: 6g

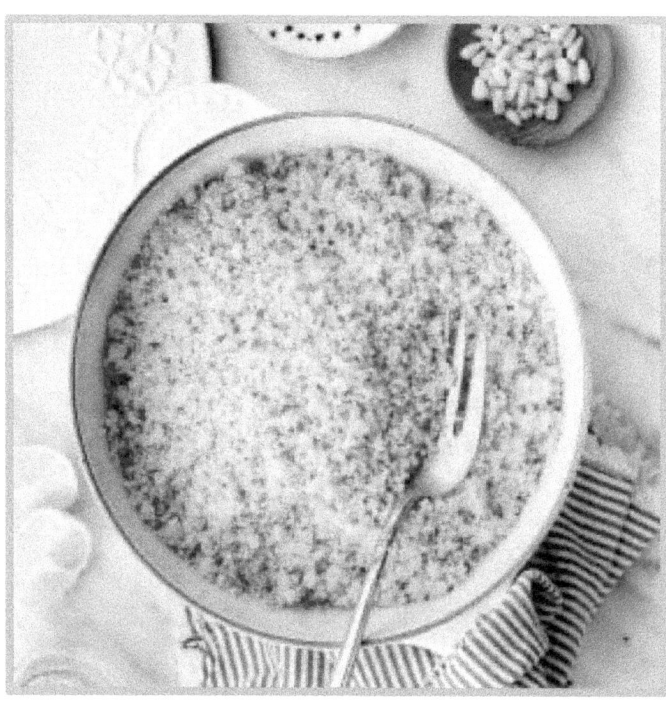

INGREDIENTS

- 1½ cups of plain rice milk
- ½ cup of water
- 1 vanilla bean, split
- ½ cup of honey
- ¼ teaspoon of ground cinnamon
- 1 cup of couscous

DIRECTIONS

1. In a large saucepan, mix the rice milk, water, and vanilla bean in a large saucepan over medium heat.
2. Bring the milk to a gentle simmer, reduce the heat to low, and let the milk simmer for 10 minutes to allow the vanilla flavor to infuse into the milk.
3. Remove the saucepan from the heat.
4. Take out the vanilla bean and, using the tip of a paring knife, scrape the seeds from the pod into the warm milk.
5. Stir in the honey and cinnamon.
6. Stir in the couscous, cover the pan, and let it stand for 10 minutes.
7. With a fork, fluff the couscous before serving.

193. Raspberry Brûlée

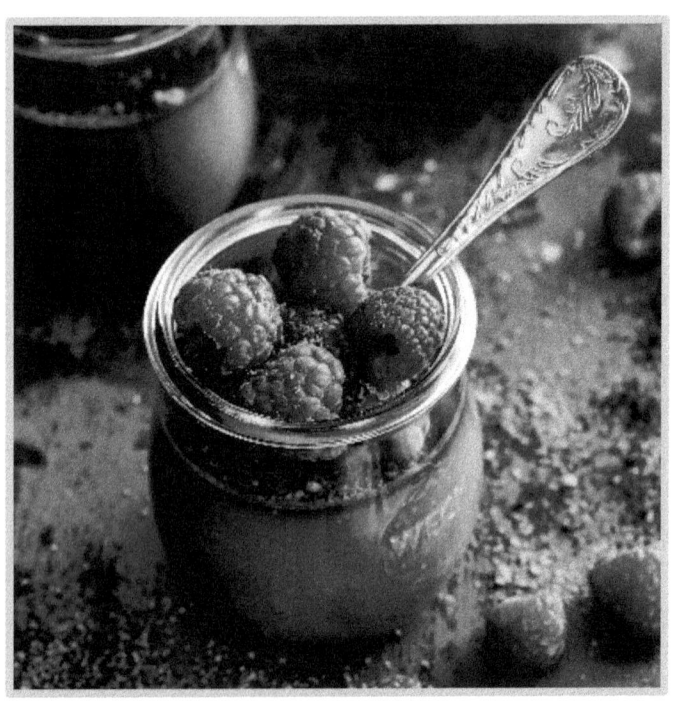

NUTRITION

Calories: 188
Fat: 13g
Carbohydrates: 16g
Phosphorus: 60mg
Potassium: 158mg
Sodium: 132mg
Protein: 3g

PREP TIME
15 min

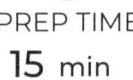

COOK TIME
1 min

SERVING
4 people

DIRECTIONS

1. Preheat the oven to broil.
2. Beat the sour cream, cream cheese, 2 tablespoons brown sugar, and cinnamon for about 4 minutes or until the mixture is very smooth and fluffy.
3. Evenly divide the raspberries among 4 (4-ounce) ramekins.
4. Get the cream cheese mixture and put a spoon over the berries and smooth the tops.
5. Store the ramekins in the refrigerator, covered, until you are ready to serve the dessert.
6. Sprinkle ½ tablespoon brown sugar evenly over each ramekin.
7. Place the ramekins on a baking sheet and broil 4 inches from the heating element until the sugar is caramelized and golden brown.
8. Remove from the oven. Let the brûlées sit 1 minute and serve.

INGREDIENTS

- ½ cup of light sour cream
- ½ cup of plain cream cheese, at room temperature
- ¼ cup of brown sugar, divided
- ¼ teaspoon of ground cinnamon
- 1 cup of fresh raspberries

194. Sweet Cinnamon Custard

PREP TIME
15 min

COOK TIME
1 min

SERVING
4 people

NUTRITION

Calories: 110
Fat: 4g
Carbohydrates: 14g
Phosphorus: 100mg
Potassium: 64mg
Sodium: 71mg
Protein: 4g

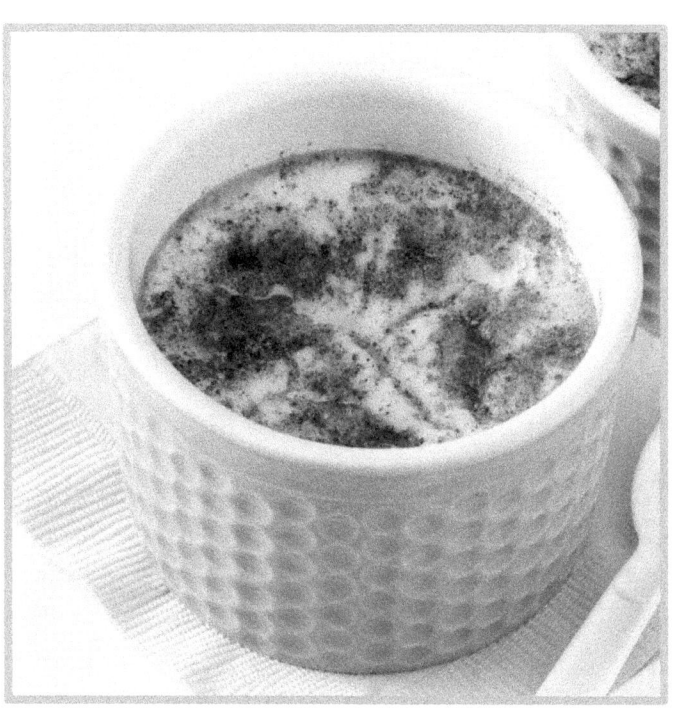

INGREDIENTS

- Unsalted butter, for greasing the ramekins
- 1½ cups of plain rice milk
- 4 eggs
- ¼ cup of granulated sugar
- 1 teaspoon of pure vanilla extract
- ½ teaspoon of ground cinnamon
- Cinnamon sticks, for garnish (optional)

DIRECTIONS

1. Preheat the oven to 325°F.
2. Lightly grease 6 (4-ounce) ramekins and place them in a baking sheet; set aside.
3. In a large bowl, whisk together the rice milk, eggs, sugar, vanilla, and cinnamon until the mixture is very smooth.
4. Pour the mixture through a fine sieve into a pitcher.
5. Evenly divide the custard mixture among the ramekins.
6. Put hot water in the sheet; make sure not to put any water in the ramekins, until the water reaches halfway up the sides of the ramekins.
7. Bake for about 1 hour or until the custards are set, and a knife inserted in the center of one of the custards comes out clean.
8. Take the custards off from the oven and take the ramekins out of the water.
9. Cool on wire racks for 1 hour and then transfer the custards to the refrigerator to chill for an additional hour.
10. Garnish each custard with a cinnamon stick, if desired.

195. Raspberry Mousse

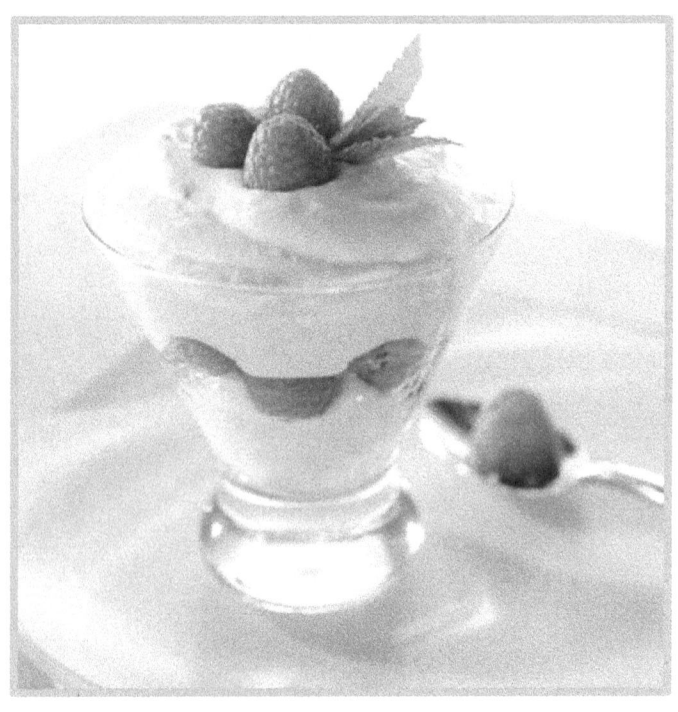

NUTRITION

Calories: 94
Carbohydrate: 20.1g
Protein: 1.1g
Sodium: 22mg
Potassium: 133mg
Phosphorus: 28mg
Dietary Fiber: 5.2g
Fat: 1.61g

PREP TIME 15 min

COOK TIME 12 min

SERVING 6 people

DIRECTIONS

1. Place the raspberries in a pot filled with the water. Cook until raspberries have softened (around 10–12 minutes).
2. Transfer the mixture into a bowl. Add the jelly powder and stir well to dissolve.
3. Once the mixture has cooled down, add in the whipping cream. Distribute the mixture into 6 dessert bowls or glasses.
4. Chill for at least a couple of hours prior to serving.
5. Garnish with a tbsp. of fresh raspberries on top of each serving.

INGREDIENTS

- 1 cup of frozen raspberries
- ¼ cup of water
- 2 tbsp of no sugar added jelly powder
- 1 ½ cup of whipping cream
- 1 pack of fresh raspberries

196. Honey Ginger Cookies

PREP TIME
15 min

COOK TIME
10 min

SERVING
30 cookies

NUTRITION

Calories: 112

Carbohydrate: 16g

Protein: 1g

Sodium: 90mg

Potassium: 18mg

Phosphorus: 13mg

Dietary Fiber: 0.4g

Fat: 5g

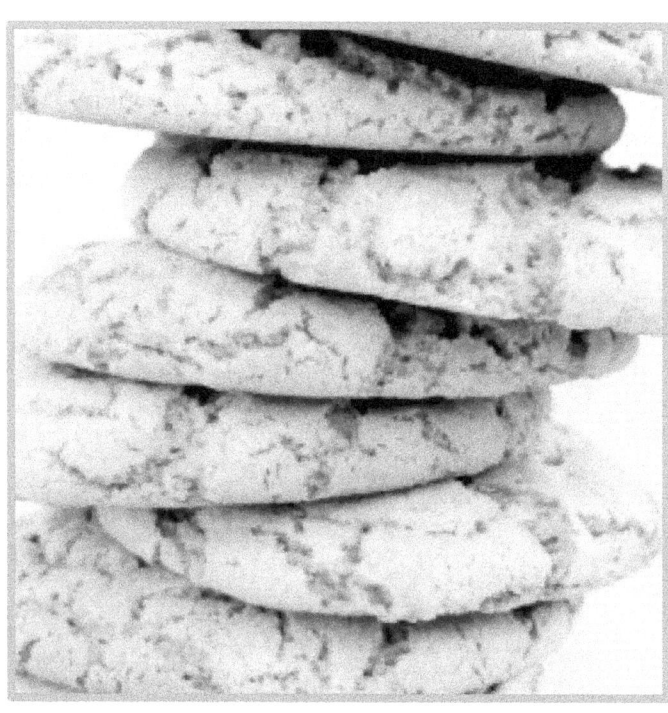

INGREDIENTS

- 2 cups of all-purpose flour
- ¾ cups of vegetable shortening
- 1 cup of white sugar
- ¼ cup of honey
- 2 tsp. of baking soda
- 1 tsp. of ginger powder
- 1 ¼ tsp. of cinnamon
- 1 tsp. of ground cloves
- A bit of icing sugar (for the top)

DIRECTIONS

1. Preheat the oven to 325°F/175°C.
2. Combine all the cream/wet ingredients in a mixing bowl and beat well.
3. In a separate bowl, sift the flour and combine it with the sugar and all the other ingredients.
4. Add the wet ingredients into the dry mixture and mix fast and well.
5. Roll into balls with your hands and place over a greased paper sheet, making sure each cookie ball is at least 1 inch apart from the other.
6. Bake for 8–10 minutes.

197. Honey Baked Pear

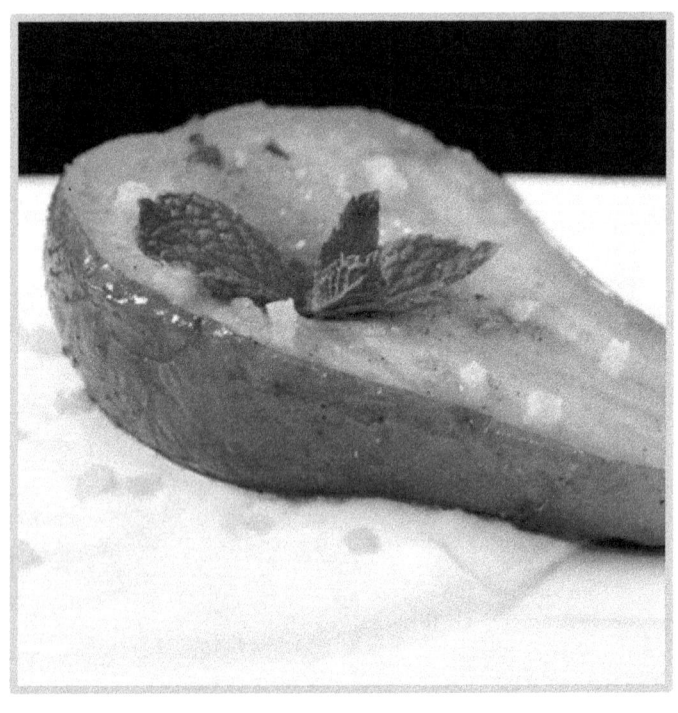

NUTRITION

Calories: 141
Carbohydrate: 23g
Protein: 0.5g
Sodium: 2mg
Potassium: 121mg
Phosphorus: 12mg
Dietary Fiber: 2.7g
Fat: 6g

PREP TIME
15 min

COOK TIME
30 min

SERVING
8 people

DIRECTIONS

1. Preheat the oven at 350°F/175°C.
2. Pour the lemon juice over the pears to avoid any darkening.
3. Mix the melted butter, spices, zest, and vanilla in a bowl. Pour over the pears.
4. Place the marinated pears in an oven-safe pan and bake for 25–30 minutes.
5. Serve warm.

INGREDIENTS

- 4 pears, peeled and halved
- ¼ cup of unsalted butter or margarine
- ¼ cup of lemon juice
- ½ tsp. of 5-spice powder
- 1 tsp. of orange zest
- 1 tsp. of vanilla extract

198. Watermelon Sorbet

PREP TIME
8 min

COOK TIME
1 min

SERVING
2 people

NUTRITION

Calories: 52

Carbohydrate: 13g

Protein: 0g

Sodium: 1mg

Potassium: 96mg

Phosphorus: 9mg

Dietary Fiber: 0.3g

Fat: 0g

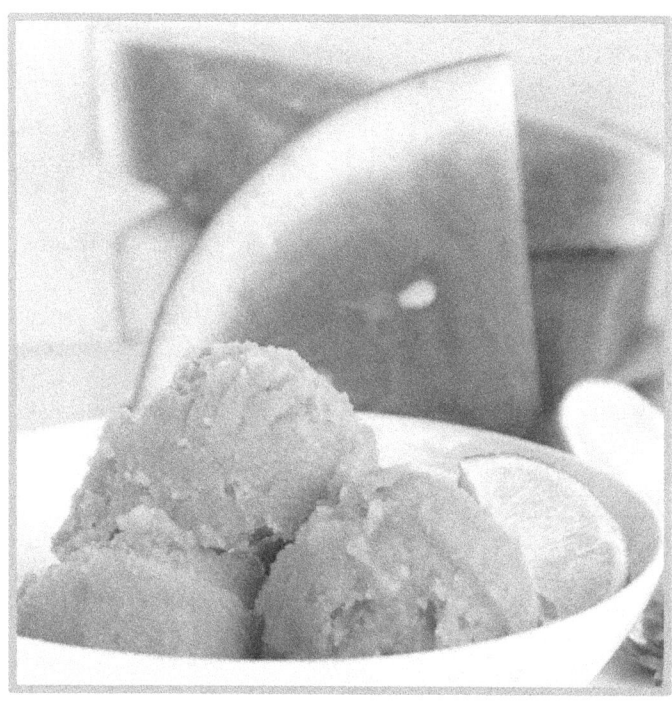

INGREDIENTS

- 1 cup of ice, crushed
- 1 cup of watermelon chunks, seeded
- 2 tbsps. of lime juice
- 1 tbsp. of sugar
- 2 small watermelon slices (for garnishing)

DIRECTIONS

1. Pulse all the ingredients except for the watermelon slices in a blender for 30 seconds to 1 minute.
2. Pour the mixture into 2 mason jars or glasses, top with the wedges, and serve chilled immediately.

199. Aunt Tula's Carrot Cake

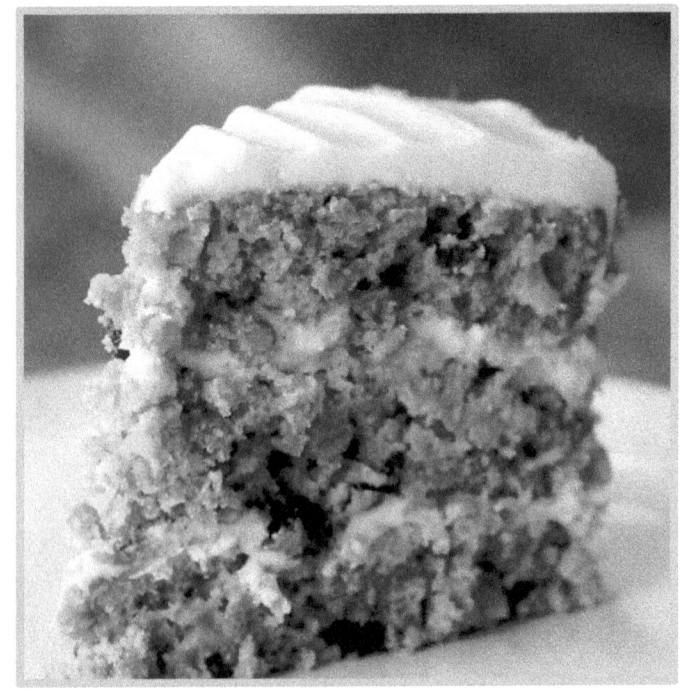

NUTRITION

Calories: 324
Carbohydrate: 34g
Protein: 4g
Sodium: 180.7mg
Potassium: 98mg
Phosphorus: 54mg
Dietary Fiber: 1g
Fat: 19g

PREP TIME
15 min

COOK TIME
50 min

SERVING
20 people

DIRECTIONS

1. Preheat the oven at 350°F/180°C.
2. In a large mixing bowl, combine all the dry ingredients, e.g., flour, sugar, and others. Slowly incorporate the oil, the beaten eggs, the vanilla, and the milk. Mix well until the mixture is uniform and slightly fluffy.
3. Pour the cake batter onto a lightly greased cake pan (around 9x11 inches)
4. Bake for 45–50 minutes
5. In a separate mixing bowl, beat the cream cheese with the icing sugar and vanilla powder to make your frosting.
6. Spread over the cooled carrot cake with a flat spatula. Slice and serve.

INGREDIENTS

- 2 cups of all-purpose flour
- 1 cup of white sugar
- 3 cups of carrot
- 1 cup of vegetable oil
- 4 large eggs, beaten
- 2 tbsp. of skimmed milk
- 8 oz. of cream cheese
- ¼ cup of unsalted butter
- 2 tsp. of cinnamon
- 1 tsp. of vanilla extract
- 2 tsp. vanilla powder
- 1 cup of icing sugar

200. Turnover Delights

PREP TIME
20 min

COOK TIME
20 min

SERVING
8 people

NUTRITION

Calories: 139.0

Protein: 2.0g

Sodium: 50.2mg

Phosphorus: 2.8mg

Potassium: 178.1mg

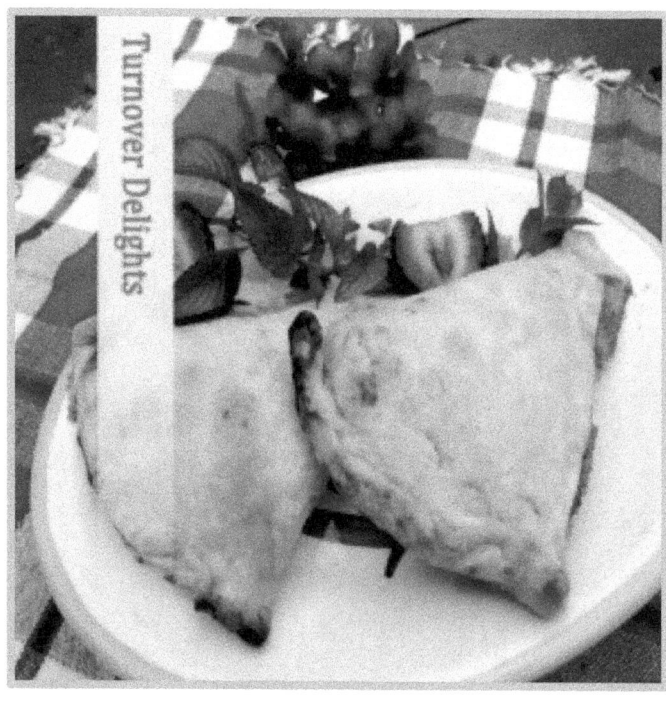

INGREDIENTS

- 1 1/4 lbs. tart apples
- 1 cup sliced strawberries
- 3 tbsp. sugar
- 1 tbsp. all-purpose flour
- 1/4 tsp. ground cinnamon
- 1/8 tsp. ground nutmeg
- 1 pkg. (2 sheets) frozen puff pastry, defrosted
- egg wash (1 egg beaten with 1 tbsp. water)

DIRECTIONS

1. Preheat oven to 400°F.
2. Peel and core apples and cut into ¾ inch dice.
3. Add the strawberries, sugar, flour, and spices.
4. Flour a board and lightly roll each sheet of pastry to a 12x12-inch square.
5. Cut each square into 4 smaller squares.
6. Brush the edges of the squares with the egg wash and place a tablespoon full of apple filling in the center.
7. Fold the pastry diagonally over apples and press edges with a fork to seal tightly.
8. Transfer to a lined sheet pan.
9. Brush top with egg wash and sprinkle with sugar. Make 2 small slits on top of each turnover.
10. Bake for 20 minutes until brown and puffed.

201. Peaches and Cream Puffs

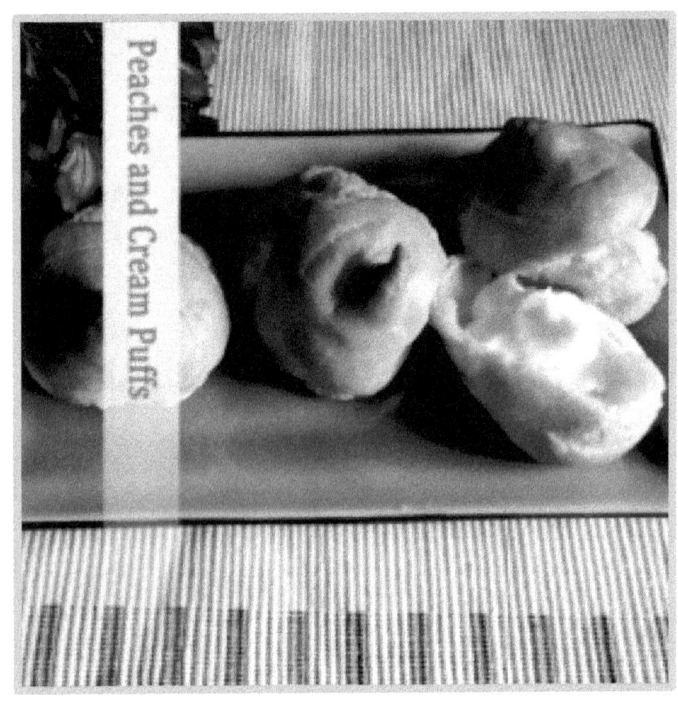

NUTRITION

Calories: 227.1

Protein: 4.8g

Sodium: 82.1mg

Phosphorus: 6.9mg

Potassium: 95.7mg

PREP TIME
30 min

COOK TIME
45 min

SERVING
12 people

DIRECTIONS

1. Preheat oven to 400°F.
2. Peel and core apples and cut into ¾ inch dice.
3. Add the strawberries, sugar, flour, and spices.
4. Flour a board and lightly roll each sheet of pastry to a 12x12-inch square.
5. Cut each square into 4 smaller squares.
6. Brush the edges of the squares with the egg wash and place a tablespoon full of apple filling in the center.
7. Fold the pastry diagonally over apples and press edges with a fork to seal tightly.
8. Transfer to a lined sheet pan.
9. Brush top with egg wash and sprinkle with sugar. Make 2 small slits on top of each turnover.
10. Bake for 20 minutes until brown and puffed.

INGREDIENTS

- 1 1/4 lbs. tart apples
- 1 cup sliced strawberries
- 3 tbsp. sugar
- 1 tbsp. all-purpose flour
- 1/4 tsp. ground cinnamon
- 1/8 tsp. ground nutmeg
- 1 pkg. (2 sheets) frozen puff pastry, defrosted
- egg wash (1 egg beaten with 1 tbsp. water)

CHAPTER 15

Frequently Asked Questions

When you are diagnosed with kidney disease, it is perfectly natural and common to have some questions regarding kidney function and renal diet. Here are the most common questions and their answers in brief:

Q: How much protein should I take daily?

A: The exact amount of protein you should take per day depends on your existing body weight, stage of renal disease, and general health status. This is something that you can figure out with your doctor or renal dietitian. However, doctors recommend approx.—1.1–1.3 gr of protein per kg of body weight daily in most cases. For example, if you weigh 143Pounds/65Kg, you can eat up to 84 grams of protein per day.

Q: Am I allowed to take extra vitamins and supplements?

A: Due to the fact that a lot of nutrient-dense foods should be avoided in a renal diet because of their high potassium or phosphorus content, it is generally suggested to take vitamins that are water-soluble and namely B-complex vitamins and vitamin C in smaller doses. However, excess supplementation may lead to side effects like stomach irritation, gas, and constipation, so make sure you do not exceed the daily-recommended dose on the package.

Q: Are alcoholic beverages ok to drink in a renal diet?

A: Drinks that contain lower amounts of alcohol than others, e.g., wine and beer, are fine to drink on a semi-regular basis, e.g., 2–3 times a week. However, heavy alcoholic drinks like vodka, rum, tequila, gin, and whiskey should be limited to 2–3 times a month, as frequent consumption will place kidneys and other vital organs under stress.

Q: How can I know if a packed food product or recipe is low in potassium?

A: When you are checking a product label or new recipe but don't know if it's actually low in potassium or not, here is a basic guideline of levels per serving:

Very low potassium levels

    Up to 35 mg/serving

Low potassium levels

    Up to 150 mg/serving

Moderate potassium levels

    Between 150–250 mg/serving

High potassium levels

    250–500 mg/serving

Very high potassium levels

    500mg+/serving

If you are checking a recipe, make sure that you calculate all ingredients' total levels to determine the amount of potassium. In this book, we made it easier for you by including recipes that are low or moderate in potassium and display the actual potassium level per serving.

Q: Do I have to limit my fluids after being diagnosed?

A: A limitation of fluids is generally recommended during the last stages of kidney damage, and it would be better to discuss it with your doctor. If you go the opposite and only drink 500ml of fluids or less per day, you risk dehydrating yourself and cause other problems.

Q: Are artificial sweeteners OK in the renal diet?

A: Artificial sweeteners that are low in carbs are generally fine to the consumer within the renal diet, with the exception of aspartame, which is linked to many health problems; sweeteners like stevia, sucralose, and xylitol are perfectly fine when consumed moderately on a regular basis.

Q: Can I follow this diet if I have a kidney transplant?

A: Although this diet is designed to help patients of nearly all stages of kidney damage, once you have a kidney transplant surgery, you may follow a similar diet afterward, but your protein requirements will be higher, as your body will need extra protein to heal damaged tissue. In addition, maybe you will need to eat higher amounts of calcium to avoid any depletion because of steroid medications. The exact diet and portions are something that you will discuss with your doctor or renal dietician post-surgery.

Best Advice to Avoid Dialysis

As specified, if you are currently in the first stages of renal damage, you can actually prevent dialysis mainly through diet, but there are other general lifestyle factors that will help. You have to follow a lifestyle that keeps your body weight under control and makes you feel healthy. Here are some tips:

Exercise on a regular basis. It is advised to be physically active to keep your heart and breathing system healthy, as renal damage can also affect their functions as well. Most doctors recommend exercising 2–3 times a week and performing mild exercises to keep yourself active but not too tired or exhausted. Three hours in total of mild exercise per week is perfectly fine for this purpose.

Monitor your blood sugar levels. Blood sugar levels and diabetes are often a side effect or even a contributing factor to renal damage. Even if you don't currently have diabetes, it is still important to monitor your blood sugar levels as they can further place you at risk of developing renal disease. Have it checked at least once every month, and if you are in pre-diabetes or full set diabetes status, make sure that you take all the medicines that your doctor prescribes for your case.

Keep your immune system balanced. When our immune systems are underactive or overactive, many types of diseases can occur due to the body's inability to fight them properly. In the case of renal disease, some autoimmune conditions like Lupus are negatively associated with the disease's progression. In this case, your doctor may prescribe steroids to keep your immune system from getting over-triggered and attacking vital organs, e.g., kidneys.

APPENDIX A

Measurement and Conversion

VOLUME

IMPERIAL	METRIC	IMPERIAL	METRIC
1 tbsp.	15ml	1 pint	570ml
2 fl. oz.	55ml	1 ¼ pints	725ml
3 fl. oz.	75ml	1 ¾ pints	1 litre
5 fl. oz. (¼ pint)	150ml	2 pints	1.2 litres
10 fl. oz. (½ pint)	275ml	2½ pints	1.5 litres
		4 pints	2.25 litres

METRIC CUPS CONVERSION

CUPS	IMPERIAL	METRIC
1 cup of flour	5 oz.	150g
1 cup of caster or granulated sugar	8 oz.	225g
1 cup of soft brown sugar	6 oz.	175g
1 cup of soft butter/margarine	8 oz.	225g
1 cup of sultanas/raisins	7 oz.	200g
1 cup of currants	5 oz.	150g
1 cup of ground almonds	4 oz.	110g
1 cup of oats	4 oz.	110g
1 cup of golden syrup/honey	12 oz.	350g
1 cup of uncooked rice	7 oz.	200g
1 cup of grated cheese	4 oz.	110g
1 stick of butter	4 oz.	110g
¼ cup of liquid (water, milk, oil etc.)	4 tablespoons	60ml
½ cup of liquid (water, milk, oil etc.)	¼ pint	125ml
1 cup of liquid (water, milk, oil etc.)	½ pint	250ml

WEIGHT

IMPERIAL	METRIC	IMPERIAL	METRIC
½ oz.	10g	6 oz.	175g
¾ oz.	20g	7 oz.	200g
1 oz.	25g	8 oz.	225g
1½ oz.	40g	9 oz.	250g
2 oz.	50g	10 oz.	275g
2½ oz.	60g	12 oz.	350g
3 oz.	75g	1 lb.	450g
4 oz.	110g	1 lb. 8 oz.	700g
4½ oz.	125g	2 lb.	900g
5 oz.	150g	3 lb.	1.35kg

OVEN TEMPERATURES

GAS MARK	FAHRENHEIT	CELSIUS
1/4	225	110
1/2	250	130
1	275	140
2	300	150
3	325	170
4	350	180
5	375	190
6	400	200
7	425	220
8	450	230
9	475	240

APPENDIX B

Dirty Dozen and Clean Fifteen

A non-profit environmental watchdog organization called Environmental Working Group (EWG) looks at data supplied by the US Department of Agriculture (USDA) and the Food and Drug Administration (FDA) about pesticide residues. Each year it compiles a list of the best and worst pesticide loads found in commercial crops. You can use these lists to decide which fruits and vegetables to buy organic to minimize your exposure to pesticides and which product is considered safe enough to buy conventionally. This does not mean they are pesticide-free, though, so wash these fruits and vegetables thoroughly.

These lists change every year, so make sure you look up the most recent one before you fill your shopping cart. You'll find the most recent lists, as well as a guide to pesticides in product, at EWG.org/FoodNews.

Dirty Dozen

- Apples
- Celery
- Cherries
- Cherry tomatoes
- Cucumbers
- Grapes
- Nectarines
- Peaches
- Spinach
- Strawberries
- Sweet bell peppers
- Tomatoes

In addition to the Dirty Dozen, the EWG added two types of produce contaminated with highly toxic organophosphate insecticides:

- Kale/Collard greens
- Hot peppers
- Clean Fifteen
- Asparagus
- Avocados
- Cabbage
- Cantaloupe
- Cauliflower
- Eggplant
- Grapefruit
- Honeydew
- Melon
- Kiwis
- Mangos
- Onions
- Papayas
- Pineapples
- Sweet corn
- Sweet peas (frozen)

CONCLUSION

Congratulations on having to transit the lines of this book from start to finish.

In this book, I have provided better insights into how the kidneys work, what could affect the functioning of the kidneys, the typical signs and symptoms associated with kidney malfunctioning, the stages of kidney disease, and likewise, the changes that must be adhered to prevent further damage and eventual kidney failure—most of which centered around dietary choices. Because we are accustomed to everyday eating, it has become increasingly important to not only watch what we eat but also how we eat most, especially if you have CKD. Being able to manage your CKD is very vital to the long term sustainability and functionality of your kidneys. A renal diet, as explained in this book, is so significant that it provides you with better oversight of what to eat, what not to eat and also, how you eat—all of which is geared toward managing your CKD and delaying the progression of the disease. This book has provided you with most of the tools needed to get you started toward a prolonged kidney function by elaborating on a variety of handpicked low sodium, potassium, and phosphorus recipes that you can have for breakfast, as snacks and appetizers, soups, and stews, vegetables, salads, meats, and desserts, coupled with the necessary nutritional information to guide your choices—which you can also use in adapting to your daily meal plans. Hence, it is my sincere desire that you found great value from this book.

Finally, I want you to take full responsibility for the health of your kidneys and overall well-being by incorporating what I have shared in this book into your daily dietary choices. I believe doing so would prevent further damage to your kidneys while also prolonging its ability to function healthily without the need for dialysis or transplant as it did for my patients.

On a lighter note, if you have found any benefit reading this book, I'd appreciate it if you could take some time to leave an honest review on amazon. Reviews encourage other readers to give independent authors like myself a chance. They help more than I can describe. And trust me, I could use all the help you provide; thanks.

I wish you all the best on your journey toward health and wellness!

CPSIA information can be obtained
at www.ICGtesting.com
Printed in the USA
LVHW061116101120
671124LV00015B/426